Cardiology

Editor

MICHAEL PEES

VETERINARY CLINICS OF NORTH AMERICA: EXOTIC ANIMAL PRACTICE

www.vetexotic.theclinics.com

Consulting Editor
JÖRG MAYER

May 2022 • Volume 25 • Number 2

ELSEVIER

1600 John F. Kennedy Boulevard • Suite 1800 • Philadelphia, Pennsylvania, 19103-2899
http://www.vetexotic.theclinics.com

VETERINARY CLINICS OF NORTH AMERICA: EXOTIC ANIMAL PRACTICE Volume 25, Number 2
May 2022 ISSN 1094-9194, ISBN-13: 978-0-323-84890-9

Editor: Stacy Eastman
Developmental Editor: Axell Ivan Jade M. Purificacion

Veterinary Clinics of North America: Exotic Animal Practice (ISSN 1094-9194) is published in January, May, and September by Elsevier, Inc., 360 Park Avenue South, New York, NY 10010-1710. Subscription prices are $296.00 per year for US individuals, $697.00 per year for US institutions, $100.00 per year for US students and residents, $345.00 per year for Canadian individuals, $707.00 per year for Canadian institutions, $359.00 per year for international individuals, $707.00 per year for international institutions, $100.00 per year Canadian students/residents, and $165.00 per year for international students/residents. To receive student/resident rate, orders must be accompanied by name of affiliated institution, date of term, and the *signature* of program/residency coordinator on institution letterhead. Orders will be billed at individual rate until proof of status is received. Foreign air speed delivery is included in all *Clinics* subscription prices. All prices are subject to change without notice. **POSTMASTER:** Send address changes to *Veterinary Clinics of North America: Exotic Animal Practice*, Elsevier Health Sciences Division, Subscription Customer Service, 3251 Riverport Lane, Maryland Heights, MO 63043. **Customer Service: Telephone: 1-800-654-2452** (U.S. and Canada); **1-314-447-8871** (outside U.S. and Canada). **Fax: 1-314-447-8029. E-mail: journalscustomerservice-usa@elsevier.com (for print support); journalsonlinesupport-usa@elsevier.com (for online support).**

Reprints. For copies of 100 or more of articles in this publication, please contact the Commercial Reprints Department, Elsevier Inc., 360 Park Avenue South, New York, New York 10010-1710. Tel.: 212-633-3874; Fax: 212-633-3820; E-mail: reprints@elsevier.com.

Veterinary Clinics of North America: Exotic Animal Practice is covered in *MEDLINE/PubMed (Index Medicus).*

Contributors

CONSULTING EDITOR

JÖRG MAYER, Dr med vet, MSc
Diplomate, American Board of Veterinary Practitioners (Exotic Companion Mammals); Diplomate, European College of Zoological Medicine (Small Mammals); Diplomate, American College of Zoological Medicine; Associate Professor of Zoological Medicine, Department of Small Animal Medicine and Surgery, University of Georgia College of Veterinary Medicine, Athens, Georgia, USA

EDITOR

MICHAEL PEES, Dr Med vet
Diplomate, European College of Zoological Medicine (Avian and Herpetology); Professor, Head, Department of Small Mammal, Reptile and Avian Diseases, University of Veterinary Medicine Hannover, Foundation, Hannover, Germany

AUTHORS

CARLOS F. AGUDELO, MVDr, PhD
Dogs and Cat Clinic, Faculty of Veterinary Medicine, VETUNI Brno, Brno, Czech Republic

HEIKE AUPPERLE-LELLBACH, PD, Dr med vet
Laboklin GmbH & Co KG, Bad Kissingen, Germany

ARGIÑE CEREZO-ECHEVARRIA, DVM
Diplomate, American College of Veterinary Pathologists; Laboklin GmbH & Co KG, Bad Kissingen, Germany

KONICEK CORNELIA, Drmedvet
Department of Small Animal Medicine, University of Veterinary Medicine Vienna, Vienna, Austria

DOMINIK FISCHER, Dr med vet
Diplomate, European College of Zoological Medicine (Wildlife Population Health); Klinik für Vögel, Reptilien, Amphibien und Fische der Justus-Liebig-Universität Gießen, Germany; Zoo Wuppertal, Wuppertal, Germany

BRENNA COLLEEN FITZGERALD, DVM
Diplomate, American Board of Veterinary Practitioners; Owner and Consultant, Avian Exclusive Veterinary Consultation, Englewood, Colorado, USA; Consultant, Medical Center for Birds, Oakley, California, USA

RACHEL FRANZISKA HEIN, Med Vet
Department for Small Mammal, Reptile and Avian Diseases, University of Veterinary Medicine Hannover, Foundation, Hannover, Germany

MICHAELA GUMPENBERGER, Dr med vet
Assistant Professor, Diagnostic Imaging, Department for Companion Animals and
Horses, University of Veterinary Medicine Vienna, Vienna, Austria

KAREL HAUPTMAN, MVDr, PhD
Jekl & Hauptman Veterinary Clinic – Focused on Exotic Companion Mammal Care, Brno,
Czech Republic

KATHRIN JÄGER, Dr med vet
Laboklin GmbH & Co KG, Bad Kissingen, Germany

VLADIMIR JEKL MVDr, PhD
Diplomate, European College of Zoological Medicine (Small Mammal); Associate
Professor, Jekl & Hauptman Veterinary Clinic – Focused on Exotic Companion Mammal
Care, Department of Pharmacology and Pharmacy, Faculty of Veterinary Medicine,
VETUNI Brno, Brno, Czech Republic

INGMAR KIEFER DrMedVet
Head of the Radiology Department, Department for Small Animals, Veterinary Teaching
Hospital, University of Leipzig, Leipzig, Germany

MARIA-E. KRAUTWALD-JUNGHANNS, ME (DVM). Prof. Drmedvet
Diplomate, European College of Zoological Medicine (Avian); Department for Birds and
Reptiles, Veterinary Teaching Hospital, University of Leipzig, Leipzig, Germany

KERSTIN MÜLLER, PD Dr
Diplomate, European College of Zoological Medicine; Small Animal Clinic, Freie
Universität Berlin, Berlin, Germany

ELISABETTA MANCINELLI, DVM
CertZooMed, Diplomate, European College of Zoological Medicine (Small Mammals);
Valley Exotics, Valley Veterinary Hospital, Gwaelod y Garth Ind Est., Cardiff, United
Kingdom

MICHAEL PEES, Dr Med vet
Diplomate, European College of Zoological Medicine (Avian and Herpetology); Professor,
Head, Department of Small Mammal, Reptile and Avian Diseases, University of Veterinary
Medicine Hannover, Foundation, Hannover, Germany

ANDRES POHL, Dr med vet
Kleintier- und Vogelpraxis Haldensleben, Germany

ANNIKA POSAUTZ, Dr med vet
Research Institute of Wildlife Ecology, Department of Interdisciplinary Life Sciences,
University of Veterinary Medicine Vienna, Vienna, Austria

LIONEL SCHILLIGER, DVM
Diplomate, European College of Zoological Medicine (Herpetology); Diplomate, American
Board of Veterinary Practitioners (Reptile and Amphibian Practice); Clinique Vétérinaire du
Village d'Auteuil, Paris, France

SILVANA SCHMIDT-UKAJ, Dr med vet
Service for Birds and Reptiles, Small Animal Internal Medicine, Department for
Companion Animals and Horses, University of Veterinary Medicine Vienna, Vienna,
Austria

NICO J. SCHOEMAKER, DVM, PhD
Diplomate, European College of Zoological Medicine (Small mammal and Avian); Division of Zoological Medicine, Department of Clinical Sciences, Faculty of Veterinary Medicine, Utrecht University, Utrecht, the Netherlands

J. MATTHIAS STARCK, PhD
Professor, Department of Biology, Ludwig-Maximilians University Munich, Planegg-Martinsried, Germany

JENS STRAUB, Dr med vet
Tierklinik Düsseldorf GmbH, Germany

VERENA STRAUSS, Mag med vet
Research Institute of Wildlife Ecology, Department of Interdisciplinary Life Sciences, University of Veterinary Medicine Vienna, Vienna, Austria

YVONNE R.A. VAN ZEELAND, MVR, DVM, PhD, CPBC
Diplomate, European College of Zoological Medicine (Avian and Small mammal); Division of Zoological Medicine, Department of Clinical Sciences, Faculty of Veterinary Medicine, Utrecht University, Utrecht, the Netherlands

JEANETTE WYNEKEN, PhD
Professor of Biological Sciences, Director, FAU Marine Lab at Gumbo Limbo Environmental Complex, Florida Atlantic University, Boca Raton, Florida, USA

Contents

The heart development, form, and functional specializations of chelonians, squamates, crocodilians, and birds characterize how diverse structure and specializations arise from similar foundations. This review aims to summarize the morphologic diversity of sauropsid hearts and present it in an integrative functional and phylogenetic context. Besides the detailed morphologic descriptions, the integrative view of function, evolution, and development will aid understanding of the surprising diversity of sauropsid hearts. This integrated perspective is a foundation that strengthens appreciation that the sauropsid hearts are the outcome of biological evolution; disease often is linked to arising mismatch between adaptations and modern environments.

Currently, there are more than 8200 amphibian species described, including the orders Anura (frogs and toads), Caudata (salamanders and newts) and Gymnophiona (caecilians). Amphibians have 3 heart chambers: 2 atria and 1 ventricle. Their heart anatomy, histology, and physiology are reviewed. The basic morphology of the heart is similar in all amphibians with some differences due to their lifestyle. Blood flow, blood mixing, and blood oxygenation show variation due to interindividual and interspecific differences. Finally, different diagnostic methods to investigate the amphibian heart are described and reported amphibian heart diseases are summarized, including genetic, congenital, infectious, and neoplastic heart diseases.

The notion that poikilotherms do not suffer from cardiovascular conditions is being increasingly challenged as diagnostic tools used in companion animal practice are applied to reptiles. However, the cause, diagnosis, and treatment of cardiac conditions in reptiles is difficult because of the scarcity of published literature. Auscultation, electrocardiography, radiography, and ultrasonography are helpful diagnostic techniques in herpetologic practice. Although the pharmacokinetics and pharmacodynamics of cardiovascular drugs are poorly understood in these animals, basic principles remain applicable; these include pharmacologic and nonpharmacologic interventions. Further research is needed to establish species-specific cardiac reference ranges and evidence-based treatment options.

Cardiovascular diseases are common in pet birds. Diagnosis is often made postmortem only. In any case, suspicious for cardiac disease, a full diagnostic work up should be applied. First indications are given by the anamnestic data. Relative predisposition to cardiovascular diseases is associated with the species, breed, age, gender, lifestyle, and diet. Clinical signs and examination can reveal further indications of cardiovascular diseases, but may be unspecific or even without any pathologic finding. Diagnostic imaging, at least radiography, and echocardiography are always recommended. Advanced imaging methods, especially angiocardiography, can be valuable but is also more invasive and expensive.

As part of the cardiovascular examination, all birds underwent clinical and echocardiographic examinations. Radiographs and blood samples were taken. Each bird was premedicated with midazolam and medetomidin and anesthetized with inhalation anesthesia using isoflurane. We performed computed tomographic angiography (CTA) after intravenous injection of 1 to 2 mL contrast agent per kg followed by a 1 mL saline solution flush. We were been able to identify the arteries that previous studies revealed to be most likely affected by atherosclerotic lesions: the aorta, both pulmonary arteries, and both brachiocephalic trunks. CTA was safe and is of potential diagnostic value in birds.

Samples of 363 Psittacidae were included in this study with a focus on cardiovascular diseases. These were identified in 28.9% of the animals, with pericarditis and/or epicarditis and myocarditis representing approximately half of all lesions and bacteria being the most common infectious cause. Cardiac lymphoma was only seen in 5 birds, whereas degenerative vascular lesions were diagnosed in 26.7% of the cases. Histopathology in the context of clinical findings and complementary examination results is the most useful tool for the evaluation of cardiac diseases.

Cardiovascular disease, including congestive heart failure, pericardial disease, and atherosclerosis, is becoming increasingly better recognized in companion birds. A wide range of medications is available to treat these conditions, including diuretics, vasodilators, positive and negative inotropes, antiarrhythmic agents, and pentoxifylline. This review systematically discusses each of these drug classes and their potential applications in avian species. Although treatment approaches remain largely empirical and extrapolated from small animal and human medicine, the management strategies presented here have the potential to both maintain quality of life and extend survival time for the avian cardiac patient.

The incidence of cardiac diseases in pet rabbits and rodents increased over the past decade as these species live longer and diagnostics methods are more precise to diagnose heart diseases even in small-sized animals. The article summarizes diagnostics of cardiac diseases in selected exotic companion mammals, particularly in rabbits, guinea pigs, chinchillas, and rats. The emphasis of the paper is given on clinical examination, thoracic radiography, electrocardiography, and echocardiography.

Information about heart diseases and their treatment is still sparce for rabbits and rodents. Dilated cardiomyopathy seems to occur more frequently in rabbits, whereas in guinea pigs pericardial effusion is often diagnosed. There are still no available therapeutic studies for heart diseases in rabbits and rodents, and treatment is often extrapolated from dogs and cats. Consideration should be given to the off-label use of drugs, mostly not licensed in the species mentioned in this article.

Cardiac disease is relatively common in middle-aged to older ferrets and may comprise acquired or congenital disorders leading to problems with conduction, contractility, or outflow. Clinical signs are often seen in advanced stages of the disease, with lethargy, hind limb weakness, ascites, hepatosplenomegaly, and respiratory distress owing to pleural effusion or lung edema being prominent features. Diagnostic workup and therapeutic intervention largely follow guidelines such as those established for dogs and cats, with feline doses often serving as a starting point for therapy.

VETERINARY CLINICS OF NORTH AMERICA: EXOTIC ANIMAL PRACTICE

FORTHCOMING ISSUES

September 2022
Exotic Animal Clinical Pathology
J. Jill Heatley and Karen E. Russell, *Editors*

January 2023
Pain Management
David Sanchez-Migallon Guzman, *Editor*

May 2023
Dermatology
Dario d'Ovidio and Domenico Santoro, *Editor*

RECENT ISSUES

January 2022
Sedation and Anesthesia of Zoological Companion Animals
Miranda J. Sadar and João Brandão, *Editors*

September 2021
Herd/Flock Health and Medicine for the Exotic Animal Practitioner
Shangzhe Xie, *Editor*

May 2021
Respiratory Medicine
Vladimir Jekl, *Editor*

SERIES OF RELATED INTEREST

Veterinary Clinics of North America: Small Animal Practice
Available at: https://www.vetsmall.theclinics.com/

THE CLINICS ARE NOW AVAILABLE ONLINE!
Access your subscription at:
www.theclinics.com

Preface

Cardiology in Exotic Pets: Challenges and Evolution

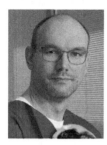

Michael Pees, Dr Med vet
Editor

About 13 years have passed since the last issue on "Cardiology in Exotic Animals" was published in *Veterinary Clinics of North America: Exotic Animal Practice*, and I had the opportunity and pleasure to join the team of authors and contribute to this emerging scientific field. Since then, a lot has happened in the world of exotic veterinary medicine, with new studies, new experiences, and of course, a huge step forward in the development of technical possibilities. I therefore feel honored to have the opportunity to introduce this new "Cardiology" issue of *Veterinary Clinics of North America: Exotic Animal Practice*, dedicated to those patients that are termed "exotic" but are seen more and more regularly in many veterinary practices.

Cardiology has undergone constant evolution, not revolution, over the past years, and knowledge in this field has increased step by step, starting from a deeper understanding of the underlying anatomy and physiology, the establishment of modern diagnostic methods as well as the standardization of traditional methods, and finally progress in the therapy of cardiac diseases. Nevertheless, in many aspects, cardiology in our exotic pets is still in its infancy, but it is growing rapidly, giving us new options for the understanding of these disease processes, and of course, for helping our patients.

This issue is intended to give an up-to-date overview on the current knowledge of the anatomy, physiology, diagnostics, and most commonly known cardiac diseases in very different animal groups and to summarize the state-of-the-art therapeutic options available for them. I wish to thank the authors who contributed to this issue and shared their experience and knowledge in the respective fields they are specializing in. I also want to thank Elsevier and Joerg Mayer for the invitation to serve as guest editor, and the Elsevier team, especially Stacy Eastman, Axell Ivan, Jade M. Purificacion, and Rajkumar Mayakrishnan, for their continuous help and assistance in the preparation of this issue.

Vet Clin Exot Anim 25 (2022) xi–xii
https://doi.org/10.1016/j.cvex.2022.02.001
1094-9194/22/© 2022 Published by Elsevier Inc.

I hope that you enjoy reading these articles, that you find interesting new options and ideas, and that the content of this issue might help you to diagnose and treat cardiovascular disorders in exotics pets.

Michael Pees, Dr Med vet
Department of Small Mammal, Reptile
and Avian Diseases
University of Veterinary Medicine
Bünteweg 7
D-30559 Hannover, Germany

E-mail address:
michael.pees@tiho-hannover.de

Comparative and Functional Anatomy of the Ectothermic Sauropsid Heart

J. Matthias Starck, PhD[a],*, Jeanette Wyneken, PhD[b]

KEYWORDS

- Atrium • Ventricle • Sinus venosus • Cavum arteriosum • Cavum pulmonale
- Cavum venosum • Right aorta • Left aorta

KEY POINTS

- The hearts of sauropsids initially develop similarly from an embryonic tube that loops on itself and during that process forms the 2 atria and the ventricular partitions. The sinus venosus remains and the embryonic outflow tract, the truncus arteriosus, becomes organized as the visceral arches. The particular outflow tracts of crocodilians and birds primarily differ from that of other sauropsids in which visceral arches contribute to each and in the formation of a complete interventricular septum.
- The ventricles of lizards, snakes, and turtles have partially separated but communicating chambers within the ventricle that can allow mixing of blood. Crocodilians have a complete intraventricular septum to form a 4-chambered heart, with 2 aortae to the body and a pulmonary trunk to the lungs. In contrast, birds have a 4-chambered heart with a right aorta to the body and a pulmonary trunk to the lungs.
- Squamates and chelonians have intracardiac shunting capacity. Shunting in crocodilians may occur outside the heart via the Foramen of Panizza.
- Pythons and at least some varanid lizards have a well-developed muscular ridge that allows some functional separation of blood flow within the ventricle (but also intracardiac shunting). The physiologic implications are the capacity to sustain higher systemic blood pressures and higher metabolic rates than other squamates.

INTRODUCTION

Sauropsids (ie, Chelonia, Lepidosauria, and Archosauria) show a remarkable diversity in morphology and function of their hearts and vascular circuits. Despite their distinct and derived features, the textbook paradigm still contextualizes sauropsid hearts as "primitive" or "transitional" to the mammalian heart. Such views are rooted in idealistic morphology and typological thinking and neglect the fascinating relationships of the

[a] Department of Biology, Ludwig-Maximilians-University Munich, Planegg-Martinsried D82152, Germany; [b] Florida Atlantic University, FAU Marine Lab at Gumbo Limbo Environmental Complex, Boca Raton, FL 33431-0991, USA
* Corresponding author.
E-mail address: starck@lmu.de

Vet Clin Exot Anim 25 (2022) 337–366
https://doi.org/10.1016/j.cvex.2022.01.001
1094-9194/22/© 2022 Elsevier Inc. All rights reserved.

sauropsid heart with the regulatory capacity of respiration, metabolism, digestion, and thermoregulation. Over the past 50 years, comparative physiologists and functional morphologists placed the sauropsid heart into modern phylogenetic context and emphasized the robust capacity of the ectothermic sauropsids' hearts. Furthermore, developmental biologists have sorted out cardiac embryogenesis, mainly in mammals and birds, as well as a few ectothermic sauropsids. The comparative data available now for ectothermic sauropsids enable evolutionary and functional understanding of their hearts through comparative morphology, physiology, and developmental biology. It is essential to recognize that all animals are the consequences of historical compromises shaped by natural selection to maximize reproduction, not health. Organisms are not optimally engineered machines, a view that is subconsciously entrenched in our thinking. In addition, because biological evolution acts much more slowly than societal changes, much disease has foundations in the mismatch of adaptations (to many environmental changes in evolutionary time) to modern environments.[1] Including an evolutionary perspective reminds us that many genetic variants interact with environments and other genes acting during development both influence the heart phenotypes and disease phenotypes.

Given the diverse fields contributing to understanding ectothermic sauropsid cardiac form and function, we provide a glossary (**Table 1**) to ease access to this literature.

One of the complications in understanding the heart morphology is that the hearts of different clades (sauropsids, mammals) arose from a common ancestral (plesiomorphic) morphology such that highly diverse heart morphology occurs in some clades but also highly convergent morphologies in others (eg, birds and mammals). Thus, basic elements of the heart are homologous in all amniotes, but homologous parts diversified independently in the various groups of amniotes. Therefore, we will occasionally refer to the basal pattern of heart anatomy of amniotes, which includes a brief perspective from mammalian heart development, where appropriate.

During the past decade, several papers presented important perspectives into a functional and evolutionary understanding of the sauropsid heart and provided new evolutionary explanations of the observed morphologic diversity. Through this literature, we understand the heart morphology of various groups of sauropsids as independently derived from a common amniote basal pattern. However, given the persistent difficulties of explaining the complex morphology of the sauropsid heart, an alternative perspective re-emerged, interpreting sauropsid hearts as remnants in amniote evolutionary history. This view assumes that the observed morphologic diversity is not related to specialized functions like shunting[2-4] or, that sauropsid hearts represent a transitional developmental position in an otherwise anagenetic evolutionary sequence.[5-7] A more moderate perspective suggests that functional and physiologic principles of adaptation may not be determined easily because of the complexity of interacting processes.[8,9]

DEVELOPMENT

During early embryogenesis, the heart develops from the primary and secondary heart fields. Precardiac cells move to the midline of the embryo and condense into bilateral endocardial tubular structures. Those endocardial tubes merge into a single tube, whereas the adjoining splanchnic mesoderm forms the epimyocardium. Once the single heart tube has formed, it has 3 layers: endocardium, myocardium, and a thin enveloping epicardium (the latter 2 from epimyocardium). The pericardium forms later from the surrounding coelomic mesenteries. The single linear heart tube, traditionally, is described with reference to the heart landmarks of basal vertebrates (eg,

Table 1
Glossary of terms

Evolutionary Terminology

Clade	A group of organisms that includes a common ancestor and all of its descendants
Plesiomorphy/plesiomorphic	An ancestral character
Apomorphy	A character that is different from the form found in ancestors; it is an innovation for that species
Symplesiomorphy	A character shared by the 2 or more taxa that occurs in their earliest common ancestor
Synapomorphy	Two or more taxa in a clade share a character with their recent common ancestor

Taxonomic Terminology

Archosaurs	Crocodilians and birds
Aves	Birds
Chelonia	Turtles, terrapins, and tortoises; also genus of the green sea turtle
Ectothermic sauropsids	Turtles, lizards, snakes, crocodilians, and amphisbaenians
Lepidosauria	Lizards, snakes, and the tuatara
Nonavian archosaurs	Alligators, caimans, crocodiles, and gharials
Rynchocephalia	The tuatara, *Sphenodon punctatus* is the sole member of this clade
Sauropsids	Turtles, tuatara, squamates, crocodilians, and birds
Serpentes	Snakes
Squamates	Lizards, snakes, and amphisbaenians (squamates are within the Lepidosauria)

Cardiac Terminology

Endocardium	Specialized endothelial cells that, during embryogenesis, form a lining on the inside of the developing heart, which is maintained throughout life.
Epicardium	A layer of mesothelial tissue that envelops the heart in all vertebrates and is the inner (visceral) layer of the pericardium
Myocardium	The heart muscle layer is composed of cardiomyocytes and fibroblasts
Pericardium	The outer parietal pericardium is composed of layers of collagen fibrils and elastin fibers and formed from mesenteries during development

(continued on next page)

Table 1 (continued)	
Outflow tract/Inflow tract	The vessels that leave the ventricle of a developing heart/vessels draining into the developing heart
Cavum/cava	Distinct cavities termed compartments within the ventricle
Conus arteriosus	Gives rise to the pulmonary artery trunk (in lower vertebrates it has spiral valve separating pulmonary from systemic flow paths); conus arteriosus differentiates into a basal (embryonic) bulbus cordis and the truncus arteriosus
Bulbus arteriosus	Embryonic distal outflow tract; bulbus arteriosus is an arterial structure containing smooth muscle
Bulbus cordis	Base of the pulmonary trunk
Truncus arteriosus	Embryonic: cranial end of the bulbus cordis (also known as the conus cordis) gives rise to the aorta and pulmonary trunk
Looped heart	Embryonic: changes shape from a simple linear tube to a more complex structure with a rightward helical loop
Sinus venosus	The first (venous) chamber of the heart
Atrium	The 2nd and 3rd chambers of the heart receiving venous blood via the sinus venosus on the right and the pulmonary vein on the left. They drain into the ventricle
Auricle	Archaic term for the atrium; contemporary the flap-like edge of the atria chamber in mammals
Ventricle	The 4th muscular chamber of the heart
Cavum venosum	Central ventricular compartment of the ventricle; receives blood from the right atrium
Cavum arteriosum	Left ventricular compartment receives blood from the left atrium; this blood primarily flows to the aortae.
Cavum pulmonale	Right-most ventricular compartment receives blood from the right atrium. This blood primarily flows to the pulmonary trunk
Bulbuslamelle	Smooth-surfaced ventricular myocardium is opposite the muscular ridge; attaches/supports the dorsal valves of the aortae
Muscular ridge	A spiraling septum within the ventricle partially separates the cavum venosum from the cavum pulmonale (also known as the horizontal septum or the Muskelleiste). It holds the ventral valves of the aortae and the dorsal valve of the pulmonary artery

(continued on next page)

Table 1
(continued)

Vertical septum/interventricular septum	A sheet-like aggregation of spongy myocardium partially separates the cavum arteriosum from the cavum venosum; located immediately caudal to the atrioventricular valves
Horizontal septum	The muscular ridge = interventricular septum
Great vessels	Pulmonary trunk and arteries, aortae
Truncus pulmonalis	Pulmonary truck is the base of the outflow from the ventricle to the pulmonary arteries
Systemic aortae	Left and right aortae
Conduction system	Low conducting atrioventricular canal muscle is present and spongy ventricular muscle serves the dual purpose of conduction and contraction
Pacemaker	Located in the right leaflet of the sinoatrial valve in Python
Sinus node/Sinuatrial node	Sinoatrial junction functions as SA in squamates. The electrical impulse was delayed between the sinus venosus and the right atrium, allowing the sinus venosus to contract and aid right atrial filling.
Cartilago cordis	Cartilaginous element located between the roots of the aortic trunk and pulmonary artery in 11 species of snakes. In Spanish terrapins (chelonians), the cartilage develops in the proximal part of the outflow tracts, aorticopulmonary septum and the pars fibros.
Major Veins to the Heart	
Postcava	Venous drainage of the viscera and ~posterior two-third of the body
Right precava	Vein draining the head and forelimbs forming to anterior sinus venous horn along right side the head and forelimbs forming to anterior sinus venous horn along right side.
Left precava	Posterior sinus horn
Landmarks	
Base	Cranial pole of the heart
Apex	Caudal pole of the heart.
Shunts and Connections	
Intracardiac shunt	Directing of the blood in the ventricle to the systemic circulation while minimizing flow to the pulmonary vessels (right to left shunt) or from the systemic circuit to include flow to the pulmonary circuit as well.

(continued on next page)

Table 1 (*continued*)	
Peripheral shunts	Shunting of blood between the aortae via the
Foramen of Panizza	A hole that connects the left and right aorta as they leave the heart of Crocodilians.
Interaortic foramen	The bases of the left and right aortae in snakes are joined by the foramen allowing blood exchange between the 2 aortae.
Pulmonary vascular shunt	Pulmonary bypass
Systemic vascular shunt	Left & right aortic flow exchange
Valves	
Aortic valves	Semilunar valves at the bases of the aortae are mesenchymal
Atrioventricular valve	Single-flapped (medial leaflets) valves that are mesenchymal valves. Single-flapped (medial leaflets) valves that are mesenchymal valves except in crocodilians that have right muscular flap valve.
Cog-tooth valve	Base of pulmonary artery in crocodilians
Pulmonary valve	Sphincter or cog valve (crocodilians) that creates resistance to or opens for pulmonary arterial flow from the ventricle.
Sinuatrial valves	The sinuatrial valves are myocardial

Chondrichthyes) as having 4 regions. Starting from venous pole to arterial pole these regions are sinus venous, atrium, ventricle, and outflow tract (conus arteriosus[a]). The developing heart tube grows asymmetrically so that it loops upon itself, resulting in the regions becoming morphologically distinct.[10] These early embryonic regions are topographically assigned (**Fig. 1**) and do not equal the developing or even the adult chambers of the heart. A contemporary and developmentally more appropriate description recognizes (from venous to arterial pole) the inflow tract, embryonic ventricle, and outflow tract.[11] In several amniote clades, these embryonic regions contribute in a different and dynamic way to the formation of the atria, ventricle, and adult outflow tracts, which are determined by craniocaudal and dorsoventral patterning of gene expression and differential cell proliferation.[12–15] It is noteworthy that most developmental insights have been gained from model species (zebrafish–*Xenopus*–chicken–mouse) while knowledge of ectothermic sauropsid heart development is limited.

---

[a] "Conus arteriosus" is a comparative anatomic term that refers to the myocardial outflow tract of basal vertebrates. It is well developed in cyclostomes and Chondrichthyes but lost in teleost fish, where it is replaced by the bulbus arteriosus. The bulbus arteriosus is an arterial structure containing smooth muscle. Unfortunately, the terminology is confusing, sometimes the term "conus arteriosus" is also used erroneously in comparative embryology. During the evolution of amniotes, the conus arteriosus differentiates into a basal bulbus cordis (not to be mistaken with the bulbus arteriosus) and the truncus arteriosus; both being transitory embryonal structures.

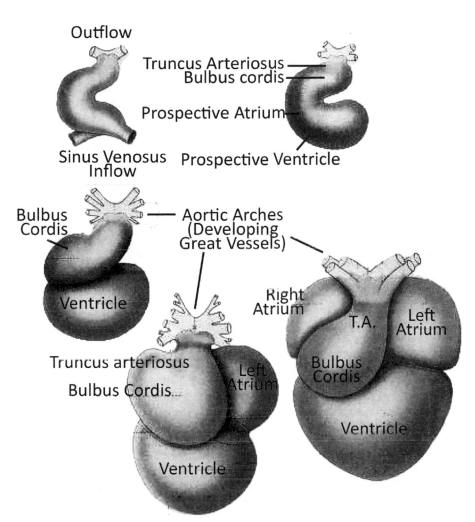

Fig. 1. Development of the sauropsid heart based on the sand lizard, *Lacerta agilis* (modified from Greil 1903). The illustrations show major stages in heart development starting with the tubular embryonic heart undergoing initial asymmetrical growth (*top left*), then looping tube so the prospective ventricle and atrium balloon to the embryo's right and aortic arches are added to the outflow (*top right*). The outflow tracks are the aortic arches, which will become the great vessels. The sinus venosus is not seen in ventral view as the forming ventricle extends ventrally and slightly caudally. The reconfiguring of the embryonic ventricle further balloons abuts the bulbus cordis; the truncus arteriosus elongates and additional aortic arches form (*middle*). The bulbus cordis is adjacent to the formed left atrium (*left bottom*). The early heart with 4 major recognizable chambers, 2 atria, the ventricle, and the sinus venosus (not seen in ventral view), has a clear bulbus cordis and truncus arteriosus nestled between the atria and the ventricle. Apoptosis has reduced the aortic arches to 3 pairs (*bottom right*). T.A., truncus arteriosus. (*Modified from* Greil 1903, publication in public domain, no copyright; downloaded from Biodiversity Heritage Library 23.06.2021).

The formation of the inflow tract and the atria appears to be similar among tetrapods and represents a conserved developmental pattern acquired in the common tetrapod ancestor. Among amniotes, however, morphologic developmental divergences begin with the looped heart (see **Fig. 1**). Separate heart chambers become recognizable at the outer curvature of the developing heart.[11,12] Ventricle formation and septation appear to proceed via differing paths in the various amniote groups.

In chelonians, *Sphenodon,* squamates, and archosaurs, the base of the outflow tract, the bulbus cordis, becomes incorporated into the ventricle. At the border between the embryonic ventricle and the outflow tract, an incomplete septum arises from the ventricle's trabeculated myocardial wall (= vertical septum) and separates the cavum arteriosum from the cavum venosum and the cavum pulmonale. Thus, the bulbus cordis contributes to the formation of the right ventricle; this process evolved independently in sauropsids and mammals. The septum includes epicardium in its core. This "trapped" epicardium develops as the vertical septum in squamates and chelonians and the anterior part of the interventricular septum in archosaurs.[16]

Other fundamental developmental processes are shortening of the outflow tract, ingrowth of the coronary arteries, separation of the pulmonary and aortic channels, and remodeling of the pharyngeal arch arteries. Early embryos of sauropsids, including birds, develop a systemic aorta (right aorta) emerging from the left-sided part of the ventricle, and supplying the main parts of the body. From the right-sided (part of the) ventricle, the pulmonary trunk, and the left aorta (= visceral aorta) arise. The pulmonary trunk divides into the pulmonary arteries supplying the lungs. The right aorta mainly supplies the digestive system. In bird embryos, the left-sided visceral aorta disappears later by apoptosis.[17] Although developmental mechanisms of these distinct patterns are becoming more clear, the evolutionary transitions resulting in the 5-chambered heart morphology of chelonians and lepidosaurs and the 4-chambered heart of the archosaurs remains to be elucidated.

Molecular studies on embryonic hearts provide some insights into potential homologies: Tbx5 expression appears to be an important molecular marker for material derived from the atrioventricular segments of the heart tube. Where expression of Tbx5 ceases, the vertical septum develops and right-sided differentiations occur. Patterning of Tbx5, in the archosaurian (crocodilians and birds) and synapsid (mammalian) lineages, likely is an important mechanism in the convergent evolution of complete ventricular septation.[18] The vertical septum (=interventricular septum) derives from the trabeculated myocardium and separates the cavum arteriosum from cavum venosum and cavum pulmonale. In crocodiles and birds, the interventricular septum separates this bulbus cordis-derived material as right ventricle from the parts of the ventricle that become the left (systemic) ventricle.

COMPARATIVE MORPHOLOGY

The postembryonic heart differs grossly between crocodilians, and the other ectothermic sauropsids (**Figs. 2–4**). In chelonians, squamates, and *Sphenodon,* the ventricle is partially divided as cava, whereas in crocodilians and birds, the ventricle is divided into left and right. The left ventricular region develops from the embryonic ventricle, whereas the right ventricular region develops by contributions from the embryonic bulbus cordis. The ventricular septum (= vertical septum, interventricular septum), be it incomplete (Chelonia, Rhynchocephalia, Squamata) or complete (Archosauria) develops at the border between the 2 regions as a myocardial infolding. In Chelonia, Rhynchocephalia, Squamata, material from the bulbus cordis also contributes to the formation of the muscular ridge and bulbuslamelle, both structures that

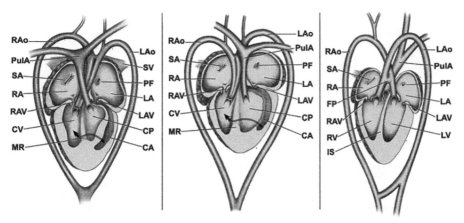

Fig. 2. Diagrams of frontal sections reptilian hearts showing the chambers, compartments, and great vessels. Note there are 3 major patterns of ventricles and outflow structures: turtles and general squamate pattern (*left*), varanid pattern (*middle*), and that of crocodilians (*right*). The pulmonary arteries (= pulmonary trunk) arise as a single structure then bifurcate. CA, cavum arteriosum; CP, cavum pulmonale; CV, cavum venosum; FP, foramen of Panizza; IS, interventricular septum (= vertical septum); LA, left atrium; LAo, left aorta; LAV, left atrioventricular valve; LV, left ventricle; MR, muscular ridge; PF, pulmonary vein foramen; PulA, pulmonary artery; RA, right atrium; RAo, right aorta; RAV, right atrioventricular valve; RV, right ventricle; SA, sinoatrial valve; SV, sinus venosus (*Courtesy of* Jeanette Wyneken, PhD, Boca Raton, Florida).

further divide the right ventricular region into the cavum venosum and the cavum pulmonale. Muscular ridge and bulbuslamelle have no equivalents in archosaurs, and thus they represent a clade-specific cardiac feature.

Sinus Venosus

In the recent literature, the sinus venosus is a largely neglected structure. It is the first part of the heart, receives venous blood from systemic return, has a myocardial wall structure, and is the primary pacemaker of myocardial contraction. Bojanus (1819)[19] described and illustrated the sinus venosus in adult European pond turtles (*Emys orbicularis*). O'Donoghue (1918)[20] described the sinus venosus of leatherback turtles (*Dermochelys coriacea*) as large and commented on similarities in snapping turtles (*Chelydra serpentina*). Benninghoff (1933)[21] described the sinus venosus of *Boa constrictor* and *Chelonia viridis* (= *C. mydas*) as large. Wyneken (2001)[22] described the sinus venosus of all extant sea turtles as a large, thinwalled chamber. Mathur (1944)[23] reported on the heart morphology of *Varanus monitor* (*Varanus monitor* is not a recognized species. We infer that Mathur likely examined *Varanus bengalensis*, a species common where he worked) including details of the sinus venosus. Despite some variability in how major veins (precava and postcava) drain into the sinus venosus, it consists of the posterior, left, and right sinus horns.[24] In a developmental and comparative study, Jensen and colleagues (2017)[25] showed that *Anolis* lizards have an extensive myocardial sinus venosus that is partially invested with atrial tissues. Joyce and colleagues (2020)[26] found smooth muscle was common in the red-eared turtle's (*Trachemys scripta*) sinus venosus and atrium. Functional mapping showed that contractions of the hearts of *Anolis* and *Python* were driven from the sinuatrial junction. The timing of the

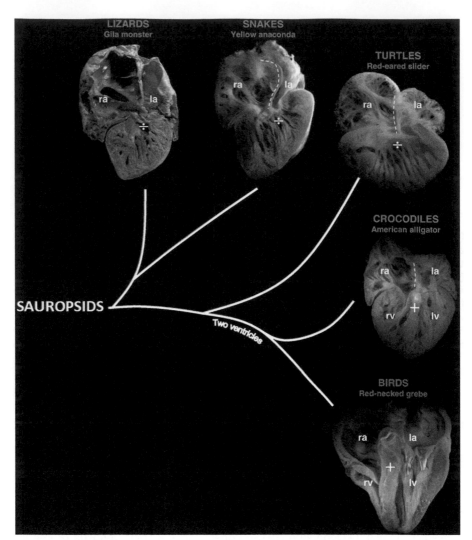

Fig. 3. Phylogenetic comparisons of dorsal halves of diastolic reptile hearts clear of blood. The left columns show representative hearts of ectothermic sauropsids: lizard (Gila monster, *Heloderma suspectum*), snake (yellow anaconda, *Eunectes notaeus*), and turtle (red-eared slider, *Trachemys scripta*); American alligator (*Alligator mississippiensis*). An endothermic sauropsid is represented by a bird, the red-necked grebe (*Podiceps grisegena*). Dashed lines represent the interatrial septum; ÷, ventricle lacks interventricular septum; +, ventricle has a complete interventricular septum; la, left atrium; ra, right atrium; rv, right ventricle; lv, left ventricle of the crocodilian and bird hearts. (*Modified from* Jensen et al. 2013; with permission from Elsevier, under license # 5147631468629; 14.09.2021).

impulses between the sinus venosus and right atrium facilitated filling from the sinus venosus before the atrium contracted.

Among archosaurs, the sinus venosus is maintained in all crocodilians (*Alligator mississippiensis*[21]; *Crocodylus niloticus*[27]) and in some birds (*Gallus*[28]; *Apteryx, Struthio, Gallus, Corvus*[29]; ostrich, pigeon[24]); in other species, it is incorporated into the right atrium.

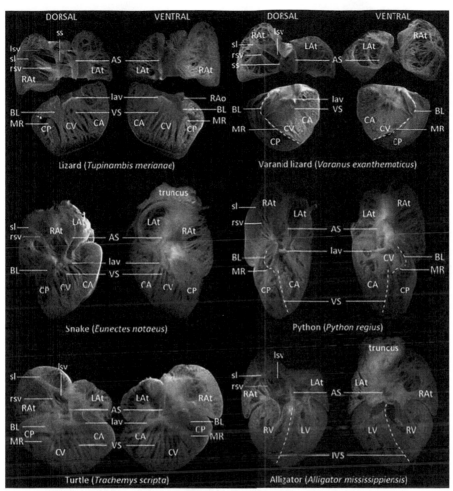

Fig. 4. Internal anatomy of dorsal and ventral halves of diastolic reptile hearts clear of blood. The left columns show representative hearts of a lizard (tegu, *Tupinambis merianae*), snake (yellow anaconda, *Eunectes notaeus*), and turtle (red-eared slider, *Trachemys scripta*); the right columns show the unique cardiac anatomy of a varanid lizard (*Varanus exanthematicus*), python (*Python regius*), and crocodilian (*Alligator mississippiensis*). Note the position of the muscular ridge (MR), the Bulbuslamelle (BL), and the vertical septum (VS); the ventricle is considered to have 3 compartments: the cavum arteriosum (CA), the cavum venosum (CV), and cavum pulmonale (CP) in all but the crocodilian. Note that the cavum pulmonale of the varanid lizard and the python are less densely trabeculated. The atrioventricular canal (dashed lines) is indicated on the dorsal halves only. AS, atrial septum; IVS, crocodilian interventricular septum; LAt, left atrium, RAt, right atrium, lav, left atrioventricular valve; lsv, left sinuatrial valve; rsv, right sinuatrial valve; L(R)V, left (right) ventricle of the crocodilian heart; RAo, right aorta; sl, suspensory ligament; ss, sinus septum. (*Modified from* Jensen et al. 2014; with permission from Elsevier, under license # 5147630468808; 14.09.2021).

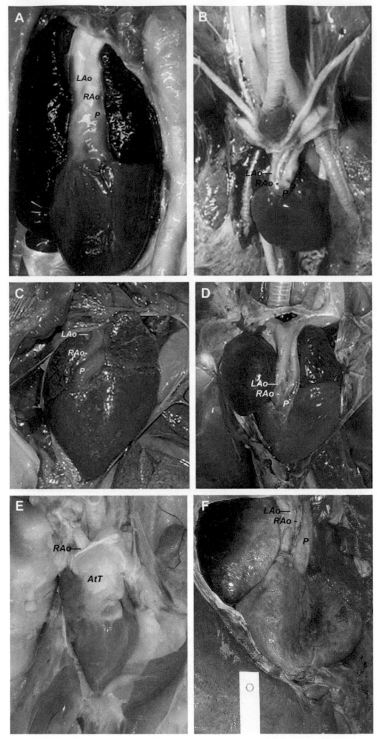

Fig. 5. Ventral views of the hearts of example sauropsids. These photos are of adult or sub-adult hearts: (*A*) the elongated heart of a Burmese python (*Python molurus*); (*B*) note the somewhat round ventricle of the red-eared slider turtle (*Trachemys scripta*); (*C*) green

Outflow Tract/Great Vessels/Truncus Arteriosus

The great vessels of sauropsids show a combination of ancestral and derived features. The adult great vessels, defined as the pulmonary trunk, and left and right aortae are derived from the embryo's truncus arteriosus. Separation of the truncus arteriosus into the aortae and the pulmonary trunk by the aortopulmonary flow divider occurs early in embryogenesis with contributions of endocardial (outflow tract cushions), neural crest, and second heart field cells. Separation of systemic and visceral aorta is primarily by fusion of the outflow tract cushions. In birds, the visceral (left) aorta disappears early in embryogenesis and the second heart field-derived aortic flow divider merges with the aortopulmonary septum (avian aortopulmonary septal complex). In mammals, the systemic (right) aorta disappears early in embryogenesis and the pulmonary flow divider merges with the aortopulmonary septum.[17] Understanding the normal patterns of separation and development is a foundation not only for understanding evolutionary convergence but also common pathologic conditions.

The interaortic septum is supported by hyaline cartilage; in older sauropsids, that cartilage may calcify.[22,30] The aortae of chelonians tend to have large bases when compared with those of other reptiles and arise dorsal and slightly to the right of the pulmonary trunk (see **Fig. 4**; **Fig. 5**). The left aorta arches dorsally and to the left supplying arteries to the abdominal viscera. The right aorta arches dorsally and slightly to the right travels caudally supplying major branches the head (carotids arteries), stomach, pancreas, spleen, and duodenum before joining the left aorta as a common dorsal aorta. In squamates, chelonians, and *Sphenodon*, the bases of the left and right aortae, topographically, appear arise from the ventricular midline or right side of the ventricle. The sauropsid pulmonary trunk gives rise to the right and left pulmonary arteries and exits the ventricular surface slightly more cranially than the aortae. In varanid lizards, the left aorta arises slightly more ventrally than the pulmonary trunk. In *Iguana iguana*, the left aorta and pulmonary trunk exit the ventricle cranioventrally but show variable levels of torsion of the 3 great vessels, such that their paths quickly become circuitous.

The morphology of the great vessels is complex because bulbus cordis, truncus arteriosus, the ventral aorta, and certain branchial arteries contribute to both the adult outflow tract and parts of the ventricle. The truncus arteriosus has a myocardial wall and is part of the heart. It is secondarily divided into the pulmonary trunk, as well as left and right aorta. Remnants of the conus arteriosus (the common cardiac outflow tract of basal vertebrates) are found at the base of the pulmonary trunk (in turtles and crocodiles; **Fig. 5**). There, the conus arteriosus derivatives act as constrictor muscles and may regulate the flow through the pulmonary trunk (see below). During embryonic development, the basal parts of the conus (bulbus cordis) form part of the ventricle ("ventricularize") and contribute to the formation of the cavum venosum, muscular ridge, and bulbuslamelle.[6,16,17,31-33] The pattern of great vessels in reptilian sauropsids clearly is derived (as compared to amphibia) and modified in the various groups. The positioning of the origin of truncus pulmonalis and aortae has considerable functional implications for those sauropsids with a 3-chambered ventricle.

◄————————————————————————————

iguana (*Iguana iguana*); (*D*) bearded dragon (*Pogona vitticeps*); (*E*) saltwater crocodile (*Crocodylus porosus*); (*F*) heart of a male leatherback sea turtle (*Dermochelys coriacea* surrounded by liver. Note the relatively short, rounded ventricle with the stout great vessels emerging from ventricle relatively more caudally than in the lizards. Also, the cut remnants of the gubernaculum cordis are present at the apex and extend to the pericardial sac. AtT, arterial trunk; LAo, left aorta; P, pulmonary trunk; RAo, right aorta (*Courtesy of* J. Wyneken, PhD, Boca Raton, Florida).

In contrast with the ectothermic sauropsids, birds lose the left aortic arch; only the right aortic arch persists and emerges from the left ventricle. The pattern observed in mammals, also which have only one (left) aorta, has independently evolved from an early amniote ancestor of sauropsids and mammals.[14,34]

Cardiac Conduction System

The morphology of the cardiac conduction system of ectotherm sauropsids is understudied. This is because, in part, no morphologic correlate of the conduction system is identifiable using macroscopic dissections or standard histology. It is known from electrocardiograms that contractions commence at the sinus venosus and continue to the atria, ventricle, and bulbus cordis.[35] Only during the past decade, with the advent of molecular markers, have the cellular building blocks of the cardiac conduction system begun to emerge. Jensen and coauthors[5,36] carried out *in situ* hybridization analysis using evolutionary conserved genetic markers to provide a 3-dimensional reconstruction of the key components of the cardiac conduction system in example squamates, archosaurs, and mammals. The authors described a molecular genetic and functionally conserved building plan where the conduction systems of adult ectothermic vertebrate hearts are similar to the embryonic systems of endothermic mammals and birds. These results indicate that primordial components of the cardiac conduction system were already present in the ancestral sauropsids (if not earlier vertebrates). The existence of a cardiac conduction system was confirmed using a different set of molecular markers and it was shown that the conduction cells are morphologically indistinct from cardiomyocytes, thus requiring molecular markers to characterize the cells.[37]

Among archosaurs, birds have an anatomically distinct pacemaking and conduction system that is, to some degree, similar (convergent) to that of mammals. Birds possess a sinus node, AV-node, AV-bundle, left and right bundle branches, and a distinct right AV-ring of Purkinje-fibers and a recurrent branch of the AV-bundle that encircles the aortic root.[21,38] Despite a superficial similarity with mammals, the morphology of the avian cardiac conduction system is a derived condition that evolved independently from the morphologic building blocks present in squamates and ectotherm archosaurs (crocodilians[5,24,25]). Thus, the evolutionary and comparative morphology of the sauropsid cardiac conduction system is characterized by certain molecular markers, but not as a distinct structure.

Gubernaculum Cordis

The gubernaculum cordis is a band of connective tissue covered with serous membrane, which attaches the apex of the heart to the pericardium in turtles, lizards, tuatara, and crocodiles. It probably is a residual of a portion of the ventral mesocardium.[39] An artery supplying the coronary arteries runs through the gubernaculum cordis in some/most chelonians,[40] Tuatara, Agamida, Iguanida, Scincida, Lacertidae, Teiidae, Helodermatidae. The heart of varanids has only a residual structure at the apex that was interpreted as a remnant of the gubernaculum cordis.[41] Most authors report the absence of a gubernaculum cordis in the snakes although de Silva (1956–1958)[42] indicated that vestiges in some species, and Webb (1969)[41] mentioned a vestigial gubernaculum cordis in some sea snakes (*Hydrophis* sp.; but see a different view on *Hydrophis platurus*[43]). Thus, it is uncommon in snakes and probably is not associated with an arterial supply. Crocodilians have a gubernaculum cordis, which is traversed by arterial trunks.[44] Therefore, the gubernaculum cordis must be considered plesiomorphic in sauropsids (shared with Amphibia). Functional implications of its (partial?) loss in snakes and varanids are unknown. In birds, a ligamentum hepatopericardium positions the heart within the pericardium and connects it with the ventral mesentery between the hepatic lobes (Braun 2003).[29,45,46] Although no other than descriptive information exists, one may speculate that the ligamentum hepato-pericardium is (partially homologous) with the gubernaculum cordis in ectotherm sauropsids.

Coronary Arterial Circulation

The coronary arterial circulation of sauropsids has been studied in 28 species from 11 families.[40] They show a well-developed coronary arterial system but describe considerable variation, especially in origin of the coronary arteries, among sauropsid clades. The level of detail in anatomic description has not been reached in any later publication; this study remains the best possible reference. More functional perspectives of myocardial perfusion in sauropsids showed that transmyocardial perfusion (nonvascular) of the alligator heart contributes a significant source of blood flow to the myocardium.[47,48] Coronary arterial morphology and blood supply to the myocardium in nonmammalian amniotes remains a poorly studied topic that requires future attention.

Blood Pressure

Sauropsid blood pressure has been measured mostly using invasive sensors (cannulas in major vessels) and often in animals recovering from anesthesia.[9] Nevertheless, 2 taxa with 5-chambered hearts, pythons and varanid lizards, stand out as having pressure separation in great vessels. Pythons and varanid lizards are exceptional in their capacities to maintain low pulmonary pressure and high systemic pressure.[49] This is unusual for ectothermic sauropsids; most have similar pressures in their great vessels. It is also noteworthy that intracardiac flow separation evolved independently in lizards (varanids) and snakes (pythons) from an ancestor endowed with the capacity for large intracardiac shunts.[24,26] For *Python regius*, the aortic walls are significantly thicker and contain more collagen than the walls of the pulmonary system.[50] Although comparative studies that include species without pressure separation are absent, this remains a singular finding, which, however, is consistent with the ventricular pressure separation in this species. Of course, archosaurs (crocodiles and birds) have complete separation of systemic and pulmonary circulations, thus separate high and low pressure circulations and high and low oxygen content of blood flow, respectively.[8]

Cardiac Shunts

The comparative morphology of the hearts of ectotherm sauropsids suggests that central shunts (intracardiac, in chelonians and lepidosaurs) or peripheral shunts (foramen of Panizza, in crocodilians) allow for bypassing the pulmonary to systemic circulations or flow to both (ie, right to left, or left to right shunt, respectively). Burggren and colleagues (2020)[9] provided an extensive review of the diversity and the history of research on cardiovascular shunting in vertebrates, and hypotheses regarding function. They conclude that cardiac and peripheral shunting may serve multiple functions depending on the physiologic condition, and suggest the need for functional contrasts, field versus laboratory studies, and selection of taxonomically appropriate species to identify adaptive significance. Indeed, many of the sometimes-contrasting results of cardiac shunting studies may result from unrecorded/unrecognized and essentially different physiologic conditions that necessarily bias results, particularly since most studies are invasive procedures into a highly sensitive system. For example, even minimally invasive procedures, such as Doppler ultrasonography on trained/acclimatized crocodiles resulted in enormous variances in measurements, making comparisons difficult because of the large sample size needed to reach statistical power (Starck, unpubl. data).

SYSTEMATIC OVERVIEW
Turtles, Terrapins, and Tortoises

In most chelonians, the heart is located topographically deep to margins of the humeral and pectoral scutes. Externally, a line extending between the shoulder joints demarks the heart position. However, in some species, it is positioned more posteriorly along the midline between humeral-pectoral and pectoral-abdominal scute lines.[30,51,52] In soft-shelled turtles (Trionychidae), the heart is displaced to the right. The shoulder girdles provide good radiographic landmarks as the base of the heart is just caudal to the level of the acromion processes and cranial to the distal procoracoid processes.[52] The chelonian heart has 4 chambers, in the traditional sense, but 6 functional chambers: sinus venosus, right and left atria, and a ventricle that is subdivided into 3 compartments termed cava; cavum venosum, cavum arteriosum, and cavum pulmonale.[22,30,52,53] The flow of blood through the heart is described in the context of the cardiopulmonary relationships during ventilation versus apnea largely based on measurements in diving species, turtles and crocodilians.[54]

Rynchocephalia

The heart of *Sphenodon punctatus* is described as largely similar to that of lizards except for having a reduced muscular ridge. Parts of the aortic valves have a cushion-like appearance that is not seen in lizards. The paired aortae exit the ventricle surface with an elevated muscular bulbus arteriosus, also not found in lizards.[24,53,55,56]

Squamata

Varanidae: Monitor lizards are the only lizards with a functionally divided ventricle. Yet, squamate reptiles have a morphologically undivided ventricle with the atrioventricular canal positioned to the left of the body midline (see **Fig. 4**). During development, the muscular ridge and bulbuslamelle form partial septa within the ventricle, but do not separate incoming atrial bloodstream. The vertical septum is formed of trabecular myocardium and located beneath the atrioventricular valve; there it functions similarly to the mammalian ventricular septum.[33] It is the electrical conduction pathway within the vertical septum coordinates flow such that atrial bloodstreams separate left side of the ventricle. In *Varanus spp.*, the cavum venosum acts as a conduit for systemic venous blood to the cavum pulmonale, during ventricular diastole. It then serves as a conduit for pulmonary venous blood in systole.

   Lacertidae: A radiological study of blood flow through the heart and great vessels of *Lacerta viridis*[57] showed that blood entering the heart from the right and left atria mix minimally in the ventricle. The blood from the lungs to the left atrium enters the left portion into the ventricle's cavum arteriosum and is sent to the right systemic arch and to both carotid arteries. The blood from the systemic circulation, entering the right atrium through the sinus venosus, is divided into 2 flow streams. One passed into the right dorsal portion of the ventricle (cavum venosum), then flowed mainly to the left systemic aorta. The other portion flowed to the dorsal portion of the ventricle, then to the ventral portion (cavum pulmonale) and to the pulmonary arteries. Substantial mixing of blood from systemic and pulmonary circuits in the heart was not observed in this study, or with other sauropsids using physiologic metrics.[26]

Snakes

The topographic position of the heart of snakes along the snout-vent length varies with respect to locomotion, habitat, phylogeny, and developmental stage.[58-63] It appears to be gravity-sensitive (ie, differs between arboreal, terrestrial, and aquatic snakes),[64–66] but the actual topographic position appears to be affected by several additional cardiovascular and behavioral factors.[58,67] Terrestrial and arboreal species tend to have hearts located closer to the head; presumably, the proximity to the pump (heart) stabilizes cephalic blood pressure when the head is raised. Purely aquatic snakes that have water pressure supporting the entire body under most circumstances have the heart located more toward the middle of their snout-vent length.

General morphology

The morphology of the snake heart has been described in sufficient detail.[23,24,52,68,69] The elongated heart is located in the pericardium. It has 5 morphologic and 6 functional chambers, that is, the sinus venosus, left and right atrium, cavum venosum, cavum arteriosum, and cavum pulmonale (see **Figs. 4** and **5**).

In snakes, the sinus venosus collects blood from the large systemic veins (postcaval vein, right precaval vein [ie, left and right anterior sinus horn], and left precaval vein [posterior sinus horn]). Myocardial contraction contributes to filling of the right atrium; the left atrium receives oxygenated blood directly from the pulmonary vein. The dominant pacemaker is a ring-like domain in the immediate vicinity of the sinuatrial junction.[25]

The left and right atrium are separated by the interatrial septum. The atrioventricular valves reach deep into the ventricle (ie, the interventricular canal). The valves have dual functions: (1) during ventricular systole, the atrioventricular valves prevent backflow from the ventricle into the atria and direct blood from the cavum arteriosum through the interventricular canal and the cavum venosum into the left and right aortae. (2) During ventricular diastole, the atrioventricular valves direct blood flow from the left atrium into the cavum arteriosum and from the right atrium into the cavum pulmonale; they also close the interventricular canal so that oxygenated and deoxygenated blood remain separated. The ventricular chambers are separated by morphologically "incomplete" septa that, however, may functionally provide a complete separation of the chambers during the heart cycle. The interventricular septum largely, but not completely, separates the cavum arteriosum from the cavum venosum and cavum pulmonale. A broad interventricular canal remains open and connects the chambers of the ventricle. However, as described earlier, the atrioventricular valves obstruct the interventricular canal during filling of the ventricle, so that the cavum arteriosum and the combined cava venosum and pulmonale are completely separated. The muscular ridge and the bulbuslamelle separate cavum venosum and cavum pulmonale; the muscular ridge derives from the embryonic outflow tract and the bulbuslamelle from the endocardial cushions. Both interact forming a potentially tight septum (in some species) that establishes high and low pressure compartments in the cavum pulmonale and cavum venosum, respectively. The truncus arteriosus embraces the pulmonary artery and the left and right aortae. It is positioned in a way that the pulmonary artery receives blood from the cavum pulmonale and the aortae receive blood from the cavum venosum. The aortic valves are semilunar valves that extend as connective tissue cushions onto the free edge of the muscular ridge and the opposite the bulbuslamelle (see **Figs. 4** and **5**; **Figs. 6** and **7**)

Functional morphology of the python heart

A generalized functional scheme for the squamate heart based on anatomic studies suggested an important role of the atrioventricular valves in directing intracardial blood flow.[68,70–72] However, the functioning of the snake heart can best be understood when using live imaging (ultrasonography[73–75]) because the action of the atrioventricular valves and the muscular ridge dynamically open and separate blood flow

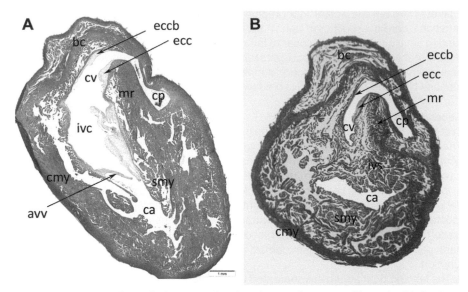

Fig. 6. Cross-section through the ventricle of *Python molurus;* paraffin-embedded, 10 μm section thickness, hematoxylin-eosin stain. (*A*) Section in a more basal position, including parts of the interventricular canal and fragments of the atrioventricular valves. (*B*) Section is located more apical (caudal) to section A, where the interventricular septum separates the cavum arteriosum from the cavum venosum and cavum pulmonale. avv, atrioventricular valves; bc, bulbus cordis; ca, cavum arteriosum; cmy, compact myocardium; cp, cavum pulmonale; cv, cavum venosum; ecc, endocard cushion; eccb, endocard cushion of bulbus lamelle; ivc, interventricular canal; ivs, interventricular septum; mr, muscular ridge; smy, spongious myocardium. Scale bar = 1 mm (original image: J.M. Starck).

during heartbeat cycle. Doppler-ultrasonography has rarely been used to analyze the pattern in blood flow in the beating heart of snakes (see **Fig. 7**).[75,76]

During early ventricular diastole, blood from both atria fills the ventricle. The left atrioventricular valve closes the interventricular canal and directs blood from the left atrium into the cavum arteriosum. The right atrioventricular valve bends caudally into the interventricular canal so that blood from the right atrium is directed into the cavum venosum and cavum pulmonale. It does not fully close the interventricular canal so that, theoretically, flow into the cavum arteriosum might be possible. There is a slight time difference between left and right, and blood from the right atrium enters the cavum venosum before the cavum arteriosum begins to fill from the left atrium. The muscular ridge is wide open and allows blood flow from the cavum venosum into the cavum pulmonale. During late ventricular diastole, blood flow from the atria has ceased. Almost all blood from the cavum venosum has crossed the muscular ridge and fills the cavum pulmonale. The interventricular canal is still closed by the flaps of the left atrioventricular valve. During early ventricular systole, the muscular ridge moves against the ventricular wall, now separating the cavum venosum and the cavum pulmonale. By moving upward, the atrioventricular valves open the interventricular canal and close the atrioventricular windows. At the same time, blood from the cavum arteriosum begins to fill the cavum venosum. In late ventricular systole, blood from the cavum pulmonale is pressed into the pulmonary artery, and blood from the cavum venosum is pumped into both aortas. During this action, the muscular ridge tightly closes the connection between the cavum venosum and cavum

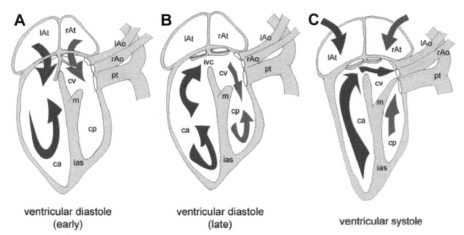

ventricular diastole
(early)

ventricular diastole
(late)

ventricular systole

Fig. 7. Pattern of blood flow in the heart of *Python regius*. (A) During early ventricular diastole, blood from the atria enters the cavum arteriosum and the cavum venosum, the atrioventricular valves close the interventricular canal, and the muscular ridge is wide open. (B)
During late ventricular diastole, blood flow from the atria has ceased, blood from the cavum
venosum crosses the muscular ridge into the cavum pulmonale, and the atrioventricular
valves close the atrioventricular windows, thereby opening the interventricular canal allowing blood flow from the cavum arteriosum into the cavum venosum. (C) During ventricular
systole, the muscular ridge separates the cavum pulmonale and cavum venosum. Blood from
the cavum pulmonale is pressed into the pulmonary trunk; blood from the cavum venosum
is pressed into the aortas. The cardiac cycle begins again by filling the atria. The arrows indicate major pattern and direction of blood flow; red color indicates systemic circulation; and
blue color indicates pulmonary circulation. (*From* Starck 2009; with permission from Wiley
and Sons under license # 5150730794725; 16.09.2021)

pulmonale (see **Fig. 7**). Thus, mixing of blood from cavum venosum and cavum pulmonale is not possible and pressure separation is established for systemic and pulmonary circulations during this stage of the heart cycle.[19,77–79]

The cardiac conduction system of snakes cannot be documented using dissection
or standard histology. However, molecular markers for the cardiac conduction system
in embryonic snakes render a positive signal in the atrioventricular canal on both sides
and in the bulbuslamelle of the ventricle close to the right part of the atrioventricular
canal as well as in the nerves in sulcus coronaries and in the interatrial septum.[37]
Although just an embryonic pattern of a molecular marker, such patterns appear to
represent a plesiomorphic feature shared with other amniotes.[5]

Aortic valves and interaortic foramina
Aortic valves have been described for several snake species of different phylogenetic
relationship.[80] The aortic valves are semilunar valves at the base of the 2 aortae. They
may vary in size and extension. No ecological correlate but a phylogenetic signal was
found in this variation. An interaortic foramen between left and right aortae was described
for 32 snake species[80] and functionally studied using Doppler ultrasonography.[81] Blood
flow through the interaortic foramina might result in an interaortic shunt of blood that
potentially alters hemodynamics and flow patterns in the systemic circulation of snakes.

Cartilago cordis
A cardiac skeletal element, the cartilage cordis (cartilage cordis), has been described
for several snake species[82] as well as other vertebrates. When present, it is located in

the aorticopulmonary septum. However, there is considerable intraspecific and interspecific variability of size and shape of the cartilago cordis. It has been described for *Python regius* but not for *Python reticularis*[82] or *Python molurus*.[83] Young (1994)[82] suggested that the cartilago cordis is best viewed as an example of the potential for chondrification that is present in the connective tissue of the aorticopulmonary septum.

Cardiac shunting in snakes

The morphology of the snake heart suggests that blood from the left (systemic) circulation can be shunted to the right (pulmonary) circulation (L-R shunt; systemic bypass) or, vice versa, pulmonary-to-systemic shunt (pulmonary bypass; **Fig. 8**).

Numerous hypotheses about the physiologic effects of shunting (or the lack thereof) have been discussed.[2–4,8,9,84–86] Although the morphology of the heart, major arteries, and the pulmonary and systemic vascular circuits suggests that various forms of shunting are possible (systemic bypass, pulmonary bypass), the occurrence of shunts is notoriously difficult to measure in live animals. Several reasons can be discussed why even carefully executed experimental studies result in conflicting outcomes.[86] (1) Most studies assume a long-term duration of shunting but ignore the possibility that shunting occurs on a beat-by-beat basis. Thus, published studies may report accurate results but reflect animals in different physiologic states thereby precluding direct comparisons among them. (2) Many important quantitative data are completely missing. We lack information about ventricle and blood volumes, and shunting volumes under different physiologic conditions. (3) Experimental studies are dominated by highly invasive studies, including open-heart surgery or perfused heart models. Although those approaches provide important basic information, it is unclear how much they reflect a normal physiologic condition. Even in noninvasive studies (eg, Doppler ultrasonography), low levels of stress, or lack of acclimatization may change the pattern of blood flow, albeit to a lesser extent than that caused by invasive surgical procedures. (4) To the best of our knowledge, capillary filtration rate and the role of the lymphatic system as a CO_2 sink have been neglected in the literature.

A recent extensive review takes an integrative approach to the adaptive value of cardiac shunting, yet minimally integrates the morphology of the cardiovascular system.[9]

Doppler ultrasonography provided evidence that in fasting/resting, *Python regius* blood is primarily (almost twice the volume) directed into the systemic circulation (24 h after feeding).[75] After feeding, the snakes show a typical postprandial increase in oxygen consumption. In association with the increased oxygen consumption, a larger blood volume is pumped through the pulmonary circulation. Although this study is one of the very few minimally invasive studies reporting blood flow shifts under different physiologic conditions, it is limited in that it studied only blood flow volume in response to digestion. Also, a beat-to-beat measurement of blood flow volume was not conducted, so that short-term regulatory changes could not be detected. It is entirely possible that different distribution of blood flow volume (shunting) may be observed under different conditions.

Archosauria

The heart of extant archosaurs (crocodiles and birds) has completely separated atria and completely separated ventricles, thus preventing cardiac mixing of blood and providing complete pressure separation of the pulmonary and systemic circulation. A sinus venosus is present in crocodiles and basal clades of birds but it is atrialized in more derived avian taxa. Crocodiles maintain the ancestral sauropsid pattern of 2 aortae; birds have the left aorta completely reduced.

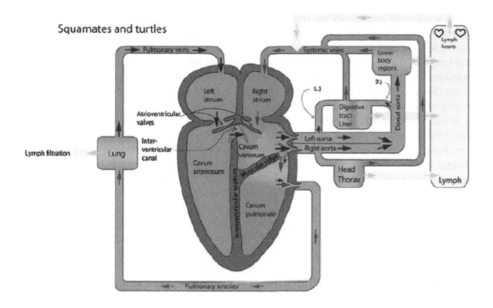

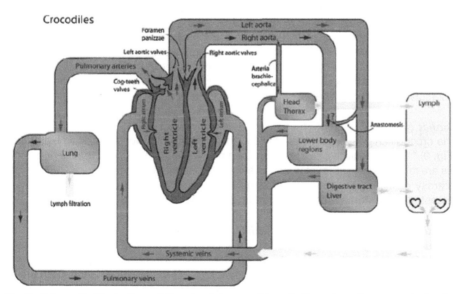

Fig. 8. Schematic illustration of the circulatory and lymphatic systems in squamates/turtles and crocodiles. Red color indicates O_2-rich, CO_2-poor blood; blue color indicates O_2-poor, CO_2-rich blood; different shades of violet stand for different degrees of mixing; lymph is drawn in yellow; and arrows indicate the direction of blood/lymph flow. (*From* Campen and Starck 2012; with permission from Springer Nature, under license # 5150731075001; 16.09.2021).

Crocodylia

The hearts of crocodilians have 5 chambers: sinus venosus, left and right atrium, and left and right ventricle. There are 2 aortae (left and right) and a common pulmonary trunk that gives rise to left and right pulmonary arteries. The separate ventricles have what may appear to be unusual outflows. The pulmonary trunk and left aorta leave the right ventricle. The left aorta's position allows the blood from the right ventricle to take an alternative route into the systemic circulation instead of going to the lungs. A connection between the left and right aortae, at their bases immediately outside the ventricle, the foramen of Panizza, remains open during diastole and allows pressure equilibration between the 2 aortae; however, its functional significance remains equivocal. We discuss each aspect below.

Among the outstanding features characterizing the crocodilian heart is the origin of the right aorta from the left ventricle, and the left aorta together with the pulmonary artery from the right ventricle. The left aorta branches into the Arteria gastroesophagea, Arteria gastrointestinalis, and the Arteria gastrosplenicointestinalis, thus it supplies esophagus, liver, stomach, and spleen. The right aorta branches into the carotids, the aorta dorsalis with the Arteria mesenterica and Arteria haemorrhoidalis, thus it supplies head, intestine, and posterior regions of the body. Left and right aortae have a connection through a window at the basis of the arterial trunk, that is, the foramen of Panizza.[87] The opening of the foramen of Panizza is rather small, and, morphology suggests, that during ventricular systole, it is covered by the flaps of the aortic valves (see **Figure 9**).[44,86,88,89] However, active changes in the diameter of the foramen might cause flow patterns to alter under different conditions.[90] Further down the circulatory system, the aortic anastomosis represents an additional connection between the 2 aortae.

The basis of the pulmonary artery is characterized by an internal lining with large connective tissue cushions (cog tooth valve), and a well-developed circular muscle (not found along the pulmonary artery).[86] The circular muscle probably represents a residue of the bulbus cordis; the cog tooth valves probably derive from the outflow tract cushions. Embryologic studies on the development of the heart of crocodiles are completely missing and early accounts[91,92] describe the heart development in insufficient detail to answer such questions.

Cardiac cartilage

The crocodilian heart has 2 well-developed cartilages composed of hyaline cartilage (**Fig. 9**).[91,93] Comparative morphologic data about the occurrence of the cartilago cordis are rare and the only systematic overview appears to be on snakes.[82] Despite that scarcity of information, one might consider the occurrence of a cartilago cordis a ancestral character that crocodiles share with other sauropsids.

Functional morphology of the crocodilian heart

The unique design of the crocodilian heart and the peripheral vascular circuits (see **Figure 8**) has evoked several functional explanations, but none has been unambiguously supported so far.[86] The current textbook paradigm[54,94] assumes key functional roles for the foramen of Panizza and the cog tooth valve suggesting that the crocodilian heart anatomy primarily supports a pulmonary bypass during diving apnea. During air breathing, the pulmonary artery is open and blood from the low pressure, right ventricle enters it. The pressure is too low for the blood to enter the left aorta. (Interestingly, it is not quite clear why the pressure is too low, or which structure would obstruct the opening of the left aorta.) The left ventricle pumps blood into the right aorta and, through the foramen of Panizza, into the left aorta. Immunohistochemistry[95–97] suggested that the foramen of Panizza and the abdominal anastomosis are under adrenergic control and proposed an active role of the foramen in exchanging blood between the right and the left aorta. During diving apnea, the cog tooth valve supposedly closes the entry into the pulmonary artery and blood is directed into the left aorta, thus bypassing the lungs. This

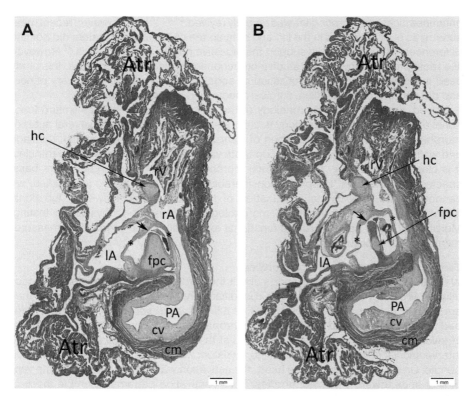

Fig. 9. Consecutive histologic sections (*A, B*) through the ventricular outflow tract including the foramen of Panizza; paraffin-embedded, 10 μm section thickness, hematoxylin-eosin stain. *Crocodylus niloticus*. *, bicuspid valve of left and right aortae, respectively; arrow, foramen of Panizza during ventricular systole; Atr, atrium; cm, constrictor muscle (bulbus cordis); cv, cog tooth valve; fpc, foraminal process of heart cartilage; hc, heart cartilage; lA, left aorta; PA, pulmonary artery; rA, right aorta; rV, right ventricle (original image: J.M. Starck).

paradigmatic view completely neglects the fact that the pulmonary and aortic valves cover the foramen of Panizza during ventricular systole so that flow through the foramen is not possible during ventricular systole.[44,86,93,98,99] Several studies suggest that flow through the foramen of Panizza occurs during ventricular diastole, that is, as retrograde flow from left to right aorta.[96,100,101] This view neglects role of the downstream abdominal anastomosis between left and right aortae. And, it neglects the observation that crocodiles enter extreme bradycardia during diving.[97,102–104] Webb (1979)[44] suggested that the foramen of Panizza is a remnant of their evolutionary history reflecting the transition from temporary pressure separation in hearts, for example, pythons and varanids, to permanent pressure separation in hearts of crocodiles and birds. However, the integrated arrangement of the crocodilian heart chambers, aortae, and the peripheral vessels has already been recognized by the comparative anatomists more than 100 years ago,[34,105,106] but their functional interpretations had been replaced by a paradigmatic focus on pulmonary bypass. Those early comparative morphologists correctly recognized that the left aorta, which emerges from the right ventricle, receives CO_2-enriched blood which is directed to the intestinal organs, mainly the esophagus, stomach, and anterior part of the small intestine. It has been suspected that in resting animals, the blood flow in the celiac artery derives from the right aorta via the abdominal anastomosis between the 2 aortae.[107] The idea that cardiovascular shunting (pulmonary bypass) enhances digestion in crocodiles was recently revived.[84,85,108–111] However, recent measurements of blood gases in the left and right aortae of American alligators did not find differences in CO_2 that would support the digestive physiology hypothesis.[27] However, like most previous physiologic studies on peripheral shunting in crocodiles, this study used invasive methods (catheterization of aortae), had only a short recovery period, and did not control for handling, surgical effects, and physiologic stress.

Indeed, the specialized morphology of the crocodilian heart still has limited functional explanations. Its morphology is unique among sauropsids with several autapomorphic characters, that is, foramen of Panizza, highly developed cardiac cartilage and well-developed bulbus cordis, cog tooth valve, and aortic origins from ventricles. It is clearly not transitory because such morphology is not found in any more basal species of Sauropsids. Despite a considerable number of (physiologic) studies, we cannot provide unequivocal explanation of the morphology. However, functional morphology requires both careful morphologic analyses and physiologic testing. Morphology alone cannot provide functional explanations and physiologic measurements cannot explain morphology.

Cardiac conduction system of crocodilians

We found only one study that reports about the cardiac conduction system in crocodilians (*Alligator mississippiensis*).[36] Crocodilians are of special interest because they are the only ectothermic vertebrates with a full ventricular septum. The authors mapped ventricular activation to document the propagation of activation along a functional atrioventricular bundle. Impulses appeared at the dorsal epicardial surface along the interventricular sulcus, a location that is consistent with an origin via an atrioventricular bundle. On the ventral side of the heart, the activation wave propagated from the ventricular apex toward the major arteries. These activation patterns resemble those of mammals and birds. However, a ventricular Purkinje network, as occurs in birds, was absent and ventricular conduction relied on the trabecular myocardium, as it does in other ectothermic vertebrates. Thus, the formation of a functional atrioventricular conduction system clearly predates the formation of an anatomically distinct Purkinje-system, which obviously developed independently in birds and mammals.

DISCLOSURE

The authors have nothing to disclose.

REFERENCES

1. Stearns SC, Nesse RM, Govindaraju DR, et al. Evolutionary perspectives on health and medicine. Proc Natl Acad Sci 2010;107(suppl. 1):1691–5.

2. Hicks JW, Wang T. Functional role of cardiac shunts in reptiles. J Exp Zoolog A Ecol Genet Physiol 1996;275(2-3):204–16.

3. Hicks JW, Wang T. The functional significance of the reptilian heart: new insights into an old question. In: Sedmra D, Wang T, editors. Ontogeny and phylogeny of the vertebrate heart. New York: Springer; 2012. p. 207–27.

4. Hicks JW. The physiological and evolutionary significance of cardiovascular shunting patterns in reptiles. Physiology 2002;17(6):241–5.

5. Jensen B, Boukens BJ, Postma AV, Gunst QD, van den Hoff MJ, Moorman AF,, Christoffels VM. Identifying the evolutionary building blocks of the cardiac conduction system. PLoS one 2012;7(9):e44231.

6. Jensen B, van den Berg G, van den Doel R, et al. Development of the hearts of lizards and snakes and perspectives to cardiac evolution. PLoS one 2013;8(6): e63651.

7. Jensen B, H Smit T. Examples of weak, if not absent, form-function relations in the vertebrate heart. J Cardiovasc Dev Dis 2018;5(3):46.

8. Burggren WW, Christoffels VM, Crossley D 2nd, et al. Comparative cardiovascular physiology: future trends, opportunities and challenges. Acta Physiol (Oxf) 2014;210(2):257–76.

9. Burggren W, Filogonio R, Wang T. Cardiovascular shunting in vertebrates: a practical integration of competing hypotheses. Biol Rev Camb Philos Soc 2020;95(2):449–71.

10. Agassiz L. Embryology of the turtle. In: Contributions to the natural history of the United States of America. Boston: Little, Brown and Company; 1857. p. 451–709.

11. Christoffels VM, Habets PE, Franco D, et al. Chamber formation and morphogenesis in the developing mammalian heart. Developmental Biol 2000;223(2): 266–78.

12. Moorman AF, Christoffels VM. Cardiac chamber formation: development, genes, and evolution Physiol Rev 2003;83:1223 67.

13. Christoffels VM, Burch JB, Moorman AF. Architectural plan for the heart: early patterning and delineation of the chambers and the nodes. Trends Cardiovasc Med 2004;14(8):301–7.

14. Jensen B, Christoffels VM. Reptiles as a model system to study heart development. Cold Spring Harb Perspect Biol 2020;12(5):a037226.

15. Jensen B, Christoffels VM, Moorman AF. An appreciation of anatomy in the molecular world. J Cardiovasc Development Dis 2020;7(4):44.

16. Poelmann RE, Gittenberger-de Groot AC, Vicente-Steijn R, et al. Evolution and development of ventricular septation in the amniote heart. PLoS One 2014; 9(9):e106569.

17. Poelmann RE, Gittenberger-de Groot AC, Biermans MW, et al. Outflow tract septation and the aortic arch system in reptiles: lessons for understanding the mammalian heart. EvoDevo 2017;8(1):1–17.

18. Koshiba-Takeuchi K, Mori AD, Kaynak BL, et al. Reptilian heart development and the molecular basis of cardiac chamber evolution. Nature 2009; 461(7260):95–8.

19. Bojanus, L.H., (1819). Anatome testudines Europaeae (Facsimile Reprints in Herpetology No. 26; Gans, C., Darevsky, I.S., and Adler, K. eds). Published by the Society for the Study of Amphibians and Reptiles. Ohio. pp. 1–185

20. O'Donoghue CH. The heart of the leathery turtle, Dermochelys (Sphargis) coriacea. With a note on the septum ventriculorum in the Reptilia. J Anat 1918;52(Pt 4):467.

21. Benninghoff A. Herz. Part III. In: Bolk L, Göppert E, Kallius E, et al, editors. Handbuch der vergleichenden Anatomieder Wirbeltiere. Band 6. Berlin & Wien: Urban & Schwarzenberg; 1933. p. 467–556.

22. Wyneken J. The anatomy of sea turtles. U.S Department Commerce NOAA Tech Memorandum NMFS-SEFSC 2001;470:1–172.

23. Mathur PN. The anatomy of the reptilian heart. Proc Indian Acad Sciences-Section B 1944;20(No. 1):1–29. Springer India.

24. Jensen B, Boukens BJ, Wang T, et al. Evolution of the sinus venosus from fish to human. J Cardiovasc Development Dis 2014;1(1):14–28.

25. Jensen B, Vesterskov S, Boukens BJ, et al. Morpho-functional characterization of the systemic venous pole of the reptile heart. Sci Rep 2017;7(1):1–12.
26. Joyce W, Crossley DA, Wang T, et al. Smooth muscle in cardiac chambers is common in turtles and extensive in the emydid turtle, *Trachemys scripta*. Anatomical Rec 2020;303(5):1327–36.
27. Conner JL, Crossley JL, Elsey R, et al. Does the left aorta provide proton-rich blood to the gut when crocodilians digest a meal? J Exp Biol 2019;222(7).
28. Quiring DP. The development of the sino-atrial region of the chick heart. J Morphol 1933;55(1):81–118.
29. Baumel JJ. Handbook of avian anatomy: nomina anatomica avium. USA: Publications of the Nuttall Ornithological Club; 1993. no. 23.
30. Farrell AP, Graperil AK, Frances ETB. Comparative aspects of heart morphology. In: Gans C, Gaunt AS, editors. Biology of the reptilia, visceral organs, 19. New York: Society for the Study of Amphibians and Reptiles; 1998. p. 375–424.
31. Greil A. Beitrage zur vergleichenden Anatomie und entwicklungsgeschichte des Herzens und des truncus arteriosus der wirbelthiere. Morphologische Jahrbuch 1903;31:123–210.
32. Bertens LM, Richardson MK, Verbeek FJ. Analysis of cardiac development in the turtle *Emys orbicularis* (Testudines: Emidydae) using 3-D computer modeling from histological sections. Anatomical Rec 2010;293(7):1101–14.
33. Hanemaaijer J, Gregorovicova M, Nielsen JM, et al. Identification of the building blocks of ventricular septation in monitor lizards (Varanidae). Development 2019;146(14):dev177121.
34. Gegenbaur C. Vergleichende Anatomie der Wirbelthiere mit Berücksichtigung der Wirbellosen, Band 2. Leipzig: Verlag von Wilhelm Engelmann; 1901.
35. Jensen B, Moorman AF, Wang T. Structure and function of the hearts of lizards and snakes. Biol Rev 2014;89(2):302–36.
36. Jensen B, Boukens BJ, Crossley DA II, Conner J, Mohan RA, van Duijvenboden K,, Christoffels VM. Specialized impulse conduction pathway in the alligator heart. Elife 2018;7:e32120.
37. Kvasilova A, Gregorovicova M, Kundrat M, et al. HNK-1 in morphological study of development of the cardiac conduction system in selected groups of sauropsida. Anatomical Rec 2019;302(1):69–82.
38. Prosheva VI, Kaseva NN. Location and functional characterization of the right atrioventricular pacemaker ring in the adult avian heart. J Morphol 2016;277(3):363–9.
39. Kingsley JS. Comparative anatomy of vertebrates. 2nd edition. Philadelphia: Blakistone Son & Co.; 1917. p. 293.
40. MacKinnon MR, Heatwole H. Comparative cardiac anatomy of the reptilia. IV. The coronary arterial circulation. J Morphol 1981;170(1):1–27.
41. Webb G. The squamate heart: a recapitulation of the literature and an examination of the structure of the heart in a number of species. Unpubl. Honors Thesis, University of New England; 1969.
42. de Silva PHDH. The heart and aortic arches in *Calotes uersicolor* (Daudin) with notes on the heart and aortic arches in *Calotes alotes* (Linne) and *Calotes nigrilabris* Peters. Spolia Zeylanica 1956-1958;28:55–68.
43. Jonnalagadda N, Tomar MPS, Putluru S, et al. Heart of yellow bellied sea snake (*Hydrophis platurus*): a gross morphological study. Int J Curr Microbiol App Sci 2018;7(3):3192–6.

44. Webb GJ. Comparative cardiac anatomy of the Reptilia. III. The heart of croco-dilians and an hypothesis on the completion of the interventricular septum of crocodilians and birds. J Morphol 1979;161(2):221–40.

45. Wolf K. *Das Herz der Vögel*. Berlin: Doctoral dissertation, Humboldt-Universität; 1967.

46. Braun S. Pathologische, pathohistologische und mikrobiologische Untersuchun-gen am Herzen und den großen Blutgefäßen von Vögeln der Ordnung Psittaci-formes. Giessen: Doctoral dissertation, Veterinary Department, University of Giessen; 2003.

47. Whittaker P, Kloner RA. Transmural channels as a source of blood flow to ischemic myocardium? Insights from the reptilian heart. Circulation 1997; 95(6):1357–9.

48. Kohmoto T, Argenziano M, Yamamoto N, Vliet KA, et al. Assessment of trans-myocardial perfusion in alligator hearts. Circulation 1997;95:1585–91.

49. Zaar M, Overgaard J, Gesser H, et al. Contractile properties of the functionally divided python heart: two sides of the same matter. Comp Biochem Physiol A Mol Integr Physiol 2007;146(2):163–73.

50. van Soldt BJ, Danielsen CC, Wang T. The mechanical properties of the systemic and pulmonary arteries of *Python regius* correlate with blood pressures. J Morphol 2015;276(12):1412–21.

51. Kik MJL, Mitchell MA. Reptile cardiology: a review of anatomy and physiology, diagnostic approaches, and clinical disease. *Semin Avian Exot Pet Med* 2005; 14(1):52–60.

52. Wyneken J. Normal reptile heart morphology and function. Vet Clin North Am Exot Anim Pract 2009;12(1):51–63.

53. Webb GJ, Heatwole H, de Bavay J. Comparative cardiac anatomy of the reptilia. II. A critique of the literature on the Squamata and Rhynchocephalia. J Morphol 1974;142(1):1–20.

54. Kardong KV. Vertebrates: comparative anatomy, function, evolution. 8th edition. New York: McGraw-Hill; 2018.

55. O'Donoghue CH. The blood vascular system of the tuatara, Sphenodon puncta-tus. Philosophical Trans R Soc Lond 1921;210:175–252. Series B, Containing Papers of a Biological Character.

56. Simons JR. The heart of the Tuatara Sphenodon punctatus. In: Proceedings of the zoological society of london146. Oxford, UK: Blackwell Publishing Ltd; 1965. p. 451–66.

57. Foxon GEH, Griffith J, Price M. The mode of action of the heart of the green liz-ard, *Lacerta viridis*. Proc Zoolog Soc Lond 1956;126(1):145–58.

58. Gartner GE, Hicks JW, Manzani PR, et al. Phylogeny, ecology, and heart position in snakes. Physiol Biochem Zool 2010;83(1):43–54.

59. Lillywhite HB, Albert JS, Sheehy CM 3rd, et al. Gravity and the evolution of car-diopulmonary morphology in snakes. Comp Biochem Physiol Part A Mol Integr Physiol 2012;161(2):230–42.

60. Anderson GE, Secor SM. Ontogenetic shifts and spatial associations in organ positions for snakes. Zoology (Jena) 2015;118(6):403–12.

61. Lillywhite HB, Lillywhite SM. Ontogenetic shifts of heart position in snakes. J Morphol 2017;278(8):1105–13.

62. McCracken HE. Organ location in snakes for diagnostic and surgical evaluation. In: Miller RE, editor. *Zoo and wildlife medicine, current therapy* 4. Philadelphia: W.B. Saunders; 1999. p. 243–8.

63. Perez D, Sheehy CM III, Lillywhite HB. Variation of organ position in snakes. J Morphol 2019;280(12):1798–807.
64. Lillywhite HB. Circulatory adaptations of snakes to gravity. Am Zoologist 1987; 27(1):81–95.
65. Lillywhite HB. Gravity, blood circulation, and the adaptation of form and function in lower vertebrates. J Exp Zoolog Part A Ecol Genet Physiol 1996;275(2-3): 217–25.
66. Seymour RS. Scaling of cardiovascular physiology in snakes. Am Zoologist 1987;27(1):97–109.
67. Seymour RS, Arndt JO. Independent effects of heart–head distance and caudal blood pooling on blood pressure regulation in aquatic and terrestrial snakes. J Exp Biol 2004;207(8):1305–11.
68. White FN. Functional anatomy of the heart of reptiles. Am Zoologist 1968;8(2): 211–9.
69. Jensen B, Abe AS, Andrade DV, et al. The heart of the South American rattlesnake, *Crotalus durissus*. J Morphol 2010;271(9):1066–77.
70. White FN. Circulation. In: Gans C, Dawson WR, editors. Biology of the reptilia, Vol. 5A physiology. London: Academic Press; 1976. p. 275–334.
71. Webb G, Heatwole H, De Bavay J. Comparative cardiac anatomy of the Reptilia. I. The chambers and septa of the varanid ventricle. J Morphol 1971;134(3): 335–50.
72. Jensen B, Nyengaard JR, Pedersen M, et al. Anatomy of the python heart. Anat Sci Int 2010;85(4):194–203.
73. Snyder PS, Shaw NG, Heard DJ. Two-dimensional echocardiographic anatomy of the snake heart (*Python molurus bivittatus*). Vet Radiol Ultrasound 1999;40(1): 66–72.
74. Schilliger L, Tessier D, Pouchelon JL, et al. Proposed standardization of the two-dimensional echocardiographic examination in snakes. J Herpetological Med Surg 2006;16(3):76–87.
75. Starck JM. Functional morphology and patterns of blood flow in the heart of *Python regius*. J Morphol 2009;270(6):673–87.
76. Schroff S, Starck JM, Krautwald-Junghanns ME, et al. Echokardiographische Untersuchungen bei Boiden: Darstellung und Blutflussmessungen. Tierärztliche Praxis Ausgabe K: Kleintiere/Heimtiere 2012;40(03):180–90.
77. Wang T, Altimiras J, Axelsson M. Intracardiac flow separation in an in situ perfused heart from Burmese python *Python molurus*. J Exp Biol 2002; 205(17):2715–23.
78. Wang T, Altimiras J, Klein W, et al. Ventricular haemodynamics in *Python molurus*: separation of pulmonary and systemic pressures. J Exp Biol 2003;206(23): 4241–5.
79. Jensen B, Nielsen JM, Axelsson M, et al. How the python heart separates pulmonary and systemic blood pressures and blood flows. J Exp Biol 2010; 213(10):1611–7.
80. Young BA, Lillywhite HB, Wassersug RJ. On the structure of the aortic valves in snakes (Reptilia: Serpentes). J Morphol 1993;216(2):141–59.
81. Young BA, Saunders M. Direct visualization of blood flow through the interaortic foramen of the eastern diamondback rattlesnake, *Crotalus adamanteus*, using echocardiography and color Doppler imaging. J Exp Zoolog 1999;284(7): 742–5.
82. Young BA. Cartilago cordis in serpents. Anatomical Rec 1994;240(2):243–7.

83. Campen R. Cardiovascular function in ectotherm sauropsids. Munich: Doctoral dissertation, Department of Biology, Ludwig-Maximilians University; 2018. p. 148.

84. Farmer CG, Uriona TJ, Olsen DB, et al. The right-to-left shunt of crocodilians serves digestion. Physiol Biochem Zool 2008;81(2):125–37.

85. Farmer CG. On the evolution of arterial vascular patterns of tetrapods. J Morphol 2011;272(11):1325–41.

86. Campen R, Starck M. Cardiovascular circuits and digestive function of intermittent-feeding sauropsids. In: Comparative physiology of fasting, starvation, and food limitation. Berlin, Heidelberg: Springer; 2012. p. 133–54.

87. Panizza B. Sulla struttura del cuore e sulla circulatione del sangue del *Crocodilus lucius*. Biblioth Ital LXX 1833;70:87–91.

88. Greenfield LJ, Morrow AG. The cardiovascular hemodynamics of Crocodilia. J Surg Res 1961;1(2):97–103.

89. Cook AC, Tran VH, Spicer DE, et al. Sequential segmental analysis of the crocodilian heart. J Anat 2017;231(4):484–99.

90. Grigg GC, Johansen K. Cardiovascular dynamics in *Crocodylus porosus* breathing air and during voluntary aerobic dives. J Comp Physiol B 1987; 157(3):381–92.

91. Rathke H. Untersuchungen über die Entwickelung und den Körperbau der Krokodile. Braunschweig: F. Vieweg; 1866. p. 1–270.

92. Reese AM. Development of the American alligator (*A. mississippiensis*). Washington DC: Smithsonian Institution Publication no. 1791; 1908. p. 1–111.

93. White FN. Circulation in the reptilian heart *(Caiman sclerops)*. Anatomical Rec 1956;125(3):417–31.

94. Kardong KV. Vertebrates: comparative anatomy, function, evolution. International edition. 3rd edition. New York: McGraw-Hill; 2002.

95. Karila P, Axelsson M, Franklin CE, et al. Neuropeptide immunoreactivity and co-existence in cardiovascular nerves and autonomic ganglia of the estuarine crocodile, *Crocodylus porosus*, and cardiovascular effects of neuropeptides. Regul Pept 1995;58(1–2):25–39.

96. Axelsson M. The crocodilian heart; more controlled than we thought? Exp Physiol 2001;86(6):785–9.

97. Axelsson M, Franklin CE. Elucidating the responses and role of the cardiovascular system in crocodilians during diving: fifty years on from the work of CG Wilber. Comp Biochem Physiol Part A Mol Integr Physiol 2011;160(1):1–8.

98. Axelsson M, Franklin CE, Löfman CO, et al. Dynamic anatomical study of cardiac shunting in crocodiles using high-resolution angioscopy. J Exp Biol 1996; 199(2):359–65.

99. Axelsson M, Franklin CE. The calibre of the foramen of Panizza in *Crocodylus porosus* is variable and under adrenergic control. J Comp Physiol B 2001; 171(4):341–6.

100. Grigg GC. The heart and patterns of cardiac outflow in Crocodilia. Proc Aust Physiol Pharmacol Soc 1989;20:43–57.

101. Axelsson M, Franklin CE. From anatomy to angioscopy: 164 years of crocodilian cardiovascular research, recent advances, and speculations. Comp Biochem Physiol A 1997;118(1):51–62.

102. Wilber CG. Cardiac responses of *Alligator mississippiensis* to diving. Comp Biochem Physiol 1960;1(2):164–6.

103. Wright JC, Grigg GC, Franklin CE. Redistribution of Air Within The Lungs May Potentiate" Fright" Bradycardia In Submerged Crocodiles (*Crocodylus porosus*). Comp Biochem Physiol Comp Physio 1992;102(1):33–6.
104. Seebacher F, Franklin CE, Read M. Diving behaviour of a reptile (*Crocodylus johnstoni*) in the wild: interactions with heart rate and body temperature. Physiol Biochem Zool 2005;78(1):1–8.
105. Hochstetter F. Über die Arterien des Darmkanals der Saurier. Gegenbaurs morphologisches Jahrbuch 1898;26:213–73.
106. Hafferl A. Handbuch der vergleichenden Anatomie der Wirbeltiere. Berlin: Bd. VI. Urban und Schwarzenberg; 1933.
107. Axelsson M, Fritsche R, Holmgren S, et al. Gut blood flow in the estuarine crocodile, *Crocodylus porosus*. Acta Physiol Scand 1991;142(4):509–16.
108. Jones DR, Shelton GRAHAM. The physiology of the alligator heart: left aortic flow patterns and right-to-left shunts. J Exp Biol 1993;176(1):247–70.
109. Jones DR. Crocodilian cardiac dynamics: a half-hearted attempt. Physiol Zoolog 1995;68(4):9–15.
110. Jones DR. The crocodilian central circulation: reptilian or avian? Verhandlungen-Deutschen Zoologischen Gesellschaft 1996;89:209–18.
111. Findsen A, Crossley DA 2nd, Wang T. Feeding alters blood flow patterns in the American alligator (*Alligator mississippiensis*). Comp Biochem Physiol Part A: Mol Integr Physiol 2018;215:1–5.

The Amphibian Heart

Silvana Schmidt-Ukaj, Dr med vet[a],*,
Michaela Gumpenberger, Dr med vet[b], Annika Posautz, Dr med vet[c],
Verena Strauss, Mag med vet[c]

KEYWORDS

- Amphibians • Amphibian heart • Amphibian cardiology • Amphibian diseases

KEY POINTS

- The class amphibia contains 3 orders: Anura (frogs and toads), Caudata (salamanders and newts), and Gymnophiona (caecilians).
- Generally, amphibians have 3 heart chambers: 2 atria and 1 ventricle.
- The basic morphology of the heart is similar in all amphibians with some differences due to their lifestyle.
- Amphibian heart diseases are only occasionally reported and include genetic, congenital, infectious and neoplastic causes.

INTRODUCTION

At present, more than 8200 amphibian species are described,[1] including the 3 orders Anura (frogs and toads), Caudata (salamanders and newts), and Gymnophiona (caecilians).

Some fields of amphibian medicine are well studied because of the amphibian role as animal models especially in the physiology of cardiovascular, musculoskeletal, renal, respiratory, reproductive, and sensory systems, as well as in evolutionary biology, environmental physiology, and in new fields like systems biology.[2,3] The most commonly studied amphibian species include the American bullfrog (*Lithobates calesbelanus*), the cane toad (*Rhinella marina*), the African clawed frog (*Xenopus laevis*), and salamanders like *Ambystoma (A)* spp.[2] Particularly in cardiovascular development and disease, the African clawed frog, *Xenopus (X)* sp, was and still is an attractive model for studies, because it shares numerous anatomic, physiologic, and genetic similarities with humans.[4]

[a] Service for Birds and Reptiles, Small Animal Internal Medicine, Department for Companion Animals and Horses, University of Veterinary Medicine, ViennaVeterinärplatz 11210 Vienna, Austria; [b] Diagnostic Imaging, Department for Companion Animals and Horses, University of Veterinary Medicine, ViennaVeterinärplatz 11210, Vienna, Austria; [c] Research Institute of Wildlife Ecology, Department of Interdisciplinary Life Sciences, University of Veterinary Medicine, ViennaSavoyenstraße 11160, Vienna, Austria
* Corresponding author.
E-mail address: Silvana.schmidt-ukaj@vetmeduni.ac.at

Vet Clin Exot Anim 25 (2022) 367–382
https://doi.org/10.1016/j.cvex.2022.01.002
vetexotic.theclinics.com
1094-9194/22/© 2022 Elsevier Inc. All rights reserved.

Generally, the amphibian heart has been studied since 1835.[5] Physiologic studies with frogs started even earlier; for example, bioelectricity started with observations by Galvani and colleagues[6] in 1793 in frog muscles, and it was shown in 1843 in a dissected frog that an electrical current accompanies each heartbeat.[7] A deeper insight into the history of electrocardiography can be obtained by the detailed review of Zywietz[8] (2003). Many fundamental studies on cardiovascular physiology were based on frog models, including Krogh's (1920) Nobel Prize work on capillary regulation and Bowditch's (1871) description of the "Treppe phenomenon," which means that an increase in the heart rate also increases the myocardial tension.[2] Therefore, the amphibians have played a major role in the development of many fields of vertebrate physiology. Further early studies in amphibians including cardiovascular studies were reviewed by Foxon[9] (1964) and Brady[10] (1964).

This was followed by ongoing research and debates about the amphibian heart as well as blood flow and blood oxygenation by various investigators. In summary, the blood flow in the amphibian heart and the vascular system can vary between species depending on their lifestyle,[9,11–16] but a deep insight into the physiology of the amphibian heart is beyond the scope of this article, which focuses on clinically important aspects of amphibian cardiology and heart diseases.

AMPHIBIAN HEART: CLINICAL ANATOMY, HISTOLOGY, AND PHYSIOLOGY

The amphibian heart is situated in the upper part of the body cavity (**Fig. 1**) and is surrounded by a pericardium. The pericardium is designed as a lymphatic space and its structure and morphology were studied in detail in *Pelophylax esculentus* by Cerra and colleagues (2003) using electron microscopy.[17]

Generally, amphibian heart morphology is similar to that of lungfishes with 3 heart chambers: 2 atria and 1 ventricle.[11,13] For gas exchange, amphibians use their lungs, skin, and buccal cavity.[9,11] Less oxygenated blood (cutaneous and buccal respiration) from the venous systems flows through the anterior and posterior vena cava and the sinus venosus into the right atrium while passing the sinuauricular valves. Oxygenated blood flows through the pulmonary vein into the left atrium. Then the blood from both atria empties into the ventricle by passing 2 pairs of auriculoventricular valves.[11,12] From there, the blood flows to the conus arteriosus, while reflux is prevented by ventriculobulbar valves[11] (**Figs. 2** and **3**). The conus arteriosus also contains a longitudinal spiral valve.[14] From there, less oxygenated blood flows through the pulmocutaneous arch into the lungs and the skin as well as oxygenated blood through the systemic

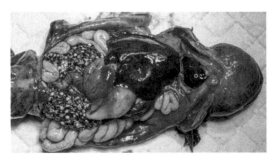

Fig. 1. Deceased axolotl (*Ambystoma mexicanum*) in ventral view. The heart (marked with an *asterisk*) is situated more cranially than the heart of most mammals and contains 2 atria and 1 ventricle. (*From* Mag. Martina Konecny, from the service for birds and reptiles, Small Animal Internal Medicine, University of Veterinary Medicine Vienna, Austria; with permission.)

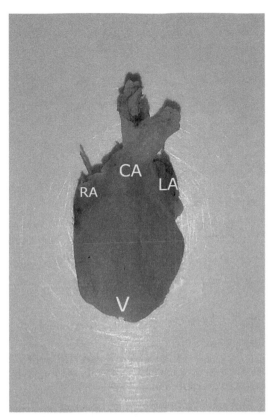

Fig. 2. Heart of a deceased giant waxy tree frog (*Phyllomedusa bicolor*), ventral view; fixed in 80% ethanol. CA, conus arteriosus; LA, left atrium; RA, right atrium; V, ventricle.

(aortic) arch to the body and the carotid arch to the head, directed by the position of the spiral valve.[11,12]

Mixing of oxygenated and less oxygenated blood is prevented by different mechanisms like the trabeculation of the ventricle wall, biphasic contraction and the ventricular portion of the atrial septum, as well as a complicated blood flow, also called "selective channeling" through the heart by some investigators.[11–13] The blood flow and blood oxygenation have been studied in amphibians by various ways and investigators. The results of older studies are summarized by Foxon (1955, 1964),[9,15] Johansen and Hanson (1968),[11] Shelton (1976),[16] and Duellman (1996)[14] demonstrating a variation in arteriovenous mixing due to interindividual and interspecific differences.

Akat (2020)[18] histologically investigated the heart of Anatolian water frogs (*Pelophylax cf. bedriagae*). The sinus venosus acts as the pacemaker of the heart; it is described as very thin walled, and it mainly includes pacemaker cells and ganglion cells. The layer of the heart wall consists of the outer layer epicardium, the middle layer myocardium, and a thin endocardium, whereas the myocardium contains the muscle fibers and connective tissue. The myocardium is the thickest layer with an outer compact layer and an inner trabecular layer. Muscle fibers have the same histologic characters in all parts of the heart (**Fig. 4**).[18] Salamander hearts and especially their muscular connections between the chambers have been studied histologically in

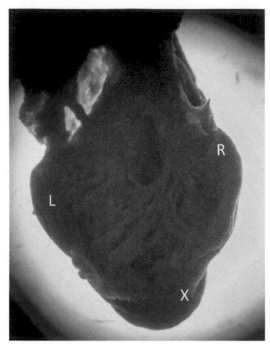

Fig. 3. Cut-section (coronal plane) of the heart of a deceased giant waxy tree frog (*Phyllomedusa bicolor*), dorsal view; fixed in 80% ethanol. Note the trabeculation of the ventricle. L, left; R, right; X, apex. 1.5× magnification.

detail by Davies and Francis[19] (1941), whereas Brady[10] (1964) gives an overview about microscopic features in frog's hearts. Serial histologic sections and 3D reconstruction techniques were also used to study heart development in *X laevis* from a linear heart tube to the appearance of atrial and ventricular chambers by Mohun and colleagues[20] (2000).

The electrical conduction system, heart innervation by the vagus nerve, and its course are described in detail by Brady[10] (1964). The amphibian heart contracts segmentally, starting in the sinus venosus, then atrial contraction follows, continued by the ventricle and the bulbus cordis.

In addition to the basic anatomy, physiology, and histology of the amphibian heart, Duellman (1996)[14] and Wright[21] (2001a) gave overviews of the lymphatic, arterial, and

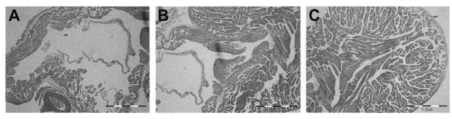

Fig. 4. The figure shows the histologic section (cut in the coronal plane) of the heart of a deceased Vietnamese mossy frog (*Theloderma corticale*), stained with hematoxylin & eosin. (*A*) A section through the atrium. (*B*) The continuation of (*A*) with the valves marked with asterisks. (*C*) The ventricle. Bar = 1 mm.

venous systems of amphibians, including the hepatic and renal portal system. Both investigators point out that interspecific variations are still poorly documented and that pharmacokinetic studies are rare. However, it is suggested to avoid administering drugs that are metabolized or excreted renally or hepatically in the hind parts of the body. Blood collection sites and amphibian hematology are described by Wright[22] (2001b). The amphibian lymph system contains lymph sacs, lymph hearts, and lymph vesicles. The lymph hearts beat independently of the heart.[21]

Species Differences

The basic morphology of the heart is similar in all amphibians with some differences due to their lifestyle.[12,14]

Normally, the right atrium is larger than the left atrium in most salamanders of the order Caudata and in anurans, but of equal size in some anurans like *X laevis*. In caecilians, either the right or the left atrium is smaller than the other.[9,14,21,23]

Atrial septation in amphibians is more diverse than in reptiles, birds, and mammals. The interatrial septum is complete (anurans and salamander genus *Siren*) or fenestrated (in caecilians and salamanders except *Siren*),[9,14] absent or modified in certain lungless species,[21,23–25] and varies between caecilian families.[9,26] Different salamander species also have different incomplete ventricular divisions.[14] Interspecies variations of the conus arteriosus, the sinus venosus, and the arches are described by Foxon (1964),[9] Johansen and Hanson (1968),[11] Duellman (1994)[14] and Wilkinson (1996).[23]

DIAGNOSTIC POSSIBILITIES OF AMPHIBIAN HEART DISEASES
Electrocardiography and Doppler Ultrasound

Bhaskar and Vinod (2006)[27] used human electrocardiography (ECG) machines for recording frog (*Phrynoderma hexadactylum*) ECG for teaching purposes. Right and left arm electrodes were positioned in ventral axillary regions, a chest electrode in the chest region near the lower ventricle, and left and right foot electrodes in ventral inguinal regions. First, the ECG shows P, R, and T waves. By removing the ventricle, R and T are lost. By removing the atria, the ECG shows no P wave anymore. Therefore, it can be shown that the R and T waves are contributed by the ventricle, whereas the P wave is contributed by the atria.

Heart rates in amphibians can be measured by various ways, but for veterinary purposes, Chai (2015, 2016)[28,20] recommends ECG, Doppler ultrasound, or a pulse oximeter in bigger amphibians (**Fig. 5**). ECG in caecilians is described by Peters and Mullen (1960).[30] A portable ECG machine was used in 1962 in wild *Caecilia guntheri*. Heart position was palpated and electrodes were positioned subcutaneously equilateral triangle about the heart.[30]

Heart rates vary with temperature and development; for example, in the frog, *Eleutherodactylus coqui* the heart begins to beat from 40 to 50 beats/min at 25°C, the heart frequency increases to 110 to 120 beats/min during development, and then after hatching it decreases again.[31] Heart rate change during development follows no general pattern and varies between species.[31,32] Aubret and Blanvilln[32] (2013) measured heart rates of frogs and salamanders (*Pelophylax esculentus, Rana dalmatina, Calotriton asper*) with different body masses and temperatures, and heart beats varied between 36 and 82 beats/min.

Endoscopy

Endoscopy allows examination of the pericardium, cardiac surface, and cardiac activity, but the small size of most amphibians is often challenging. Equipment, patient

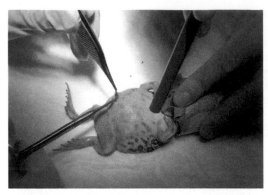

Fig. 5. Clinical picture of monitoring the heart rate of a Pacman frog (*Ceratophrys cranwelli*) during isoflurane anesthesia and surgery with a Doppler ultrasound probe.

preparation, and general procedure in amphibians, which are similar to reptiles, are described by Chai[28] (2015). Generally, the following basic equipment is listed by the investigator: a 1.9-mm integrated telescope, a 2.7-mm-diameter, 18-cm length, 30° oblique rigid telescope with a 4.8-mm operating sheath, an endovideo camera and monitor, a xenon light source and light cable, a 1- or 1.7-mm endoscopic biopsy forceps and grasping forceps, and a carbon dioxide (CO_2) insufflator with silicone tubing or air or saline instead. The investigator recommends that endoscopic procedures should not last more than 10 minutes, because CO_2 insufflation dries out the organs and mucosa of amphibians. The investigator prefers tricaine methanesulfonate (MS-222) for sedation or anesthesia. Amphibians have an undivided pleuroperitoneal cavity. For this reason coelioscopy allows visualization of nearly all coelomic organs, including the heart, from one entry. Therefore, animals are placed in dorsal recumbency and the surgical field in the midcoelom is prepared aseptically with diluted povidone-iodine solution (1:10) in sterile saline or 0.75% chlorhexidine solution. When accessing the coelom with a paramedian skin and abdominal membrane incision, glands, lymph hearts, and blood vessels, especially the midventral vein, should be avoided. After endoscopy, the coelomic membrane and the skin are closed in one layer with simple interrupted sutures. The investigator recommends monofilament nylon as suture material and removal of sutures after 4 to 8 weeks.[28]

Endoscopy is also used in experimental medicine; for example, Marshall and colleagues[33] (2017) investigated cardiac repair after endoscopy-guided heart resection in *X laevis* and therefore developed an endoscopy-guided approach with a 3-mm paramedian skin incision beneath the sternum. Patient preparation and general procedure are similar to Chai[28] (2015). Analgesia was performed with butorphanol (1 mg/kg) and meloxicam (0.4 mg/kg), both injected into the lymph sacs.[33]

Diagnostic Imaging

Radiology and ultrasonography are readily available, quite cheap, noninvasive, and in general useful for diagnosing and monitoring amphibian diseases. Both can usually be performed without anesthesia. Most radiographs can be obtained by placing amphibians directly on the cassette (most frogs or salamanders, for example), whereas a radiolucent box may be used to hinder the patient from escaping from the scene. More delicate or aquatic species can be placed in a moistened, narrow plastic bag. Anyhow, always 2 orthogonal views are taken. The dorsoventral view is performed in perpendicular beam, whereas the lateral view should be done with horizontal beam technique (**Fig. 6**; see **Fig. 9**). High-resolution digital mammography or dental films improve diagnostic possibilities especially in small amphibians (see **Fig. 6**). However, because the heart is mostly situated in the region of the shoulder girdle or even close to the throat and not surrounded by sufficient fat or aerated lung, it cannot be differentiated on plain images (see **Fig. 6**). Routine angiography is not performed in amphibian patients. Therefore, ultrasonography is the most feasible diagnostic imaging tool in amphibian heart investigations.[34,35]

Most ultrasonographic examinations can be carried out by placing the amphibians in water-filled plastic containers or plastic (freezer) bags when attaching a high-frequency transducer to the surface of the water or the container (**Fig. 7**).[34,35] Less delicate amphibians can be manually fixated gently while the transducer is coupled with some gel or only water to the soft skin at the region of the heart, cranioventral of the body. No further preparation of the patient is required. Furthermore, calm handling encourages cooperation of the animals.

2D and 3D echocardiography are described in detail by Dittrich and colleagues[36] (2018) in the axolotl (*Ambystoma mexicanum*). Owing to the small size of most amphibian patients, high-megahertz transducers have to be used. **Fig. 8** provides a longitudinal view of a frog's heart in systole and diastole. The ventricle is identified by its hyperechoic thick muscles and trabeculation, whereas the atria have a paper-thin hyperechoic wall.

Pericardial effusion may be the most obvious pathologic finding[37] (**Fig. 9**), while Doppler sonography may be needed to observe abnormal blood flow or determine blood velocity.[38,39]

Barely any more literature about echocardiography in amphibian patients exists because under clinical circumstances veterinarians or biologists most likely focus on hepatic, gastrointestinal, or renal disorders as well as monitoring the reproductive status and embryonal development.

Some other studies focus on the extraordinary regeneration potentials in axolotls. Recently myocardial repair was documented sonographically.[40]

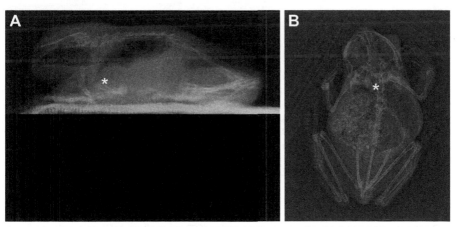

Fig. 6. Lateral (*A*) and dorsoventral (*B*) radiographs of 2 different Australian green tree frogs (*Litoria caerulea*), the first one being performed in horizontal beam technique. Owing to the lack of fat, the heart is not differentiable in plain images. An asterisk points out the cardiac location. Note the different image quality: (*A*) performed with a digital cassette system; (*B*) exposed on a high-resolution detector system.

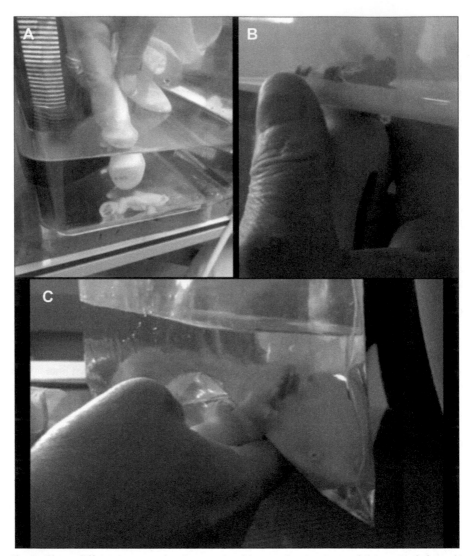

Fig. 7. Three different approaches in sonographic examination in amphibians. Both frogs (*A* and *B*) were placed in a plastic box. While the African clawed frog (*Xenopus laevis*) (*A*) is submerged in water and the transducer is placed through the water on or near the frog, the European fire-bellied toad (*Bombina bombina*) (*B*) is placed on a wet paper towel with the transducer attached to the bottom of the box with some gel. The axolotl (*Ambystoma mexicanum*) (*C*) on the other hand is submerged in a freezer bag and the transducer is attached to the thin plastic outer surface. This technique can even be used to perform radiographs easily.

Contrast-enhanced computed tomography (CT) as well as MRI can provide multiplanar and detailed images, but they are compromised by higher costs, potential need of anesthesia, and less availability. Furthermore, the small size of lots of amphibians hinders acceptable image resolution (**Fig. 10**). Therefore these cross-sectional imaging tools may barely be used in patients, although outstanding cardiac function

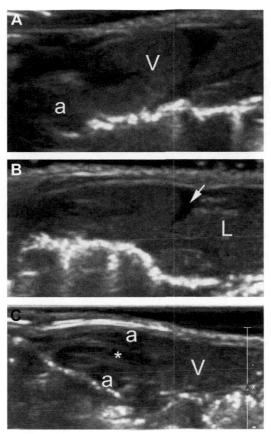

Fig. 8. Echocardiography in an Australian green tree frog (*Litoria caerulea*), long axis view, (*A*) in diastole, (*B*) and (*C*) in systole. The ventricle (V) has prominent trabeculae and a thick muscle, whereas the atria (*A*) are thin walled. In (*C*) part of the truncus arteriosus (*asterisk*) is seen as well. Mild normal pericardial fluid is present (*arrow*). The head of the animal points to the left. The liver (L) is adjacent to the cardiac ventricle.

studies with MRI in few axolotls (*A mexicanum*) exist.[41] High-detail anatomic studies are provided by contrast-enhanced micro-CTs performed in deceased species.[42]

Necropsy and Histopathology

The procedure of necropsy and collecting samples for histopathology in amphibians is described by Pessier and Pinkerton[43] (2003). The investigators emphasize timely necropsy (refrigerated and within 4–6 hours postmortem) and a thorough history of the animal. After an external examination including the skin, the animal is placed in dorsal recumbency and the coelomic cavity is opened and investigated. Diagnostic histopathology is strictly recommended because amphibians often show nonspecific gross pathologic findings. Samples for histopathology in general should always contain samples of the heart, as well as the skin, lung and gill, lymph heart, liver, kidney, spleen, stomach, intestine, and brain. For small amphibians, the heart can be sampled and fixed whole in formalin, whereas in larger amphibians, the atria and ventricle can be incised and examined. In the authors' experience, adhesions between the heart

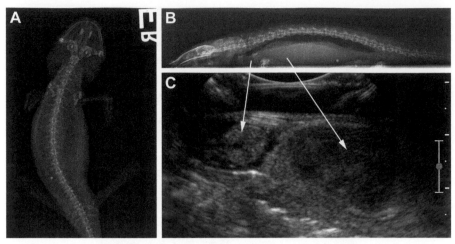

Fig. 9. Dorsoventral (*A*) and lateral (*B*) radiographs and corresponding sonographic (*C*) image of an axolotl (*Ambystoma mexicanum*) suffering from severe hepatomegaly and mild pericardial effusion. Note that mild fluid accumulation is normal within the pericardial sac in amphibians. In this case it was subjectively twice as much fluid as normally observed.

and liver are common, often as the result of bacterial epicarditis. Samples for further investigations, like for cytology, parasitology, bacteriology, mycology, or virus isolation, can be collected similar to other animal species. In cases of septicemia, suggested samples are aseptically collected heart blood for bacterial culture. After removal and dissection of the visceral organs, the musculoskeletal system, peripheral nerves, and bones are investigated and sampled, followed by the brain and the sensory organs.

AMPHIBIAN HEART DISEASES

Comprehensive postmortem studies in amphibians are rare, and heart diseases are only occasionally reported. Recently, Flach and colleagues[44] (2020) investigated 73

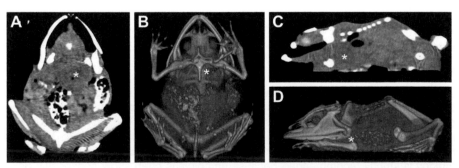

Fig. 10. Horizontal (*A*) and sagittal (*C*) multiplanar reconstruction in soft tissue window of a CT in a deceased Gunther's triangle frog (*Cornufer guentheri*) as well as 3D models (*B* - view from dorsal, *D* - view from left lateral). The heart (marked with an *asterisk*) is barely visible on plain images and only mildly more hypodense than the adjacent organs. In the 3D models only the location of the heart is marked, whereas it is not detectable without contrast enhancement.

captive caecilians postmortem between 2007 and 2017. Unfortunately, in 35 cases the cause of death could not be determined and in 13 cases the animals were autolytic. The major cause of death was dermatitis (22 cases). Heart lesions were described in only one case (*Geotrypetes seraphini*) but were not described in detail.

The following heart diseases could be found in the literature.

Genetic Cardiac Diseases in Amphibians

In axolotl, *A mexicanum,* a recessive lethal mutant gene results in an absence of embryonic heart function. The heart never begins to beat, therefore embryos do not begin to eat and die.[45–48] This mutation is in the focus of scientists studying developmental cardiovascular biology.[2]

Congenital Cardiac Diseases in Amphibians

Elkan[49] (1976) described an ectopic location of the heart in a captive-bred African clawed frog, *X laevis,* due to a pectoral defect. The same species is used in the frog embryo teratogenesis assay-Xenopus, which is an established method for testing developmental toxicity by different chemicals inducing malformations like numerous heart anomalies.[50]

Infectious Causes

Infectious causes of heart diseases in amphibians comprise different bacterial, fungal, viral, and parasitic pathogens.

Green[48] (2001) stated that carditis (epicarditis, myocarditis) is reported rarely in amphibians, but possibly occurs because of the widespread prevalence of gram-negative bacillary septicemias, although there are no bacterial diseases specific to the heart.

The same investigator mentioned that systemic chlamydial infections can cause granulomatous endomyocarditis. Chlamydia are gram-negative, coccoid, obligate intracellular pathogens, and chlamydiosis is frequently reported in anurans. Clinical signs include depigmentation, petechiation and sloughing of skin, abdominal swelling, accumulation of fluid in lymphatic sacs, and lethargy. Histology shows marked histiocytic or granulomatous inflammation mainly in the liver, and also in the spleen, lungs, heart, and kidneys.[51]

Mycobacteriosis is an infectious disease of amphibians, known since the early nineteenth century. Mycobacteria are gram-positive, acid-fast bacilli, and different mycobacterial species can be found in certain amphibians. Mycobacteria usually cause chronic granulomatous infections, when affecting nearly all tissues including the skin, intestine, lung, liver, kidney, spleen, and heart. Unfortunately, clinical signs are often unspecific.[48,51–54]

Cunningham and colleagues[55] (1996) investigated unusual and mass mortalities of the common frog (*Rana temporaria*) in Great Britain and mainly found skin ulcerations with or without necrosis of distal limbs and systemic hemorrhages. Possible causes were bacteria like *Aeromonas hydrophila* and viruses like iridovirus, poxvirus, and adenovirus. Of the 32 investigated hearts 25 were histologically without any abnormalities, but others showed pericardial inflammation, focal myocardial necrosis, congestion, and intramyocardial hemorrhage. Bollinger and colleagues[56] (1999) also found an iridovirus (Regina virus) as the cause of high mortalities in larval and adult tiger salamanders (*Ambystoma tigrinum diaboli*) in Canada in 1997. Salamanders developed a generalized viremia and intracytoplasmic inclusions were found in the heart.

Batrachochytrium dendrobatidis (Bd) and *Batrachochytrium salamandrivorans* (Bsal) are 2 important pathogen chytrid fungi responsible for high morbidity and mortality in free-ranging and captive amphibians.[57] Voyles and colleagues[57] (2009) investigated which pathophysiologic changes lead to mortality in Bd-infected frogs and found that chytridiomycosis disrupts cutaneous osmoregulation that results in cardiac arrest and death. Other systemic fungal infections like *Mucor amphibiorum* sometimes also cause cardiac granulomas.[48]

Pathogenic helminths affecting the amphibian heart include trematodes and nematodes. Helminths like trematodes can be found encysted in the myocardium and the pericardium. Large numbers are often found in wild amphibians and can cause pericarditis, adhesions between the epicardium and pericardium, and hydropericardium and subsequently can lead to death.[48] Nematodes, like *Rhabdias* spp larvae, migrate through the body including the heart muscle and frequently disperse hematogeneously.[58]

Cardiac Neoplasias in Amphibians

Spontaneous neoplasms in amphibians are rarely reported either because of extraordinary regenerative capacity, anticancer secretory products, and cytoproctectives[59] or because of inadequate research of amphibian neoplasms.[60] Green and Harshbarger[61] (2001) as well as Stacy and Parker[59] (2004) and Hopewell and colleagues[60] (2020) have reviewed amphibian neoplasms, but no heart neoplasia was included. In the review by Balls[62] (1962) a hemangioma of the heart in a *Hyla arborea* originally reported by Stolk (1958) is included. The neoplasm was found on the ventricle and consisted of a network of dilated blood vessels.

SUMMARY

Although the amphibian heart has been studied since 1835 and some detailed physiologic studies exist, the clinical context is often missing. Diagnostic tools for amphibian heart diseases are similar to those of other animal species, but unfortunately, heart diseases in amphibians are still reported rarely and large postmortem studies are lacking. This article reviewed clinically important aspects of amphibian cardiology and summarized reported heart diseases. We intend to stimulate clinical veterinary research in amphibians affected by heart diseases.

CLINICS CARE POINTS

- Amphibians have 3 heart chambers: 2 atria and 1 ventricle. The basic morphology of the heart is similar in all amphibians with some differences due to their lifestyle.
- The cardiovascular system of amphibians includes the arterial, venous, and lymphatic system. It is suggested to avoid administering drugs in the hind parts of the body, because they may metabolized or excreted renally or hepatically, due to the renal and hepatic portal system.
- Amphibian heart diseases include genetic, congenital, infectious, and neoplastic heart diseases, but they are only occasionally reported. Diagnostic tools for amphibian heart diseases are similar to those of other animal species.

ACKNOWLEDGMENTS

The authors want to thank Dr. Robert Riener from the Aqua Terra Zoo (Haus des Meeres) Vienna, Austria, for necropsy samples, as well as Mag. Martina Konecny from the service for birds and reptiles, Small Animal Internal Medicine, University of Veterinary Medicine Vienna, Austria for her photographic skills.

DISCLOSURE

The authors have nothing to disclose.

REFERENCES

1. Frost D. and the American Museum of Natural History. Amphibian Species of the World 6.1, an Online Reference. Available at: http://amphibiansoftheworld.amnh.org. Accessed June 9, 2021.
2. Burggren WW, Wartburton S. Amphibians as animal models for laboratory research in physiology. Ilar J 2007;48(3):260–9.
3. Hopkins WA. Amphibians as models for studying environmental change. Ilar J 2007;48(3):270–7.
4. Hempel A, Kühl M. A matter of the heart: the african clawed frog Xenopus as a model for studying vertebrate cardiogenesis and congenital heart defects. J Cardiovasc Dev Dis 2016;3(2):21.
5. Mayer AFJC. Analecten für vergleichende Anatomie *1*. Bonn (Germany): Mayer AFJC; 1835. p. 1–114. Available at: https://digitale-sammlungen.ulb.uni-bonn.de/ulbbnfb/content/titleinfo/5177020. Accessed June 10, 2021.
6. Galvani L, Valli E, Carminati B, et al. Abhandlung über die Kräfte der thierieschen Elektrizität auf die Bewegung der Muskeln. Prag: Calve JG; 1971:1-219. Available at: https://digitale-sammlungen.de/de/views/bsb00006413?page=1. Accessed June 10, 2021.
7. Matteucci C. Sur un phenomene physiologique produit par les muscles en contraction. Ann Chim Et Phys 1842;6:339.
8. Zywietz C. A brief history of electrocardiography- progress through technology. Hannover (Germany): Biosigna Institute for Biosignal Processing and Systems Research; 2003.
9. Foxon GEH. Blood and respiration. In: Moore JA, editor. Physiology of the Amphibia. London (UK): Academic Press; 1964. p. 151–200.
10. Brady AJ. Physiology of the amphibian heart. In: Moore JA, editor. Physiology of the Amphibia. London (UK): Academic Press; 1964. p. 211–50.
11. Johansen K, Hanson D. Functional anatomy of the hearts of lungfishes and amphibians. Am Zool 1968;8(2):191–210.
12. Heinz-Taheny KM. Cardiovascular physiology and diseases of amphibians. Vet Clin North Am Exot Anim Pract 2009;12(1):39–50.
13. Stephenson A, Adams JW, Vaccarezza M. The vertebrate heart: an evolutionary perspective. J Anat 2017;231(6):787–97.
14. Duellman WE, Trueb L. Biology of Amphibians. Baltimore (MD): Johns Hopkins Univ. Press; 1994. p. 1930.
15. Foxon GEH. Problems of the double circulation in vertebrates. Biol Rev 1955;30(2):196–228.
16. Shelton GEH. Gasexchange, pulmonary blood supply, and the partially divided amphibian heart. In: Davies PS, editor. Perspectivse in experimental biology. Oxford (UK): Pergamon Press; 1976. p. 247–59.
17. Cerra MC, Amelio D, Tavolaro P, et al. Pericardium of the frog, Rana esculenta, is morphologically designed as a lymphatic space. J Morphol 2003;257(1):72–7.
18. Akat E. A histological study on heart of *Pelophylax cf. Bedriagae* (Anura: Ranidae). Russ J Herpetol 2020;27(3):123–6.
19. Davies F, Francis ETB. The heart of the salamander (*salamandra salamandra l.*), with special reference to the conduction (connecting) system and its bearing on

the phylogeny of the conducting systems of mammalian and avian hearts. Biol Sci 1941;578(231):99–130.

20. Mohun TJ, Leon LM, Weninger WJ, et al. The morphology of heart development in Xenopus laevis. Dev Biol 2000;218:74–88.

21. Wright KM. Anatomy for the clinician. In: Wright KM, Whitaker BR, editors. Amphibian medicine and captive husbandry. Malabar (FL): Krieger Publishing Company; 2001. p. 27–8.

22. Wright KM. Hematology. In: Wright KM, Whitaker BR, editors. Amphibian medicine and captive husbandry. Malabar (FL): Krieger Publishing Company; 2001. p. 129–46.

23. Wilkinson M. The heart and aortic arches of rhinatrematid caecilians (Amphibia: Gymnophiona). Zool J Linn Soc 1996;118(2):135–50.

24. Benninghoff A. Das Herz. In: Bolk L, Göppert E, Kallius E, et al, editors. Handbuch der vergleichende Anatomie der Wirbeltiere. Berlin (Germany): Urban & Schwarzenberg; 1933. p. 467–555.

25. Putnam JL, Kelly DL. A new interpretation of interatrial septation in the lungless salamander, Plethodon glutinosus. Copeia 1978;1978:251–4.

26. De Bakker D, Wilkonson M, Jensen B. Extreme variation in the atrial septation of caecilians (Amphibia: Gymnophiona). J Anat 2014;226(1):1–12.

27. Bhaskar A, Vinod A. Demonstrating of the origin of ECG waves. Adv Physiol Educ 2006;30(3):128.

28. Chai N. Endoscopy in amphibians. Vet Clin North Am Exot Anim Pract 2015;18(3): 479–91.

29. Chai N. Surgery in amphibians. Vet Clin North Am Exot Anim Pract 2016;19(1): 77–95.

30. Peters JA, Mullen RK. Electrocardiography in caecilia guentheri (Peters). Physiol Zool 1966;39(3):193–201.

31. Fritsche R. Ontogeny of cardiovascular control in amphibians. Amer Zool 1997; 37:23–30.

32. Aubret F, Blanvilln G. A non-invasive method of measuring heart rates in small reptiles and amphibians. Herpetol Rev 2013;44(3):421–3.

33. Marshall L, Vivien C, Girardot F, et al. Persistent fibrosis, hypertrophy and sarcomere disorganisation after endoscopy guided heart resection in adult Xenopus. PLoS One 2017;12(3):e0173418.

34. Stetter MD. Diagnostic imaging of amphibians. In: Wright KM, Whitaker BR, editors. Amphibian medicine and captive husbandry. Malabar (FL): Krieger Publishing Company; 2001. p. 253–72.

35. Schildger B, Triet H. Ultrasonography in Amphibians. J Exot Pet Med 2001;10(4): 169–73.

36. Dittrich A, Thygesen MM, Lauridsen H. 2D and 3D echocardiography in the axolotl (Ambystoma mexicanum). J Vis Exp 2018;29:141.

37. Heidbrink S. Ultraschall beim Axolotl. Proceeding 46. Arbeitstagung der AG Amphibien- und Reptilienkrankheiten, Gera, 11.-13.11.2016, 67-78.

38. Willens S, Dupree SH, Stoskopf MK, et al. Measurements of common iliac arterial blood flow in anurans using doppler ultrasound. J Zoo Wildl Med 2006;37(2): 97–101.

39. Holtze S, Lukac M, Cizelj I, et al. Monitoring health and reproductive status of olms (Proteus anguinus) by ultrasound. PLoS one 2017;12(8):e0182209.

40. Ditttrich A, Lauridsen H. Cryo-injury induced heart regeneration in the axolotl and echocardiography and unbiased quantitative histology to evaluate regenerative progression. J Vis Exp 2021;(171):e61966.

41. Sanches PG, Veld RCO, de Graaf W, et al. Novel axolotl cardiac function analysis method using magnetic resonance imaging. PLoS One 2017;12(8):e0183446.
42. Metscher BD. MicroCT for comparative morphology: simple staining methods allow high-contrast 3D imaging of diverse non-mineralized animal tissues. BMC Physiol 2009;9(1):1–14.
43. Pessier AP, Pinkerton M. Practical gross necropsy of amphibians. J Exot Pet Med 2003;12(2):81–8.
44. Flach EJ, Feltrer Y, Gower DJ, et al. Postmortem findings in eights species of captive caecilian (amphibia: gymnophiona) over a ten-year period. J Zoo Wild Med 2020;50(4):879–90.
45. Lemanski LF. Morphology of developing heart in cardiac lethal mutant mexican axolotls, Ambystoma mexicanum. Dev Biol 1973;33:312–33.
46. Davis LA, Lemanski LF. Induction of myofibrillogenesis in cardiac lethal mutant axolotl hearts rescued by RNA derived from normal endoderm. Development 1987;99(2):145–54.
47. Smith SC, Armstrong JB. Heart development in normal and cardiac-lethal mutant axolotls: a model for the control of vertebrate cardiogenesis. Differentiation 1991; 47(3):129–34.
48. Green DE. Pathology of Amphibia. In: Wright KM, Whitaker BR, editors. Amphibian medicine and captive husbandry. Malabar (FL): Krieger Publishing Company; 2001. p. 451–3.
49. Elkan E. Pathology in the Amphibia. In: Lofts B, editor.: Physiology of the Amphibia, 3. Volume. New York·Academic Press Inc.273-312.
50. Dumont JN, Bantle JA, Linder G. The history and development of FETAX (ASTM standard guide, E-1439 on conducting the frog embryo teratogenesis Assay-Xenopus). In: Linder G, Krest S, Sparing D, et al, editors. Multiple stressor effects in relation to declining amphibian populations. West Conshohocken (PA): ASTM International; 2003. p. 3–22.
51. Densmore CL, Green DE. Diseases of amphibians. Ilar J 2007;48(3).235–54.
52. Martinho F, Heatley JJ. Amphibian mycobacteriosis. Vet Clin North Am Exot Anim Pract 2012;15(1):113–9.
53. Chai N. Mycobacteriosis in Amphibians. In: Miller ER, Fowler ME, editors. In: fowler's Zoo and wild animal medicine current therapy, ume 7. Missouri: Elsevier Saunder; 2012. p. 224–30.
54. Milnes EL, Delnatte P, Lentini A, et al. Mycobacteriosis in a Zoo Population of Chinese Gliding Frogs (Rhacophorus dennysi) due to Mycobacterium marinum. J Herpetol Med Surg 2020;30(1):14–20.
55. Cunningham AA, Langton TES, Bennett PM, et al. Pathological and microbiological findings from incidents of unusual mortality of the common frog (Rana temporaria). Philos Trans R Soc Lond B Biol Sci 1996;351:1539–57.
56. Bollinger TK, Mao J, Schock D, et al. Pathology, isolation, and preliminary molecular characterization of a novel iridovirus from tiger salamanders in Saskatchewan. J Wildl Dis 1999;35(3):413–29.
57. Voyles J, Young S, Berger L, et al. Pathogenesis of Chytridiomycosis, a cause of catastrophic amphibian declines. Science 2009;326:582–5.
58. Williams RW. Observations on the life history of Rhadias sphaerocephala Goodey, 1924 from Bufo marinus L., in the Bermuda Islands. J Helminthol 1960; 34(1/2):93–8.
59. Stacy BA, Parker JM. Amphibian oncology. Vet Clin North Am Exot Anim Pract 2004;7(2):673–95.

60. Hopewell E, Harrison SH, Psey R, et al. Analysis of published amphibian neoplasia case reports. J Herpetol Med Surg 2020;230(3):148–55.
61. Green DE, Harshbarger JC. Spontaneous neoplasia in amphibia. In: Wright KM, Whitaker BR, editors. In: Amphibian medicine and captive husbandry. Malabar (FL): Krieger Publishing Company; 2001. p. 335–400.
62. Balls M. Spontaneous neoplasms in amphibia: a review and descriptions of six new cases. Cancer Res 1962;22:1142–54.

Heart Diseases in Reptiles
Diagnosis and Therapy

Lionel Schilliger, DVM, DECZM (Herpetology), DABVP (Reptile and Amphibian Practice)

KEYWORDS

- Reptile • Cardiology • Diagnosis • Therapy • Ultrasonography • Radiography
- Electrocardiography

KEY POINTS

- Cardiopulmonary function in reptiles is strongly influenced by temperature, stress, and the method of physical restraint. Clinicians should therefore be mindful of these aspects when examining reptile patients.
- Heart sounds in reptiles are muffled and difficult to auscultate. The use of a digital or a pressure-sensitive acoustic stethoscope allows for a more sensitive diagnosis of heart murmurs, especially in snakes and monitor lizards whose heart is not surrounded by osseous structures.
- Ultrasonography and Doppler examination are the diagnostic tools of choice for the evaluation of reptilian heart diseases.
- ECG in reptiles can provide diagnostic information. However, it is limited by the absence of species-specific cardiac parameters and low electric amplitudes that provide readings of poor diagnostic quality.
- Little to no information exists on cardiovascular treatment or the pharmacologic actions of cardiac drugs in reptiles.

DIAGNOSIS

Numerous cardiovascular conditions have been described in reptiles. These include cardiomyopathy, septic endocarditis, valvular insufficiency, myocarditis, pericardial effusion, infarcts, atherosclerosis, aneurysms, gout, arterial calcification, thrombus, parasitic infestation, congenital heart defects, and tumors.[1] As in any species, the clinician should always conduct a full examination to evaluate for concurrent disease and determine if cardiac disease is primary or secondary.[1,2] Cardiopulmonary function in reptiles is strongly influenced by external conditions and stimuli, including temperature, stress, and the method of physical restraint. Clinicians should therefore ensure that they are conducting a physical examination once the reptile is calm and within its

Clinique Vétérinaire du Village d'Auteuil, 35 rue Leconte de Lisle, Paris 75016, France
E-mail address: Dr.L.Schilliger@club-internet.fr

Vet Clin Exot Anim 25 (2022) 383–407
https://doi.org/10.1016/j.cvex.2022.01.003
1094-9194/22/© 2022 Elsevier Inc. All rights reserved.

preferred optimal temperature (which is measured using an infrared thermometer).[3] The method of restraint should be consistent across patients of a same species and mimic their natural resting position, or the position in which cardiac parameters were established for that species.[1–3]

Physical Examination

Clinical signs of cardiovascular diseases in reptiles mirror those seen in mammals, although certain differences exist because of differing cardiovascular anatomy and physiology between both taxonomic classes. Signs include cardiomegaly (evidenced by swelling around the cardiac region) (**Fig. 1**), cyanosis (**Fig. 2**), peripheral edema (eg, around the mandibular region) (**Fig. 3**), pulmonary edema, and ascites (**Fig. 4**).[1–4] Decreased cardiac output can result in exercise intolerance, syncope, tachycardia, cyanosis, decreased peripheral perfusion, and arrhythmias.[1] Ataxia and head tilt may be observed in the case of brain anoxia secondary to heart failure, atherosclerosis, or arteriosclerosis (**Fig. 5**).[4–6]

Congestive heart failure (CHF) results in chronic, excessive compensatory mechanisms to maintain cardiac output and blood pressure. Its pathophysiology is probably similar across vertebrate taxa, with some differences between mammals and reptiles, mainly in terms of anatomic structure, physiologic regulation, and the relative influences of neural (autonomic) versus humoral (kallikrein-kinin, renin-angiotensin, endothelin) systems.[7] Noncrocodilian reptiles possess a single ventricle with a different mechanism of blood ejection, which allows them to shunt blood from right to left under certain natural or pathologic conditions.[8–12] These features influence the pathophysiology of heart failure, notably edema formation. Clinical signs of CHF include pulmonary edema and coelomic effusion (caused by increased preload) and cardiac remodeling, such as cardiomegaly (caused by increased afterload). Pitting edema is uncommon. Unlike in mammals, coughing is not a feature of CHF because reptiles lack a true diaphragm.[8]

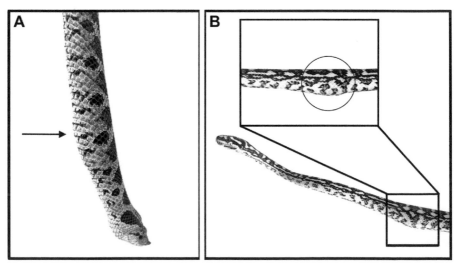

Fig. 1. Cardiomegaly in a southern hog-nosed snake (*Heterodon simus*) (*A, arrow*) and in a jungle carpet python (*Morelia spilota cheynei*) (*B, circle*). (*Courtesy of* Clément Paillusseau.)

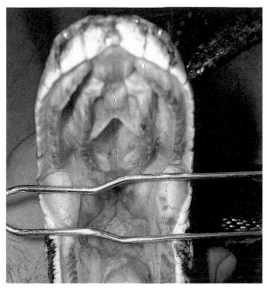

Fig. 2. Cyanotic mucous membranes in a Burmese python (*Python bivittatus*) suffering from a left atrioventricular insufficiency.

Auscultation

Heart sounds in reptiles are muffled and difficult to auscultate with a standard stethoscope. A digital stethoscope (eg, ThinklabsOne, Thinklabs, Centennial, CO) or a pressure-sensitive acoustic stethoscope (eg, Ultrascope, Parker Medical Associates LLC, Charlotte, NC) is used to diagnose heart murmurs, especially in large snakes (eg, boids) and in large lizard species where the heart lies in the midcoelomic region (varanids), as opposed to within a bony pectoral girdle (eg, iguanids, agamids, lacertids, chameleons, skinks) (**Fig. 6**).[1–3]

A continuous Doppler ultrasonic probe (8 MHz) is used as an adjunct to cardiac auscultation to measure heart rate (HR) and estimate cardiac rhythm in all species.

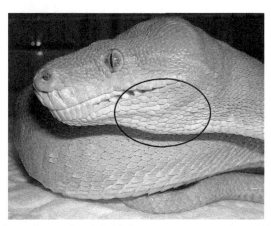

Fig. 3. Edema in the gular region (*circle*) in a green tree python (*Morelia viridis*) with congestive heart failure.

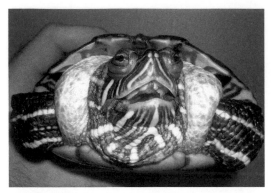

Fig. 4. Ascites in a red-eared slider (*Trachemys scripta elegans*) with congestive heart failure.

The probe is placed with an acoustic coupling gel at the level of the heart or large efferent arteries (**Fig. 7**).[1]

Blood Pressure Measurement and Pulse Oximetry

As in mammals, the autonomic nervous system in reptiles regulates blood pressure: the parasympathetic outflow reduces blood pressure via the acetylcholine neurotransmitter, whereas the sympathetic outflow increases blood pressure via adrenaline and noradrenaline neurotransmitters.[7] The oculocardiac reflex is exploited as an effective short-term method of restraint for large noncooperative lizards (eg, iguanids and monitors). This method involves applying gentle pressure on the closed eyelids for

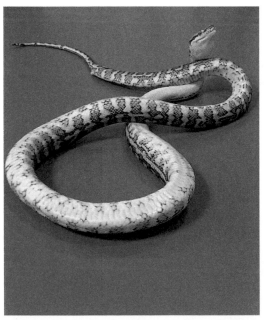

Fig. 5. Postural abnormalities (ataxia and circling) in a McDowell carpet python (*Morelia spilota mcdowelli*) with brain anoxia secondary to heart failure and decreased blood perfusion secondary to atherosclerosis.

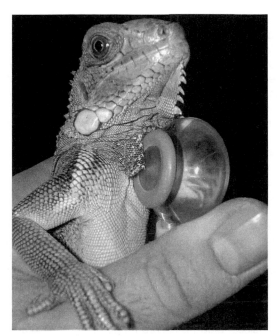

Fig. 6. Use of a pressure-sensitive acoustic stethoscope (Ultrascope®) in a juvenile green iguana (*Iguana iguana*).

30 seconds to 2 minutes to stimulate the vagal nerve and thereby reduce HR and blood pressure.[13] In mammals, two additional antagonist hormonal systems mediate blood pressure: the kallikrein-kinin system (hypotensive) and the renin-angiotensin system (hypertensive). The importance of these systems in nonmammalian vertebrates is poorly understood. In snakes, the bradykinin ligand is structurally different from its mammalian counterpart and its effects on cardiovascular function is species-dependant.[7] The physiology of the renin-angiotensin system has been described in some reptile species, indicating that angiotensin receptors cannot be classified as

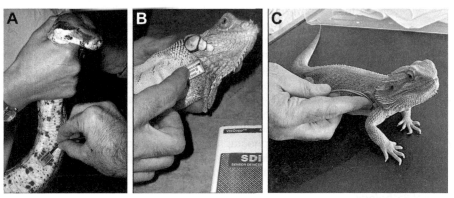

Fig. 7. Use of a continuous Doppler ultrasonic probe (8 MHz) as an adjunct to cardiac auscultation in a constrictor boa (*Boa imperator*) (*A*), in a green iguana (*Iguana iguana*) (*B*), and in a bearded dragon (*Pogona vitticeps*) (*C*).

AT_1 or AT_2 receptors seen in mammals. Blood pressure regulation is not necessarily dependent on body temperature; for example, constant blood pressure in slider turtles (*Trachemys scripta*) is observed during warming and cooling phases, indicating barostatic regulation because of hysteresis of HR as body temperature changed.[14]

Blood pressure is measured either directly or indirectly. Direct measurement is achieved through catheterization of the carotid or femoral artery and requires sophisticated equipment; however, it produces the most reliable measurement. Indirect measurements are more suited for general practice, because they are performed using a sphygmomanometer on the forelimb or tail. In medium- and large-sized turtles and lizards, the cuff is placed on the proximal front limb with the sensor above the brachial artery, in the palmar region of the radius-ulna, or at the proximal level of the tail in large specimens. In snakes, the cuff is placed caudal to the cloaca (coccygeal artery) (M.K. Lichtenberger, personal communication, 2006).[15]

Significant differences between invasive and noninvasive blood pressure measurements have been observed in green iguanas (*Iguana iguana*).[15] Comparative studies between both techniques are therefore warranted and results obtained using sphygmomanometers should be interpreted with caution. For example, in three boid species (boa constrictors, carpet pythons, and reticulated pythons), an oscillometric unit (MDE Escort Multiparameter Monitor, Medical Data Electronics, Arleta, CA) overestimated systolic arterial blood pressure, and underestimated diastolic and mean arterial blood pressure.[16] Nevertheless, blood pressure range using noninvasive techniques have been described across many species. Chelonians have the lowest mean arterial pressure (15–40 mm Hg), whereas in some lizards (eg, chameleons) it is closer to that of mammals (60–80 mm Hg). In green iguanas, mean arterial pressure is 40 to 50 mm Hg; less than 1% isoflurane anesthesia, the average systolic pressure is 43 ± 7 mm Hg and average diastolic pressure is 29 ± 4 mm Hg.[15] In snakes, indirect systolic blood pressures have been reported between 40 and 90 mm Hg (M.K. Lichtenberger, personal communication, 2006) and the average blood pressure increases in proportion to animal length.[17] In arboreal snakes, blood pressure increases in proportion to the distance between the heart and the head; this relationship is less pronounced in terrestrial snakes (eg, *Python bivittatus*), because they are less affected by variations in gravitational force.[17]

Reptilian hemoglobin generally has lower oxygen affinities compared with that of mammals and reptilian red blood cells can deliver oxygen to tissues even at low blood oxygen levels. In theory, pulse oximetry can be used to monitor oxygen saturation levels in response to treatment; however, its use has not been validated in reptiles.[18] Results should always be interpreted with caution because pulse oximeters are designed and calibrated for use in mammals, which have a different hemoglobin structure and oxygen hemoglobin dissociation curve compared with reptiles. In green iguanas, oxygen saturation is lower in pulse-oximetry compared with arterial blood gas analysis.[19] Pulse oximetry is used to measure relative change in oxygen saturation during treatment, although care should be taken to maintain a constant environmental temperature, because this influences oxygen saturation. The sensor is placed in the cloaca or esophagus. Similarly, capnography is not validated for reptiles, and results are particularly difficult to interpret in species with cardiac right-to-left shunting where mixing of deoxygenated and oxygenated blood occurs.

Clinical Pathology

Blood levels of creatine kinase and lactate dehydrogenase can increase following damage to cardiac muscle, such as myocarditis or infarcts.[20] This must be differentiated from other causes, because increased plasma creatine kinase can also result from skeletal muscle damage (eg, traumatic injuries), intramuscular injections of caustic drugs (eg, enrofloxacin), and loss of body condition. In mammals, cardiac troponins (troponin I and troponin T) are regulatory proteins that control calcium-mediated interaction between actin and myosin; both are used to detect myocardial damage. Unfortunately, the use of cardiac troponins to measure myocardial damage in reptiles has not been evaluated, although they might be of use to assess progression of cardiac dysfunction.

Several lactate dehydrogenase isoenzymes are described in reptiles, although their diagnostic utility has not yet been described.[20] Dyslipidemias are known to occur in reptiles, such as hypercholesterolemia associated with atherosclerosis in a bearded dragon.[6] Hypocalcemia, commonly seen in cases of nutritional disorders, can affect striated cardiac muscle and be visualized as electrocardiographic abnormalities.[1,20] A complete blood count and blood smear are highly valuable in certain cases; leukocytosis, lymphocytosis, and heterophilia can indicate infections (eg, vegetative or septic endocarditis) and abnormal red or white blood cells can lead to a diagnosis of hematopoietic neoplasia.[18]

Electrocardiography

General principles
The application and interpretation of electrocardiography (ECG) in reptiles follows the same principle as in mammals. The main challenge associated with ECG in reptiles is related to the low electric amplitudes (typically <1.0 mV) that frequently generate ECGs of poor diagnostic value.

Standard reference ranges are only available for some species, including red-eared sliders (T scripta elegans),[21] green iguanas (I iguana),[22] Moreau tropical house geckos (Hemidactylus mabouia),[23] Gomera giant lizards (Gallotia bravoana),[24] bearded dragons (Pogona vitticeps),[25] Russell vipers (Daboia russelli), Indian spectacled cobras (Naja naja),[26] constrictor boas (Boa constrictor imperator), green anacondas (Eunectes murinus), California king snakes (Lampropeltis getulus californiae), rat snakes (Pantherophis obsoletus),[27] corn snakes (Pantherophis guttatus),[28] ball pythons (Python regius),[22] and one species of crocodilian (American alligators [Alligator mississippiensis]).[29] ECG readings are also available for several species in the order squamata, but were obtained in the 1960s and might therefore not be accurate.[30] Examples of reference values are given for the corn snake (P guttatus) (Table 1) and the bearded dragon (P vitticeps) (Table 2).

ECG readings are influenced by lead placement, environmental temperature, and stress. It is therefore of critical importance that readings are taken in the same conditions as when the reference range was established. ECG reading should ideally be recorded when the reptile is calm, in its preferred optimal temperature zone, and with a constant HR.

The AliveCor Veterinary Heart Monitor (AliveCor Inc, San Francisco, CA) provides an easier alternative for the placement of ECG electrodes in reptiles.[31] It consists of a single-lead ECG recorder with two electrodes that are connected to a smartphone case. The ECG is used wirelessly to monitor, record, analyze, and transfer recordings. This device is not as accurate as gold standard ECG measurement using standard electrodes but should rather be considered as an anesthetic monitoring tool (M.S. Higareda, unpublished data); results should ideally be confirmed with a standard ECG. A study of 12 healthy green iguanas showed significant differences between the R wave amplitude compared with those obtained from two standard ECGs (Seiva Praktik Veterinary, and CardioStore).[32]

Table 1
Electrocardiogram amplitudes and interval durations (lead II) in corn snakes (*Pantherophis guttatus*) recorded at 25 and 50 mm/s and 1 and 2 mV/cm (n = 29)

Parameters	Amplitudes (mV)	Durations (s)
P wave	0.107 ± 0.045	0.064 ± 0.016
T wave	0.180 ± 0.127	N/A
R wave	1.061 ± 0.395	0.107 ± 0.019
PR interval	N/A	0.259 ± 0.059
RT interval	N/A	0.585 ± 0.145

Abbreviation: N/A, not available.

ECGs were obtained at a temperature of 22°C–24°C immediately after removing snakes from their vivaria heated at 26°C–30°C. No Q, R, or SV waves could be observed.

Data from Lewis M, Bouvard J, Eatwell K, et al. Standardisation of electrocardiographic examination in corn snakes (*Pantherophis guttatus*). Vet Rec 2020;186(9):1-8.

Table 2
ECG measurements (recorded at 25 mm/s and 0.5 mV/cm), heart rate, and mean electric axis in bearded dragons (*Pogona vitticeps*) (n = 52)

	Mean or (Median)	Range	Standard Deviation or (Interquartile Range)
Weight (g)	335	66–517	140
Age (mo)		4–30	
Snout-vent length (cm)	18.9	11.5–23.0	3.0
Cloacal temperature (°C)	32.7	27.7–37.9	2.0
Ambient temperature (°C)		26–35	
Heart rate (beats/min)	90	24–170	39
R-R interval (mS)	(723)	353–2520	(533–1020)
P-wave duration (mS)	56	30–100	13
P-wave amplitude (mV)	0.03	0.01–0.06	0.01
PR interval (mS)	145	75–253	38
SV-wave duration (mS)	(57.5)	30–125	(50–67)
SV-wave amplitude (mV)	0.03	0.01–0.07	0.01
SV-R interval (mS)	243	130–440	62
QRS duration (ms)	85	60–120	15
R-wave amplitude (mv)	0.23	0.08–0.57	0.11
S-wave amplitude (mV)	0.04	0.01–0.13	0.02
QT interval (mS)	355	120–980	139
T-wave amplitude (mV)	0.04	0.01–0.14	0.02
Mean electric axis		+60–+110	

ECGs were performed at room temperature as soon as the lizards were removed from the vivaria heated at 26°C–32°C with a daytime basking area at 45°C.

Data from C. Hunt. Electrocardiography of the Normal Inland Bearded Dragon (*Pogona vitticeps*). Submitted in part fulfilment of the requirements for the Royal College of Veterinary Surgeons (RCVS) Diploma in Zoological Medicine 2013. Unpublished data).

Electrode placement

Correct electrode placement is essential to avoid erroneous ECG readings. The electrodes are attached to the reptile using self-adhering skin electrodes or alligator clips. Placement varies according to species. In snakes, the cranial limb leads (negative yellow and positive red leads) are placed approximately two heart lengths cranial to the heart, slightly to the left side at the level of the junction between the dorsal and ventral scales. The caudal limb leads (neutral green and positive black leads) are also placed two heart lengths caudal to the heart, but on the right lateral side (**Fig. 8**A).[26] This provides the equivalent tracings of lead II in mammals. A second placement scheme is possible by placing the cranial leads cranial to the heart on each side of the body (red lead on the right side and yellow lead on the left side), whereas the caudal leads are placed caudal to the heart (green lead on the left side and black lead on the right side) (**Fig. 8**B).[33] A third option includes following Einthoven triangle: the yellow lead is placed one heart length cranial to the heart on the right side, and the red lead is placed 60% to 75% of the snout-to-vent distance from the head, on the left side. The green lead is placed on the right side, across from the positive lead (**Fig. 8**C).[3,34]

In chelonians, the two red and yellow cranial electrodes are placed in the cervical region, lateral to the neck, and the green and black caudal leads are placed on the skin of the knees or caudally to the pelvic limbs (**Fig. 9**).[21,33] In a study involving a cohort of 72 turtles and tortoises (representing 20 species), adhesive electrodes were placed on the plastron and clamp electrodes to the skin folds. ECG waves could be detected in 41 (57%) animals and complete P, QRS, and T complexes were observed in only 19 (26%) animals.[35]

In lizard species where the heart is situated within the pectoral girdle, the cranial electrodes are placed on the lateral cervical region (red lead on the right, yellow lead on the left) and the caudal electrodes are placed on the lateral body wall just caudal to the elbow (green lead on the left, black on the right) (**Fig. 10**A).[25] The caudal electrodes can also be placed on the lateral body wall just cranial to the stifle, with the stifle flexed against the body wall (**Fig. 10**B).[25] In lizard species where the heart is caudal to the pectoral girdle (ie, varanids), the traditional four-limb placement is used (ie, one lead on each limb, proximally up to the elbows and knees) (**Fig. 11**A).[30,33] The same configuration applies to crocodilians (**Fig. 11**B).[1,30,33]

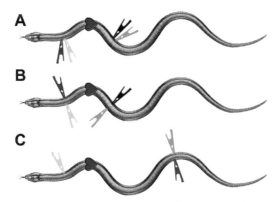

Fig. 8. ECG electrode placement in snakes. (*A*) According to Karthik M, Rajkumar K, Krishna MK, et al, 2013. (*B*) According to Kharin S and Shmakov D, 2009. (*C*) According to Mitchell MA, 2009 and Bogan JE, 2017. Figure illustrated by Pierre Morice.

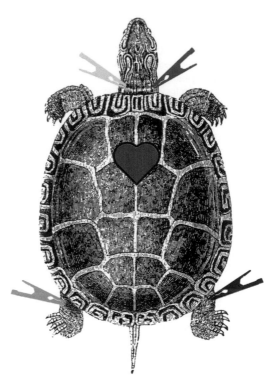

Fig. 9. ECG electrode placement in chelonians according to Holz RM and Holz P, 1995 and Kharin S and Shmakov D, 2009. Figure illustrated by Pierre Morice.

If using the AliveCor Veterinary Heart Monitor in snakes, juvenile crocodilians, and varanids, the two electrodes are placed on either side of the cardiac region in the longitudinal axis with the animal in dorsal recumbency (**Fig. 12**). In lizard species where the heart is located at the base of the neck, one electrode is placed immediately cranial to the cardiac region and the other is placed caudally, at the level of the coelomic cavity. In chelonians, each front limb is placed on an electrode.[31]

Interpretation

The interpretation of ECG readings in reptiles follows the same principles as that in mammals, with analogous P, QRS, and T complexes (**Fig. 13**). Compared with similar-sized mammals, reptile ECGs display P-wave pleomorphism, substantially reduced Q and S deflections, and prolonged QT intervals.[21–30] In a review of ECG recordings in three reptile species kept at 35°C to 37°C, HR was on average four-fold lower, atrial and ventricular conduction (longer P- and QRS-wave durations) two-fold slower, and PR intervals and QT intervals four-fold longer compared with that of mammals and birds.[22]

Findings specific to reptiles include the SV wave, which represents the depolarization of the sinus venosus and the caudal vena cava.[1] It is preceded by the T wave (ventricular repolarization) and followed by the P wave (atrial depolarization). The SV wave is of low amplitude (typically ≤ 0.1 mV) and is difficult to separate from the T wave. It can also be obscured by background skeletal muscle activity. The mean electrical axis is difficult to determine because of low voltage potential and is of limited value.

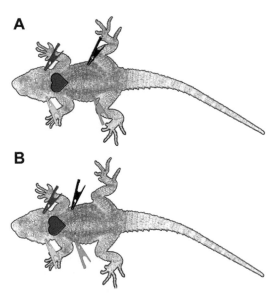

Fig. 10. Two options for ECG electrode placement (*A, B*) in nonvaranid lizards. According to Hunt, 2013. Figure illustrated by Pierre Morice.

Widened QRS complexes and prolonged QT intervals have been observed in a green iguana with aortic stenosis and atrioventricular dilatation.[36] Tall and wide QRS complexes were reported in a carpet python (*Morelia spilota variegata*) with atrioventricular valve insufficiency. Increased PR intervals associated with decreased QT intervals are described in a carpet python with atrioventricular valve insufficiency.[37] A first-degree atrioventricular block was diagnosed in a bearded dragon with hypertensive heart disease and severe atherosclerosis.[5]

Diagnostic Imaging

Radiography

Radiography is of considerable diagnostic value in general herpetologic practice, but of limited use when it comes to reptile cardiology. This is caused by anatomic features that limit x-ray penetration and the absence of standard reference parameters.[38]

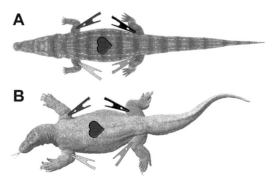

Fig. 11. ECG electrode placement in crocodilians (*A*) and varanids (*B*) according to Mullen RK, 1967 and Kharin S and Shmakov D, 2009. Figure illustrated by Pierre Morice.

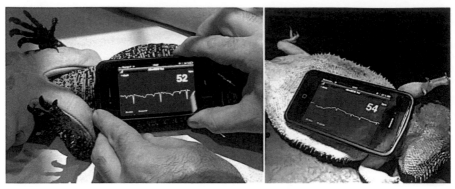

Fig. 12. Use of a single-lead ECG recorder (AliveCor Veterinary Heart Monitor®) connected to a smartphone case in a varanid (*Varanus indicus*) (*left*) and in a bearded dragon (*Pogona vitticeps*) (*right*).

Radiography is of most use in snakes, where the position of the lungs around the heart provides sufficient contrast to evaluate the shape and size of the cardiac silhouette (**Fig. 14**).[1,39] In contrast, the heart cannot be visualized in chelonians and crocodilians because it is superimposed by other visceral organs and is masked by osteoderms.[40] The utility of cardiac radiography is also limited in lizard species where the heart is obscured by the bony pectoral girdle.[41] The absence of reference parameters is overcome to a certain extent by performing and comparing radiographs during routine health evaluations.

As with any radiographic examination, a dorsoventral and a horizontal lateral view should be captured. In chelonians, a craniocaudal view is useful, but this is mostly indicated for visualizing lung fields.[1,40] The potential for normal physiologic variations in heart size should be taken into consideration when assessing cardiac enlargement. In Burmese pythons (*P bivittatus*), ventricular myocardium can increase by up to 40% within 48 hours of feeding as a result of increased metabolic demands and subsequent oxygen consumption.[42] Great vessels should always be assessed in addition to the heart, because mineralization is observed secondary to hypervitaminosis D_3 or other metabolic disturbances.[1]

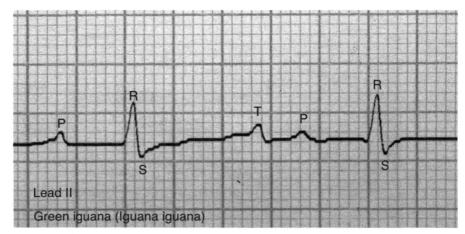

Fig. 13. Typical ECG complex in reptiles. SV wave is absent. P, P wave; R, R wave; T, T wave.

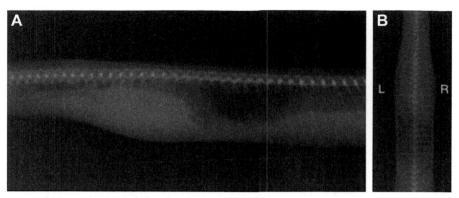

Fig. 14. Enlarged cardiac silhouette (cardiomegaly) causing deviation of the trachea toward the left side in a Southern hognose snake (*Heterodon simus*). Laterolateral (*A*) and dorsoventral (*B*) incidences. (*Courtesy of* Clément Paillusseau.)

Echocardiography
General principles. Ultrasound is a safe and noninvasive tool of great diagnostic utility in reptile cardiology, especially when paired with Doppler examination. Echocardiography has substantially contributed to current knowledge on reptile cardiac anatomy and physiology. It is challenging in crocodilians, chelonians, and many species of lizards, because of the presence of osseous structures (eg, pectoral girdle, plastron, osteoderms) that impede ultrasound penetration.

Standard reference parameters for echocardiographic evaluations are being progressively established; standardizations and/or reference ranges are available for Burmese pythons (*P bivittatus*),[43] ball pythons (*P regius*),[44,45] red-tailed boas (*B constrictor*),[46] bearded dragons (*P vitticeps*),[47] green iguanas (*I iguana*),[48] red-eared sliders (*T scripta elegans*),[49] Hermann tortoises (*Testudo hermanni*), Russian tortoises (*Testudo horsfieldii*),[50] and giant Aldabra tortoises (*Aldabrachelys gigantea*).[51] Typical cardiac parameters include longitudinal and transverse ventricular and atrial lengths measured during diastole and systole, transverse and longitudinal fractional shortenings, diastolic and systolic areas and volumes, and ventricular wall thicknesses and velocities.

Most ultrasound machines used in small animal practice are suitable for reptiles. If available, an epicardiac transducer can also be used to obtain high-resolution images of the heart.[1,50,52]

Snakes. In boids, three views are recommended for a complete cardiac evaluation.[43] First, a ventral approach (**Fig. 15**A) involves placing the probe ventral to the heart to view the organ from the caudal ventricular apex to the cranial atria, the sinus venosus, the atrioventricular junctions, and the three arterial trunks. A first short-axis transapical section shows the outline of the apical myocardium and the pericardium as an echogenic line (**Fig. 16**). By moving the probe cranially, a transventricular subarterial short-axis section allows visualization of the three ventricular subchambers (the cavum venosum, the cavum arteriosum, and the cavum pulmonale), the interventricular (vertical) septum located between the cavum arteriosum and the cavum venosum, and the muscular ridge (horizontal septum) marking the separation between the cavum venosum and the cavum pulmonale (**Fig. 17**). By moving the probe cranially, the resulting transarterial short-axis section shows the two aortic arches of equal diameter and the pulmonary trunk of larger diameter (known as the "Mickey-Mouse-head" section)

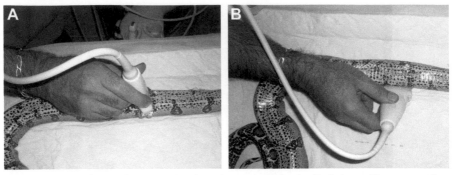

Fig. 15. Echocardiographic examination in a true red-tailed boa (*Boa constrictor constrictor*). (*A*) Ventral approach (short-axis section). (*B*) Left lateral approach (long-axis section).

(**Fig. 18**). By slightly moving the probe toward the right, a transatrial short-axis section is obtained, showing the opening of the sinus venosus into the right atrium and both sinoatrial valves (**Fig. 19**). Long-axis sections are visualized by rotating the probe 90° in relationship to the previous position. These show both atrial cavities opening into the single ventricle. The left atrioventricular junction is observed by orientating the ultrasound plane ventrodorsally from the right to the left. The right atrioventricular junction is observed by orientating the ultrasound plane ventrodorsally from left to

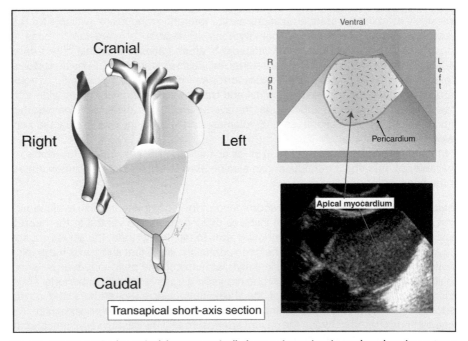

Fig. 16. Transventricular apical (or transapical) short-axis section in snakes showing a transversal section of the apical myocardium. Figure illustrated by Dominique Tessier. (From Schilliger, et al. 2006, with the permission of the Journal of herpetological Medicine and Surgery.)

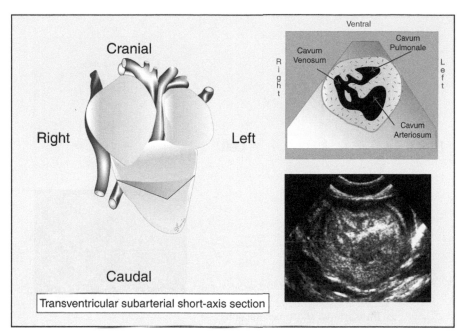

Fig. 17. Transventricular subarterial short-axis section in snakes showing the three cava (cavum pulmonale, cavum venosum, cavum arteriosum), the muscular (horizontal) ridge, and the vertical septum. Figure illustrated by Dominique Tessier. (From Schilliger, et al. 2006, with the permission of the Journal of herpetological Medicine and Surgery.)

right. The monocuspid atrioventricular valves can also be visualized in this view (**Fig. 20**).[43]

The second (right intercostal) and third (left intercostal) involve placing the probe laterally on either side of the body to view the three arterial trunks, both atria, and the single ventricle (**Fig. 15**B).[43] Reference values are provided for the ball python (*P. regius*) (**Table 3**).[44]

Chelonians. In chelonians, the optimal view is obtained through the left or right cervical windows that enable visualization of base to apex inflow and outflow (**Fig. 21**). Fractional shortening is calculated by measuring ventricular size, wall thickness, and outflow tracts. Pulsed-wave Doppler is used to record diastolic biphasic atrioventricular flow and the systolic ventricular outflow. This enables calculation of early diastolic (E) and late diastolic (A) wave peak velocities, E/A ratio, ventricular outflow systolic peak and mean velocities and gradients, velocity-time integral, acceleration and deceleration times, and ejection time.[49] Reference values are provided for the red-eared slider (*T scripta elegans*) (**Table 4**).[49]

Lizards. In lizard species where the heart is located at the base of the neck, the probe is positioned cranial or caudal to the bony pectoral girdle, although this window is narrow and can restrict visualization of the entire heart in certain species (eg, chameleons). Images of better diagnostic quality are obtained by placing the probe in the left or right axillary region, either in sternal (eg, iguanids) (**Fig. 22**) or in lateral recumbency (eg, agamid lizards) (**Fig. 23**).[47,48] In varanids, the heart is located more caudally comparatively with other species, and can therefore be easily accessed via a ventral approach, caudal to the sternum and slightly on the right side (**Fig. 24**).[1,52] The left and

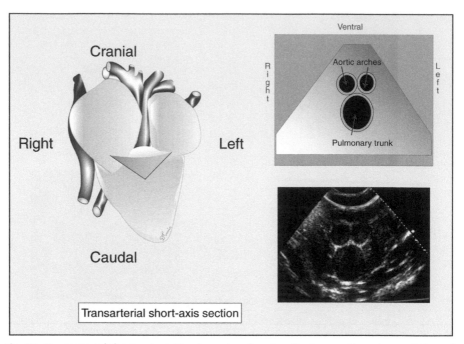

Transarterial short-axis section

Fig. 18. Transarterial short-axis section in snakes showing the two aortic arches and the pulmonary trunk. Figure illustrated by Dominique Tessier. (From Schilliger, et al. 2006, with the permission of the Journal of herpetological Medicine and Surgery.)

right axillary regions allow for more complete visualization of cardiac structures. From the left axillary approach, a long-axis view shows the atria, the single ventricle, the interatrial septum, and the atrioventricular valve leaflets (**Figure 25**). In the long-axis view, the diameters of both atria are measured during diastole. The right axillary window allows for the evaluation of pulmonary artery flow. Both right and left views can reveal pericardial effusion or valvular insufficiency. With standardized imaging planes, the diameter of the cardiac chambers, fractional area change, and fractional shortening (in the longitudinal and transverse planes) is calculated. Reference values are provided for the bearded dragon (*P vitticeps*) (**Table 5**).[47]

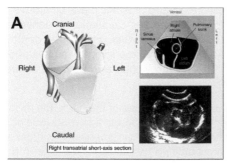
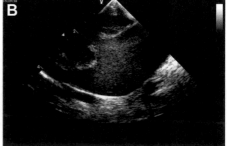

Fig. 19. (*A*) Transatrial short-axis section in snakes. Figure illustrated by Dominique Tessier. (*B*) This short-axis view shows the right atrium, the sinoatrial valves, and the sinus venous. ([*A*] *From* Schilliger, et al. 2006, with the permission of the Journal of herpetological Medicine and Surgery.)

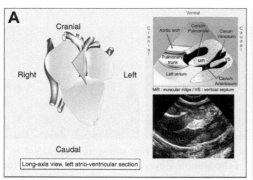 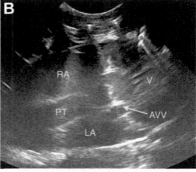

Fig. 20. (A) Long-axis section of the left atrioventricular junction in snakes. Figure illustrated by Dominique Tessier. (B) The monocuspid atrioventricular valves can also be visualized in this view. AVV, atrioventricular valve; LA, left atrium; PT, pulmonary trunk; RA, right atrium; V, ventricle. ([A] From Schilliger, et al. 2006, with the permission of the Journal of herpetological Medicine and Surgery.)

Table 3
Cardiac measurements (medians and reference ranges) in ball pythons (*Python regius*) by sex (n = 20)

		Median			Reference Range
	Parameter (units)	Male	Female		Total Population
	Heart rate (bpm)	64	62	64	56–76
	Longitudinal fractional shortening (%)	30.50	25.15	26.69	25.18–31.82
	Transversal fractional shortening (%)	31.90	31.95	31.90	26.6–34.20
	Measurements (cm)				
Ventricular systole	Pulmonary trunk diameter	0.44	0.53	0.49	0.35–0.63
	Left aortic arch diameter	0.32	0.30	0.32	0.25–0.38
	Right aortic arch diameter	0.35	0.31	0.33	0.29–0.40
	Ventricular length	1.71	1.80	1.76	1.55–2.08
	Ventricular width	1.28	1.35	1.30	1.19–1.57
	Ventricular height	1.07	1.09	1.07	1.00–1.27
	Left atrial length	**2.05**	**2.36**	**2.33**	**1.82–2.49**
	Left atrial width	0.67	0.75	0.70	0.44–0.98
	Right atrial length	2.21	2.32	2.27	1.83–2.70
	Right atrial width	0.87	0.86	0.86	0.61–1.08
	Total heart length	3.73	4.13	4.05	3.37–4.57
Ventricular diastole	Pulmonary trunk diameter	0.32	0.36	0.35	0.24–0.46
	Left aortic arch diameter	0.29	0.26	0.28	0.22–0.36
	Right aortic arch diameter	0.31	0.29	0.30	0.22–0.37
	Ventricular length	2.56	2.52	2.55	2.13–2.78
	Ventricular width	1.95	2.02	1.97	1.65–2.14
	Ventricular height	1.27	1.30	1.30	1.10–1.58
	Left atrial length	1.11	1.27	1.21	0.90–2.18
	Left atrial width	0.59	0.64	0.62	0.45–0.92
	Right atrial length	**1.24**	**1.60**	**1.44**	**1.04–1.87**
	Right atrial width	0.78	0.77	0.77	0.56–0.90
	Total heart length	3.62	3.93	3.72	3.03–4.96

Significant differences between sex (P < .05) are reported in bold.
   Data from Paillusseau C, Gandar F, Schilliger L, et al. Two-dimensional echocardiographic measurements in the ball python (Python regius). J Zoo Wildl med 2019;50(4):976-82.

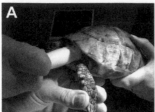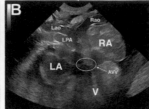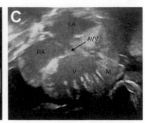

Fig. 21. Placement of an ultrasound probe (left cervicobrachial ultrasound window) in a spur-thighed tortoise (*Testudo graeca*) (*A*). Echographic view of the heart in a sulcated tortoise (*Centrochelys sulcata*) (*B*) LA, left atrium; RA, right atrium; V, ventricle; LPA, left pulmonary artery; LAo, left aortic arch; RAo, right aortic arch, (*C*) AVV, atrioventricular valve; M, myocardium, and in a red-eared slider (*Trachemys scripta elegans*) (*C*). LAO, left anterior oblique; LPA; M; RAO, right anterior oblique.

THERAPY

The pharmacokinetics and pharmacodynamics of cardiovascular drugs are poorly understood in reptiles. Unfortunately, reptiles suffering from cardiac disease are often diagnosed post mortem and thus rarely subject to therapeutic trials. Further research is therefore urgently needed to provide evidence-based recommendations for the treatment of cardiac pathologies in reptiles.

Nonpharmacologic Interventions

As with mammals, nonpharmacologic management of cardiovascular disease relies on reducing cardiac stress. Interventions include reducing metabolic rates by maintaining the reptile at the lower end of its preferred optimum temperature zone, and reducing stress by minimizing handling and keeping the patient isolated. Care should also be given to maintain an adequate diet, because overfeeding has been attributed to death in snakes with cardiomyopathy.[1]

Pharmacologic Interventions

In mammals, cardiac therapy is chosen based on the desired effect on heart contractibility and HR, vasoconstriction or vasodilatation, or increasing or reducing blood

Table 4
Mean and range for two-dimensional echocardiographic parameters of adult female red-ear slider terrapins (*Trachemys scripta elegans*)

Parameters	Mean ± Standard Deviation	Range
Ventricular long axis (diastole) (mm)	14.08 ± 2.02	10.70–17.03
Ventricular long axis (systole) (mm)	9.90 (interquartile)	8.67–11.32
Ventricular short axis (diastole) (mm)	22.61 ± 5.15	14.76–28.80
Ventricular short axis (systole) (mm)	12.11 ± 2.01	9.57–15.00
Fractional shortening (%)	44.41 ± 8.09	33.06–52.97
Ventricular wall thickness (diastole) (mm)	6.75 (interquartile)	5.83–10.33
Ventricular wall thickness (systole) (mm)	7.62 ± 2.20	5.07–11.43
Ventricular outflow tract (systole) (mm)	4.79 ± 0.97	3.53–5.67
Main arteries (mm)	5.04 ± 0.79	4.10–6.00

Data from Poser H, Russello G, Zanella A, et al. Two-dimensional and Doppler echocardiographic findings in healthy non-sedated red-eared slider terrapins (*Trachemys scripta elegans*). Vet Res Commun 2011;35:511-520.

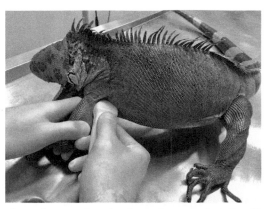

Fig. 22. Placement of an ultrasound probe (lateral approach, left axillary ultrasound window) in a green iguana (*Iguana iguana*) in sternal recumbency.

volume. The cornerstone of managing CHF rests on reducing the volume of extracellular fluid and reducing preload through the use of diuretics and vasodilators. Although extrapolation from mammals to reptiles is hazardous because of significant differences in size, metabolism, anatomy, and physiology, basic principles remain applicable. Oxygen supplementation should be instituted for animals with dyspnea, especially in the presence of pulmonary edema. Response to oxygen therapy is, however, difficult to assess in species capable of large right-to-left cardiac shunting when pulmonary vasculature is bypassed.

Inotropes and chronotropes
Inotropes are a group of drugs that alter the contractility of the heart. Positive inotropes, such as pimobendane, are commonly used in small animal cardiology and increase survival time and quality of life in the treatment of canine dilated cardiomyopathy. Digoxin is another positive inotrope that increases the cytosolic calcium concentration by inhibiting Na/K ATPase pumps in myocardial cells. Digoxin is also used for its effect in decreasing HR (negative chronotrope) and is mainly indicated for atrial fibrillation. β-Blockers (eg, atenolol, propranolol) and calcium channel

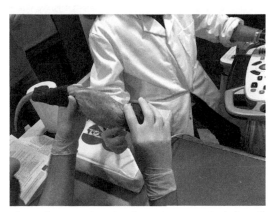

Fig. 23. Placement of an ultrasound probe (lateral approach, left axillary ultrasound window) in a bearded dragon (*Pogona vitticeps*) in lateral recumbency.

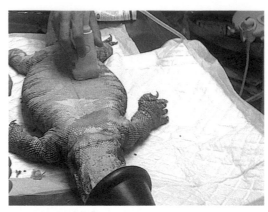

Fig. 24. Placement of an ultrasound probe (ventral approach, short-axis section of the heart) in a varanid (*Varanus salvator*) in dorsal recumbency.

blockers (eg, diltiazem) are negative inotropes that are mainly indicated in the treatment of hypertrophic cardiomyopathy in cats and supraventricular arrhythmias. β-Blockers are uncommonly used for treatment of supraventricular tachycardia and atrial fibrillation in reptile because of their unknown effectiveness in this taxon. The use of atropine (0.04 mg/kg intravenous [IV]) and glycopyrrolate (0.01 mg/kg IV) to counter the negative chronotropic effects of vagal stimulation of the heart was unsuccessful in the green iguana (*I iguana*).[53] In a study of 15 nonanesthetized healthy juvenile green iguanas, atenolol administered at 1 mg/kg IV significantly reduced resting HR, but did not significantly affect mean arterial blood pressure at the midpoint of the HR range. Failure to alter the baroreceptor reflex function in this instance suggests that atenolol is of little use in regulating blood pressure.[19]

Little evidence exists on the efficacy of cardiac chronotropes in reptiles. In the previously mentioned study of 15 nonanesthetized green iguanas, administration of methylatropine (1 mg/kg IV) increased resting HR but did not significantly affect mean arterial blood pressure.[19]

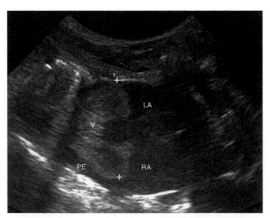

Fig. 25. Echocardiographic examination in a bearded dragon (*Pogona vitticeps*). V, ventricle; RA, right atrium; LA, left atrium; PE, pericardial effusion.

Table 5
Cardiac measurements from two-dimensional echocardiographic evaluation in bearded dragons (*Pogona vitticeps*)

Cardiac Measurements (cm)	Ventricular Systole	Ventricular Diastole
Left atrium diameter	0.81–0.96	N/A
Right atrium diameter	1.03–1.25	N/A
R + L atrium diameter	1.89–2.17	N/A
Ventricular transversal length	1.54–1.88	1.86–2.17
Ventricular longitudinal length	1.03–1.23	1.36–1.58

Abbreviation: N/A, not available.
   Data from Silverman S. *et al.* Standardization of the two-dimensional transcoelomic echocardiographic examination in the central bearded dragon (*Pogona vitticeps*). J Vet Cardiol 2016 ; 18(2):168-78.

Angiotensin-converting enzyme inhibitors
In mammals, angiotensin-converting enzyme (ACE) inhibitors block the formation of angiotensin II, which normally promotes venous and arterial vasoconstriction. In addition, ACE inhibitors suppress the production of aldosterone, which normally causes renal sodium and fluid retention. The combined effect of ACE inhibitors therefore reduces preload and afterload through venous and arterial vasodilation, and reduction of blood volume. Enalapril and benazepril are commonly used in dogs and cats because of their longer half-life, but it is unknown if this is also the case in reptiles. In American alligators, captopril and enalapril have been used to inhibit the pressor response to exogenous angiotensin I and angiotensin II at a dose of 0.5 µg/kg/h and 300 µg/kg/h, respectively.[54] Both ACE inhibitors failed to alter baseline blood pressure, significantly reduced the response to angiotensin I, but not angiotensin II. When combined with spironolactone and furosemide, enalapril administered at 0.5 to 0.7 mg/kg every 24 hours per os managed Cl IF in a spiny tailed monitor (*Varanus acanthurus*) (L.A. Clayton, C.A. Hadfield, S.R. Gore, and colleagues, unpublished data).

Diuretics
Diuretics reduce fluid overload and decrease edema and effusions by promoting water excretion. In mammals, furosemide is the diuretic of choice. It is a loop diuretic that acts by inhibiting sodium, potassium, and chloride cotransporters in the ascending limb of the loop of Henle of the kidney. Although reptiles lack a loop of Henle, furosemide has been successfully used to cause diuresis in chelonians and ophidians.[55–58] The mechanism of action is thought to involve its effect on the sodium/potassium pumps located in the urinary bladder or in the terminal rectum (many species of reptiles reflux urine from the cloaca into the rectum to absorb water in conjunction with NaCl).[58] Furosemide should be used with caution in reptile patients with renal disease, because it can cause dehydration and visceral gout. Biochemical parameters including potassium, phosphorus, and major nitrogenous waste product (ammonia, urea, or uric acid) should be monitored and treatment adapted accordingly. Furosemide (two doses at 5.2 mg/kg intramuscular, 3 weeks apart) was successfully used for the treatment of peripheral edema in a spur-thighed tortoise (*Testudo graeca*) with atrial dilatation and pericardial effusion.[59] The peripheral edema resolved within 12 hours after each injection. Treatments with furosemide (2 mg/kg/8–12 hours subcutaneous for three doses) were considered to improve quality of life in two lizards (a 6-year-old bearded dragon and a 13-year-old green iguana) suffering from

CHF.[60] However, furosemide (5 mg/kg/d intramuscular) was unsuccessful at managing atrioventricular insufficiency with secondary pulmonary edema and pericardial effusion in a carpet python (*M spilota variegata*).[37]

There is little to no information available on the use and efficacy of other diuretics in reptiles. Hydrochlorothiazide has been used as a diuretic in lizards with renal disease (S.J. Divers, personal communication). Methylated xanthines (aminophylline and theophylline) have successfully induced diuresis in different species (*Testudo* sp, *T scripta elegans*, *I iguana*, *Eublepharis macularius*, and *P vitticeps*). Their diuretic effect is apparently caused by increased rates of excretion of sodium and chloride ions by renal tubules, in addition to their positive inotropic effect on cardiac and renal functions (increased renal blood flow and increased glomerular filtration rate).[61] Spironolactone is an aldosterone antagonist and a weak diuretic in mammals that can either be used alone or in conjunction with furosemide to offset the loss of potassium. Nothing is known about its potential use in reptiles.

CLINICS CARE POINTS

- Care should be taken to consider ambient temperature and stress when performing clinical examinations of reptiles, because these can influence cardiopulmonary parameters and distort results. For this reason, reference ranges should be used with caution in instances where the environmental conditions under which they were established are not described.

- Clinical signs of cardiovascular diseases in reptiles include lethargy, cardiomegaly, cyanosis, peripheral edema, pulmonary edema, and ascites. Unlike in mammals, coughing is not a feature of chronic heart failure in reptiles. Pitting edema is uncommon because of the unique cardiovascular system of reptiles.

- The most useful diagnostic tools for reptile cardiology include ECG and ultrasound. Although frustratingly rare, most cardiac reference ranges have been established using these tools.

- No licensed drugs are currently available in reptile cardiology.

ACKNOWLEDGMENTS

Acknowledgments: my mentor in cardiology, Pr Valérie Chetboul, DVM, PhD., Dip. ECVIM (CA), my colleague Clément Paillusseau, DVM, Dip. ECZM (Herpetology) for sharing some of his pictures, and Jesse Bonwitt, DM, B.V.Sc., M.Sc., M.R.C.V.S. for proofreading this article.

DISCLOSURE

The author has nothing to disclose.

REFERENCES

1. Schilliger L, Girling S. Cardiology. In: Divers S, Stahl S, editors. Mader's reptile and amphibian medicine and surgery. St Louis: Elsevier; 2019. p. 669–98.
2. Wyneken J. Normal reptile heart morphology and function. Vet Clin North Am Exot Anim Pract 2009;12:51–63.
3. Mitchell MA. Reptile cardiology. Vet Clin North Am Exot Anim Pract 2009;12: 65–79.
4. Schilliger L, Chetboul V, Damoiseaux C, et al. Restrictive cardiomyopathy and congestive heart failure in a McDowell's carpet python (*Morelia spilota mcdowelli*). J Zoo Wildl Med 2016;47:1001–104.

5. Schilliger L, Paillusseau C, Gandar F, et al. Hypertensive heart disease in a central bearded dragon (*Pogona vitticeps*) with severe atherosclerosis and first-degree atrioventricular block. J Zoo Wildl Med 2019;50:482–6.
6. Schilliger L, Lemberger K, Chai N, et al. Atherosclerosis associated with pericardial effusion in a central bearded dragon (*Pogona vitticeps*). J Vet Diagn Invest 2010;22:789–92.
7. Breno MC, Presoto BC, Borgheresi R, et al. Characteristics of neural and humoral systems involved in the regulation of blood pressure in snakes. Comp Biochem Physiol 2007;147:766–78.
8. Farrell AP, Gamperl AK, Francis ETB. In: Gans C, Gaunt A, editors. Comparative aspects of heart morphology. Ithaca: Society for the Study of Amphibians and Reptiles; 1998. p. 375–424.
9. Kardong KV. The circulatory system. In: Kardon KV, editor. Vertebrates, comparative anatomy, function, evolution. 5th edition. New York: McGraw-Hill; 2009. p. 445–95.
10. Hicks JW. The physiological and evolutionary significance of cardiovascular shunting patterns in reptiles. News Physiol Sci 2002;17:241–5.
11. Starck JM. Functional morphology and patterns of blood flow in the heart of *Python regius*. J Morphol 2009;270:673–87.
12. Burggren W, Johansen K. Ventricular haemodynamics in the monitor lizard *Varanus exanthematicus*: pulmonary and systemic pressure separation. J Exp Biol 1982;96:343–54.
13. Barten S, Simpson S. Lizard taxonomy, anatomy, and physiology. In: Divers S, Stahl S, editors. Mader's reptile and amphibian medicine and surgery. St Louis: Elsevier; 2019. p. 63–82.
14. Galli G, Taylor EW, Wang T. The cardiovascular responses of the freshwater turtle (*Trachemys scripta*) to warming and cooling. J Exp Biol 2004;207:1471–8.
15. Martinez-Jimenez D, Hernandez-Divers SJ. Emergency care of reptiles. Vet Clin Exot Anim 2007;10:557–85.
16. Chinnadurai SK, Wrenn A, DeVoe RS. Evaluation of noninvasive oscillometric blood pressure monitoring in anesthetized boid snakes. J Am Vet Med Assoc 2009;234:625–30.
17. Enok S, Saly C, Abe AS, et al. Intraspecific scaling of arterial blood pressure in the Burmese python J Exp Biol 2014;217:2232–4.
18. Schilliger L, Selleri P, Frye FLFL. Lymphoreticular neoplasm and leukemia in a red-tail boa (*Boa constrictor constrictor*) associated with concurrent inclusion body disease. J Vet Diagn Invest 2011;23:159–62.
19. Hernandez SM, Schumacher J, Lewis SJ, et al. Selected cardiopulmonary values and baroreceptor reflex in conscious green iguanas (*Iguana iguana*). Am J Vet Res 2011;72:1519–26.
20. Heatley JJ, Russel KE. Clinical chemistry. In: Divers S, Stahl S, editors. Mader's reptile and amphibian medicine and surgery. St Louis: Elsevier; 2019. p. 319–32.
21. Holz RM, Holz P. Electrocardiography in anaesthetized red-eared sliders (*Trachemys scripta elegans*). Res Vet Sci 1995;58(1):67–9.
22. Boukens BJD, Kristensen DL, Filogonio R, et al. The electrocardiogram of vertebrates: evolutionary changes from ectothermy to endothermy. Prog Biophys Mol Biol 2019;144:16–29.
23. Germer CM, Tomaz JM, Carvalho AF, et al. Electrocardiogram, heart movement and heart rate in the awake gecko (*Hemidactylus mabouia*). J Comp Physiol B 2015;185:111–8.

24. Martinez-Silvestre A, Mateo JA, Pether J. Electrocardiographic parameters in the Gomeran giant lizard, *Gallotia bravoana*. J Herp Med Surg 2003;13(3):22–5.

25. Hunt D. Electrocardiography of the normal inland bearded dragon. Thesis submitted in part fulfilment of the requirements for the Royal College of Veterinary Surgeons (RCVS) Diploma in Zoological Medicine. London: Royal College of Veterinary Surgeons; 2013. p. 42p.

26. Karthik M, Rajkumar K, Krishna MK, et al. Electrocardiographic parameters of free living Russel's viper (Daboia russelii) and Indian spectacled cobra (Naja naja). In: Proceedings Annual Conference AAZV 2013:174-180.

27. Valentinuzzi ME, Hoff HE, Geddes LA. Observations on the electrical activity of the snake heart. J Electrocardiol 1969;2:39–50.

28. Lewis M, Bouvard J, Eatwell K, et al. Standardisation of electrocardiographic examination in corn snakes (*Pantherophis guttatus*). Vet Rec 2020;186(9):1–8.

29. Heaton-Jones TG, King RR. Characterization of the electrocardiogram of the American Alligator (*Alligator mississippiensis*). J Zoo Wildl Med 1994;25:40–7.

30. Mullen RK. Comparative electrocardiography of the Squamata. Physiol Zool 1967;40:114.

31. Schilliger L, Chai N, Chetboul V, et al. Smartphone based ECG monitor: feasibility and applications in herpetological medicine. Proc Annu Conf ARAV 2014;128–30.

32. Cermakova E, Piskovska A, Trhonova V, et al. Comparison of three ECG machines for electrocardiography in green iguanas (*Iguana iguana*). Vet Med (Praha) 2021;66(02):66–71.

33. Kharin S, Shmakov D. A comparative study of contractility of the heart ventricle in some ectothermic vertebrates. Acta Herpetol 2009;4:57–71.

34. Bogan JE. Ophidian cardiology: a review. J Herp Med Surg 2017;27(1–2):62–77.

35. Nogradi AL, Balogh M. Establishment of methodology for non-invasive electrocardiographic measurements in turtles and tortoises. Acta Vet Hung 2018;66(3):365–75.

36. Clippinger T. Aortic stenosis and atrioventricular dilatation in a green iguana (*Iguana iguana*). Proc Am Assoc Zoo Vet 1993;342–4.

37. Rishniw M, Carmel BP. Atrioventricular valvular insufficiency and congestive heart failure in a carpet python. Aust Vet J 1999;77:580–3.

38. Holmes SP, Divers SJ. Radiography: general principles. In: Divers S, Stahl S, editors. Mader's reptile and amphibian medicine and surgery. St Louis: Elsevier; 2019. p. 486–90.

39. Comolli L JR, Divers SJS. Radiography: snakes. In: Divers S, Stahl S, editors. Mader's reptile and amphibian medicine and surgery. St Louis: Elsevier; 2019. p. 503–13.

40. Holmes SP, Divers SJ. Radiography: chelonians. In: Divers S, Stahl S, editors. Mader's reptile and amphibian medicine and surgery. St Louis: Elsevier; 2019. p. 514–27.

41. Holmes SP, Divers SJ. Radiography: lizards. In: Divers S, Stahl S, editors. Mader's reptile and amphibian medicine and surgery. St Louis: Elsevier; 2019. p. 491–502.

42. Andersen B, et al. Physiology: postprandial cardiac hypertrophy in pythons. Nature 2005;434(7029):37–8.

43. Schilliger L, Tessier D, Pouchelon J-L, et al. Proposed standardization of the two-dimensional echocardiographic examination in snakes. J Herpetological Med Surg 2006;16:76–87.

44. Paillusseau C, Gandar F, Schilliger L, et al. Two-dimensional echocardiographic measurements in the ball python (*Python regius*). J Zoo Wildl Med 2019;50(4): 976–82.
45. Bagardi M, Bardi E, Manfredi M, et al. Two-dimensional and Doppler echocardiographic evaluation in twenty-one healthy *Python regius*. Vet Med Sci 2021. https://doi.org/10.1002/vms3.426.
46. Conceicao MEBAM, Monteiro OB, Andrade RS, et al. Effect of biometric variables on two-dimensional echocardiographic measurements in the red-tailed boa (*Boa constrictor constrictor*). J Zoo Wildl Med 2014;45(3):672–7.
47. Silverman S, Sanchez-Migallon Guzman D, Stern J, et al. Standardization of the two-dimensional transcoelomic echocardiographic examination in the central bearded dragon (*Pogona vitticeps*). J Vet Cardiol 2016;18:168–78.
48. Gustavsen KA, Saunders AB, Young BD, et al. Echocardiographic and radiographic findings in a cohort of healthy adult iguanas (*Iguana iguana*). J Vet Cardiol 2014;16:185–96.
49. Poser H, Russello G, Zanella A, et al. Two-dimensional and Doppler echocardiographic findings in healthy non-sedated red-eared slider terrapins (*Trachemys scripta elegans*). Vet Res Commun 2011;35:511–20.
50. Prutz M, Hungerbuhler S, Lass M, et al. Contrast echocardiography for analysis of heart anatomy in tortoises. Tierarztl Prax Ausg K Kleintiere Heimtiere 2015;43: 231–7.
51. Campolo M, Oricco S, Cavicchio P, et al. Echocardiographic evaluation of four giant Aldabra tortoises (*Aldabrachelys gigantea*). Vet Rec Open 2019;6:1–6.
52. Hochleitner C, Sharma A. Ultrasonography. In: Divers S, Stahl S, editors. Mader's reptile and amphibian medicine and surgery. St Louis: Elsevier; 2019. p. 543–9.
53. Pace L, Mader D. Atropine and glycopyrrolate, route of administration and response in the green iguana (*Iguana iguana*). Proc Annu Conf ARAV 2002;79.
54. Silldorff EP, Stephens GA. Effects of converting enzyme inhibition and alpha receptor blockade on the angiotensin pressor response in the American alligator. Gen Comp Endocrinol 1992;87:134–40.
55. Cipolle MD, Zehr JF. Renin release in turtles: effects of volume depletion and furosemide administration. Am J Physiol 1985;249:R100–5.
56. Uva B, Vallarino M. Renin-angiotensin system and osmoregulation in the terrestrial chelonian *Testudo hermanni* Gmelin. Comp Biochem Physiol A Comp Physiol 1982;71:449–51.
57. Stephens GA, Robertson FM. Renal responses to diuretics in the turtle. J Comp Physiol B 1985;155:387–93.
58. LeBrie SJ, Boelcskevy BD. The effect of furosemide on renal function and renin in water snakes. Comp Biochem Physiol C 1979;63C:223–8.
59. Redrobe SP, Scudamore CL. Ultrasonographic diagnosis of pericardial effusion and atrial dilation in a spur-thighed tortoise (*Testudo graeca*). Vet Rec 2000; 146:183–5.
60. Simone-Freilicher E, Sullivan P, Quinn R, et al. Two cases of congestive heart failure in lizards. Proc Exoticscon 2015;505–9.
61. Girling SJ, Hynes B. In: Girling SJ, Raiti P, editors. Cardiovascular and haemopoietic systems. 2nd edition. Cheltenham: BSAVA - British Small Animal Veterinary Association; 2004. p. 243–60.

Heart Disease in Pet Birds – Diagnostic Options

Konicek Cornelia, Drmedvet[a],*,
Maria-E. Krautwald-Junghanns, ME (DVM). Prof. Drmedvet. Dipl ECZM (avian)[b]

KEYWORDS

- Birds • Cardiovascular disease • Atherosclerosis • Parrots • Diagnostic imaging
- Echocardiography • ECG • Clinical examination

KEY POINTS

- Cardiovascular diseases are very common in pet birds, antemortem diagnostic remains challenging
- Diagnosis is based on the combination of anamnestic data, clinical examination, and imaging methods
- Echocardiography is a particularly valuable tool in evaluating the avian heart
- Advanced imaging diagnostics (Computed Tomography (CT)/Angiography/ Magnetic Resonance Imaging (MRI)) may allow diagnosing earlier stages of vascular pathologies, especially when technology improves and further research is conducted

INTRODUCTION

Cardiovascular disease Is frequently encountered in avian practice and poses a serious threat to the quality of life and longevity of many avian species.[1]

In regard to psittacine birds only, high prevalence of cardiac diseases could be found during postmortem examinations, whereby 36% of 104 investigated *Psittaciformes* had macroscopic lesions in the heart and/or the major vessels, even more lesions were found during histopathology.[2]

Even up to date, antemortem diagnosis of cardiovascular diseases in avian practice remains challenging. Thus, most of the described cardiovascular lesions are identified during postmortem examinations only.

Frequently described cardiovascular lesions in pet birds are atherosclerosis, pericardial effusions, pericarditis, myocarditis, dilatation or hypertrophy of the ventricles and valvular endocarditis.[3,4] Right ventricular or biventricular heart failure seems to

[a] Department of Small Animal Medicine, University of Veterinary Medicine Vienna, Veterinärplatz 1, Vienna 1210, Austria; [b] Department for Birds and Reptiles, Veterinary Teaching Hospital, University of Leipzig, An den Tierkliniken 17, Leipzig 04103, Germany
* Corresponding author.
E-mail address: cornelia.konicek@vetmeduni.ac.at

Vet Clin Exot Anim 25 (2022) 409–433
https://doi.org/10.1016/j.cvex.2022.01.004
vetexotic.theclinics.com
1094-9194/22/© 2022 Elsevier Inc. All rights reserved.

be more common than left ventricular heart failure.[5] Myxomatous degeneration or atrioventricular (AV) valve endocardiosis has been recently reported in Amazon parrots (*Amazona aestiva*) due to inadequate management in captivity.[6]

Although uncommon in pet birds, bacterial endocarditis was recently described in an Umbrella cockatoo (*Cacatua alba*) after recurrent cloacal prolapse[7]; and lately, a coarctation-like obliterative arteriopathy of the right brachiocephalic artery was even found in a Spix's macaw (*Cyanopsitta spixii*).[8]

DIAGNOSTIC APPROACH
Anamnestic Data

Relative predisposition to cardiovascular diseases is given by the species, breed, age, gender, lifestyle, and diet.[9]

Beaufrère and colleagues described several risk factors for developing atherosclerotic diseases in psittacine birds[10]: African gray parrots, Amazon parrots, and cockatiels seem to be particularly susceptible, in contrast to cockatoos and macaws. The reasons for the different predispositions among species are speculated to be associated with their various lifestyles, dietary requirements, stress, and genetics. A higher incidence of atherosclerosis was also noted in birds of 20 years and older and in the female sex, especially in association with reproductive diseases.

The predisposition to the development of atherosclerosis in female psittacine birds likely relates to the profound effects of estrogen on lipid, protein, and calcium metabolism in reproductively female active birds.[9] Still, the association with female sex should not be applied to all species, for instance in Quaker parrots the male sex seems to be more prone to atherosclerotic lesions.[11]

In addition to age, female sex, and species, risk factors for the development of atherosclerosis also include high-calorie and fat diets, dyslipidemia (eg, hypercholesterolemia), and limited physical activity.[9]

Thus, lack of exercise, years of malnutrition, and old age may lead to the first suspicion of cardiovascular diseases.[12–15]

In addition, medical history data on previously diagnosed noninfectious and infectious diseases that can cause secondary changes to the heart should be collected.

Clinical Symptoms

In companion birds, many cases are likely subclinical and go unrecognized for many years until well advanced.[9]

The clinical symptoms may be rather unspecific like symptoms of apathy/weakness and possibly central nervous disorders such as paresis or rigidity of one or more limps or "seizure disorders," as well as behavioral changes like disorientation or confusion are described. Visual impairments, like blindness or anisocoria can also occur.[9]

Persistent exercise intolerance is also a common reason for presentations and occurs regularly in both mammals and birds in connection with existing heart disease. However, due to the poor housing conditions with little free flight in many of the birds living in captivity, this symptom is noticed only rarely or late.[9,16]

Respiratory distress is also a common presentation of birds with underlying cardiovascular diseases. Signs of congestion (eg, right heart failure or pericardial effusion) can lead to coelomic effusion and liver swelling.[15] Due to the accumulation of free fluid in the coelom and the lack of a diaphragm, there is no longer adequate ventilation. As a result, typical signs of shortness of breath such as open-mouth breathing and tail wobbling can be observed.[9] The typical "heart cough" in mammals cannot be observed in birds.

Furthermore, bluish discoloration of the skin around the eyes in birds that do have featherless areas in that region (like gray parrots, **Fig. 1**) as well as recurring or untreatable skin diseases such as axillary dermatitis, feather plucking, or focal feather loss are described in connection with atherosclerotic changes.[9,17]

Clinical signs can have a subtle, insidious onset, with owners reporting progressively declining activity level, reduced appetite, and waning interest in activities, toys, and vocalizations that were historically of interest to the bird.[9] Unfortunately, in advanced stages, acute death may also occur.[18]

In birds with congestive heart failure peripheral venous congestions may be recognized by distension of the jugular and cutaneous ulnar veins, edema is rarely found, most often appearing as swelling of the periorbital region or of the hocks and feet.[9] In hospitalized patients receiving subcutaneous fluids, the first indication of circulatory compromise may be delayed absorption (>48h).[9]

Clinical Examination

A baseline diagnostic work-up is appropriate in any patient presenting with clinical signs consistent with cardiovascular diseases, to begin to assess overall systemic health status.[9] Standard examination methods for heart disease, as found in mammals, are partly lacking or hard to evaluate due to numerous physiologic peculiarities in birds. For instance, arterial pulses can't always be palpated or thoroughly assessed, strongly depending on the size and the cooperation of the patient. It is best palpated at the medial aspect of the proximal antebrachium (superficial ulnar artery), in addition, the relative warmth of each extremity can also be subjectively assessed.[9] Auscultation of the avian heart only plays a subordinate role due to many limitations; still it can provide subjective information of the rate, sound quality, and the rhythm. Particularly due to the rapid heart rate, individual heartbeats can hardly be noticed by the examiner. For this reason, muffled heart sounds, or heart murmurs are very difficult to characterize. In the case of cardiogenic pulmonary edema, increased respiratory noise is heard on auscultation in a calm bird, but characteristic "crackles" and "wheezes" are generally absent except in severe cases.[9]

Hematology

Although specific changes in the blood count have no diagnostic value in case of heart diseases, increases in the leukocyte count, heterophily, or lymphopenia have been

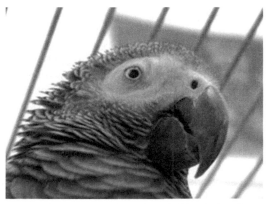

Fig. 1. African gray parrot (*Psittacus erithacus*) with bluish discoloration of the skin surrounding the eyes. A clinical finding, often associated with cardiovascular disease.

described in connection with cardiovascular diseases, especially with atherosclerosis.[14,19] Leukocytosis with a left shift, toxic changes of heterophiles may be associated with bacterial endocarditis.[7]

Biochemistry

Especially plasma lipid levels may offer some observational data pertinent to population-level risk factors for cardiovascular diseases.[9] Particular an association between total cholesterol and HDL values among certain psittacine genera in regard to their prevalence of atherosclerotic lesions can be seen.[9] Still, the connection between atherosclerosis and changes in plasma lipid levels in individual birds and the diagnostic value has not yet been adequately proven.[20] Changes in plasma lipids, such as total cholesterol and total triglycerides, as well as HDL-C and LDL-C may be noticed in an individual bird, but single measurement results should be interpreted with caution. As, until now, dyslipidemias are yet incomplete characterized or not statistically linked to cardiovascular disorders.[21]

In human medicine lipoprotein ratios, especially total cholesterol/HDL cholesterol is used as a risk predictor of heart diseases. Lipoprotein ratio and non-HDL concentrations are not commonly measured or reported in parrots, non–HDL-C can be easily obtained, in people, it is a powerful risk factor to atherosclerotic diseases, its usefulness in psittacine birds should be further explored; therefore, reference intervals and ratios should also be reported whenever reporting on lipoprotein reference intervals.[21]

Blood Pressure Measurement

Direct/invasive blood pressure measurement is regarded as the "gold standard" technique, providing the most accurate readings. For indirect measurements—depending on the size of the bird, the product used and the authors' experience -either Doppler devices[22] or oscillometric devices[23] are recommended. Unfortunately, there is poor agreement between invasive and noninvasive blood pressure measurements in birds.[24,25] Using noninvasive techniques in psittacine birds, even high variabilities between the readings from different cuff placement sites on the same individual have been reported.[25] More precise results from indirect blood pressure measurements seemed to be obtained from larger bird species.[26] The accuracy of the used method must be, therefore, assessed critically. Reference values for direct blood pressure measurements are available for selected species of psittacine birds, see **Table 1**. Regarding indirect measurements, a systolic blood pressure over 200 mm Hg in the nonanesthetized animal is noted by some authors as hypertensive.[9,22,27,28]

Because of these technical issues, the significantly higher arterial blood pressure of birds compared with mammals, and the lack of scientific data on hypertension in birds, blood pressure measurement plays a subordinate role for assessing heart diseases in birds. Still, blood pressure measurements could be useful to detect chronic hypertension.[29] Single measurements should not be overinterpreted, but repeated measurements of an individual bird in accordance with other diagnostic methods could be valuable for the detection and the therapeutic progress of cardiovascular diseases.

Electrocardiography

For recording an electrocardiogram in birds, both the use of needle electrodes and the use of so-called spring electrodes have been described in the literature.[30–32] As in human medicine, the position of the leads is based on the scheme of Einthoven.[30] In this way, 3 leads are measured, the QRS complex being negative in the second and third lead in birds. A recording speed of 100 to 200 mm/s is necessary. Clinicians have to be

Table 1
Reference values for direct blood pressure measurements (mm HG) in selected species of pet birds, measurements were taken under Isoflurane anesthesia

	Application Side	Systolic	Mean	Diastolic	Ref.
Amazona ventralis	deep radial artery	132.9 ± 22.1	116.9 ± 20.5	101.9 ± 20	Schnellbacher RW et al,[69] 2012
Amazona ventralis	superficial ulnar artery	163 ± 18	155 ± 18	148 ± 18	Acierno MJ et al,[24] 2008
Cacatua spp.	brachial artery		143 ± 4		Curro TG et al,[70] 1994

Values are reported as mean ± standard deviation

aware of the different characteristics of the avian electrocardiography (ECG) compared with small animals.[33] Due to the patient's high susceptibility to stress, the result of the ECG in the awake bird may be falsified and should, therefore, be classified as an exercise ECG.[34]

An ECG is in principle useful to evaluate heart rate and rhythm, but one should remember that electrical activity does not ensure mechanical (pumping) activity. The ECG can actually remain relatively normal in birds, with severe cardiopulmonary compromise or even cardiac arrest from anesthetic overdose.[27] It is also important to keep in mind, that arrhythmias can be explained by extracardiac and cardiac causes, as well as changes in the autonomic nervous system. It is, therefore, important to rule out metabolic abnormalities by measuring sodium, potassium, calcium, hematocrit (hypoxia), if possible the acid–base status and glucose.[33] Changes in the P waves and/or QRS complex can suggest the enlargement of the cardiac chambers and a low voltage ECG is pointing toward the possibility of pericardial effusion, ascites or obesity.[33]

Nevertheless, the application to awake birds is difficult due to the frequent lack of cooperation on the part of the patient. Problems may occur with the connection of the leads to the skin and—as already mentioned—stress may cause alterations of the recorded ECG. Therefore, ECG, for the detection of heart disease in birds, is still infrequently used in birds in comparison to mammals.

Reference values for various bird species have been established in past years, studies of electrocardiograms in pigeons,[35] African Grey parrots, and amazons[36,37] as well as some macaw species,[38,39] meanwhile also numerous studies on birds of prey[40–42] are available; see also **Table 2**.

Imaging Procedures

Radiography

In a native radiograph the position, size, and shape of the heart silhouette as well as the radiopacity of the major vessels can be assessed.[15] A clear radiographic depiction of the apex of the heart is normal in some bird species (eg, cockatoos). In other species, a clear view of the apex of the heart indicates the presence of an air sac rupture as a result of trauma, as the air surrounding the heart works as a contrast medium. In such cases, echocardiographic imaging is limited.

For measuring the heart size in the radiograph, various reference values are described, see **Table 3**.

A rare radiographic finding is microcardia in birds and it is usually associated with severe dehydration of the patient. In these cases, the heart seems greatly diminished in size and is often separated from the sternum. Far more common, an enlarged heart shadow is found in the X-ray image (**Fig. 2**) which gives the first indication of an existing cardiovascular problem. An enlarged heart shadow can have many etiologies such as cardiac hypertrophy, cardiac dilatation, pericardial effusions, aneurysms, inflammations, or neoplasms.[14,15,43,44] However, the differentiation of these causes can only be conducted by further diagnostic means.

Additional radiographic findings, such as liver enlargement, coelomic effusion, pathologies of the respiratory tract can be recognized as secondary changes or primary causes of cardiovascular diseases.[15,43] Asymmetrical changes of the heart silhouette, due to neoplasia or congenital disorders, are rare in birds. There must be substantial changes in the morphology of the heart, to be radiographically evident.

Increased radiopacity of the heart is sometimes seen with inflammatory changes; however, this is not always easy to assess.[15,43]

Table 2
Electrocardiographic reference intervals for selected pet bird species

	Psittacus Erithacus	Amazona spp.	Cacatua spp.	Ara spp.	Ancdorhynchus Hyacinthus	Ara Chloroptera	Ara Glaucogularis	Ara Rubrogenys
Heart rate (b/min)	340–600	340–600	231–571	222–545	283 ± 65	280 ± 97	269 ± 49	389 ± 85
P (s)	0.012–0.018	0.008–0.017	0.01–0.03	0.01–0.025	0.015–0.025	0.015–0.025	0.015–0.02	0.015–0.02
P (mV)	0.25–0.55	0.25–0.6			0.18–0.4	0.075–0.3	0.18–0.45	0.12–0.5
PR (s)	0.040–0.055	0.042–0.055		0.035–0.08	0.05–0.075	0.04–0.07	0.05–0.06	0.035–0.075
QRS-complex (s)	0.010–0.016	0.010–0.015	0.015–0.03	0.010–0.05	0.015–0.025	0.013–0.025	0.012–0.025	0.015–0.022
R(mV)	0.00–0.20	0.00–0.65	0.00–0.30	0.00–0.35	0.04–0.08	0.02–0.2	0.02–0.25	0.04
(Q)S(mV)	0.90–2.20	0.70–2.30	0.40–1.90	0.40–1.60				
QT (s)	0.048–0.070	0.050–0.078	0.07–0.13	0.05–0.11	0.08–0.1	0.08–0.11	0.075–0.11	0.075–0.09
T(s)	0.015–0.035	0.020–0.035			0.035–0.075	0.04–0.07	0.05–0.06	0.035–0.075
T(mV)	0.18–0.60	0.30–0.80	0.25–1.00	0.20–0.90	0.1–0.7	0.1–0.45	0.3–0.8	0.3–0.55
Ref.	Nap AM et al,[36] 1992	Nap AM et al,[36] 1992	Oglesbee BL et al,[39] 2001	Cglesbee BL et al,[39] 2001	Casares M et al,[38] 2000	Casares M et al,[38] 2000	Casares M et al,[38] 2000	Casares M et al,[38] 2000

Table 3
Reference values for radiographic measurements of the psittacine heart

	Amazona Aestiva	Cyanopsitta Spixii	Psittacus Erithacus	Poicephalus Senegalus	Amazona Amazonica	Eolophus Roseicapilla
BW (g)	393 ± 37.7		501 ± 45	143 ± 11	357 ± 38	
Sternal length (mm)	65.03 ± 3.8[a]		71 ± 3	46 ± 2	66 ± 4	51.1 ± 2.3
Cardiac width (mm)	21.82 ± 1.3	19.9 ± 1.3	27 ± 2	18 ± 1	25 ± 1	21.9 ± 1.3
Cranial coelom width (mm)	50.61 ± 1.7	37.7 ± 1.5	49 ± 4	31 ± 3	46 ± 3	36.9 ± 2.1
Cardiac width: Cranial coelom width (%)		53 ± 3	56 ± 4	57 ± 4	54 ± 3	50–65
Cardiac width: coracoid width (%)			593 ± 48	624 ± 53	599 ± 51	570–743
Reference	Silva et al,[71] 2020	Rettmer et al,[72] 2011	Straub et al,[73] 2002	Straub et al,[73] 2002	Straub et al,[73] 2002	Schnitzer et al,[74] 2021

The width of the cardiac silhouette is measured at its widest point; at the same level, the width of the cranial coelom is measured. The coracoid width is measured caudal to the shoulder joint. Values are reported as mean ± standard deviation.
[a] Measurements were taken from birds in right recumbency

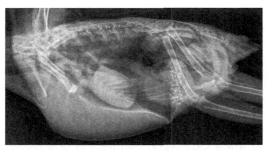

Fig. 2. Radiograph of a galah (*Eolophus roseicapilla*) in lateral projection. An enlarged cardiac silhouette, with increased radio-opacity can be easily identified on the radiograph. The clear radiographic depiction of the apex of the heart is normal for cockatoo species. For detailed information on the underlying pathology, echocardiography will be necessary.

Pathologies of the great vessels, such as atherosclerotic lesions, are only visible on the X-ray image if they are very pronounced. Radiographic findings, such as increased radio-opacity (**Fig. 3**) can be considered subjectively. Further radiographic presentations that can be assigned to avian atherosclerosis are Increased radiopacity of the heart and the caudal lungs, due to congestion.[15,43] In well-advanced atherosclerosis, due to the calcification of the vessels, there is more obviously increased radiodensity as well as focal or linear mineralization of the great vessels, most often the aorta and/or the pulmonary trunk.[29] Nevertheless, the lack of such radiopacity in the great vessels, does not rule out the possible presence of atherosclerotic lesions.

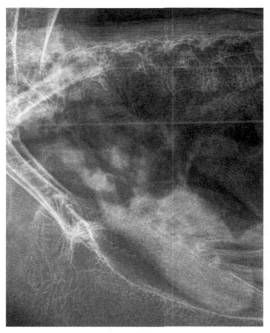

Fig. 3. Cardiac radiograph of a blue-and-gold-macaw (*Ara ararauna*) in lateral projection with subjectively increased radioopacity of the major vessels.

Angiocardiography

More detailed information of the cardiovascular tract can be obtained after the administration of intravascular contrast agent. PEES et al. (2006)[14] described the implementation of an angiocardiography of the bird under isoflurane anesthesia. The examination can be performed either by real-time fluoroscopy in or by computed tomography (CT). Using angiocardiography, the brachiocephalic trunk, the aorta, pulmonary arteries and veins, and the caudal vena cava can be visualized.[45] Therefore, angiocardiography can provide useful information especially for diagnosing changes in the heart vessels such as stenoses, dilatations, and aneurysms.[14,15,46] Still, up to date, there are only a few case reports on the use of angiocardiography in avian medicine.[19,47,48]

Using high-quality angiographic techniques to either diagnose arterial luminal stenosis or detect atheromatous plaque are likely to become the diagnostic test of choice, as soon as limitations in resolution artifacts are resolved through technological advances.[29]

Echocardiography

Echocardiography in birds is a useful intra vitam technique for morphologic and functional cardiac assessment.[44] Usually, an echocardiographic investigation is performed after a radiographic examination has revealed a suspicion of heart disease. Echocardiography allows for the depiction of cardiac structures in motion and detailed imaging of its internal structures.[17] A further advantage of echocardiography in comparison to the other imaging methods is the ability to hold the patient in an upright position during the examination. Therefore, at present, it is considered to be the superior imaging modality to assess cardiovascular diseases compared with conventional radiography.

Technique

As birds have a significantly higher heart rate than mammals of the same weight, some authors recommend performing the examination under anesthesia. Examination while awake or under sedation only is particularly advisable for severely ill animals for which general anesthesia is associated with a higher risk. Due to anatomic peculiarities, the established method of choice in birds is the B-mode method (2D echocardiography) and reference values are already available for various species; see **Table 4**.

To assess the avian heart, 2 coupling sides are described:[44]

- The *ventromedian approach*: 2 horizontal longitudinal views present the chambers, the interventricular septum and the valves of the heart (**Fig. 4**)
- The *parasternal approach* - useable in birds with enough space between the last rib and the pelvic bones: the heart is shown in semitransverse views which may be helpful for the examination of the valves and the vessels.

Morphology

Using B Mode echocardiography the size of the chambers, the relation of both ventricles, the wall thickness of the interventricular septum, and the contractility of the ventricles can be assessed subjectively and by taking measurements, as well as the morphology and the function of the left AV valves, the aortic valves and the right muscular AV valve.[44]

The most frequent pathologic findings involving the avian heart through echocardiography are pericardial effusion and hypertrophy or dilatation of the right ventricle (**Fig. 5A**). The latter 2 changes are often associated with right-sided cardiac insufficiency. In such cases, the right ventricle can appear almost as large as the left, with

Table 4
Reference values measured and calculated values for pet bird species, in comparison with birds of prey and pigeons (adapted from Krautwald-Junghanns et al, 2011 [17]; with permission)

		Psittacus Erithacus	Amazona spp.	Cacatua spp.	Diurnal Birds of Prey[a]	Columbiformes Parasternal Approach
			Ventromedian Approach			
Body weight [g]		433 ± 55	353 ± 42	426 ± 162	720 ± 197	434 ± 52
left ventricle	Systolic length [mm]	22.5 ± 1.9	21.1 ± 2.3	19.0 ± 1.3	14.7 ± 2.8	17.9 ± 1.0
	Diastolic length [mm]	24.0 ± 1.9	22.1 ± 2.2	19.9 ± 1.6	16.4 ± 2.7	20.1 ± 1.4
	Systolic width [mm]	6.8 ± 1.0	6.7 ± 1.2	6.4 ± 1.7	6.3 ± 1.1	5.2 ± 0.4
	Diastolic width [mm]	8.6 ± 1.0	8.4 ± 1.0	8.3 ± 1.5	7.7 ± 1.2	7.4 ± 0.6
	Fractional shortening [%]	22.6 ± 4.4	22.8 ± 4.2	25.6 ± 7.0	n/k	27.2 ± 4.5
right ventricle	Systolic length [mm]	9.2 ± 1.4	9.4 ± 1.8	10.3 ± 1.2	12.7 ± 2.7	n/k
	Diastolic length [mm]	11.5 ± 1.9	10.3 ± 1.3	11.3 ± 2.3	13.9 ± 2.5	9.9 ± 0.8
	Systolic width [mm]	2.8 ± 0.9	3.1 ± 0.7	2.3 ± 0.0	2.1 ± 0.6	n/k
	Diastolic width [mm]	4.8 ± 1.1	5.2 ± 1.3	3.5 ± 0.5	2.5 ± 0.8	4.0 ± 0.5
	Fractional shortening [%]	40.8 ± 11.9	34.1 ± 3.7	33.3 ± 10.3	n/k	n/k
Inter-ventricular septum	Systolic thickness [mm]	2.9 ± 0.5	2.2 ± 0.1	1.9 ± 0.3	1.9 ± 0.6	3.8 ± 0.1
	Diastolic thickness [mm]	2.5 ± 0.3	2.1 ± 0.4	1.7 ± 0.4	1.9 ± 0.5	3.3 ± 0.2
Reference		Pees M et al,[51] 2004	Pees M et al,[51] 2004	Pees M et al,[51] 2004	Boskovic M et al,[75] 1999	Schulz M,[76] 1995

Values are reported as mean ± standard deviation. n/k: not known.
[a] Accipitriformes, Falconiformes, Strigiformes

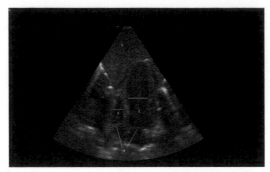

Fig. 4. B- Mode echocardiographic image of an avian heart using the ventromedian approach, presenting the chambers (1 right ventricle, 2 left ventricles), the interventricular septum, and the atrioventricular valves (4) of the heart. In addition, parts of the liver parenchyma (3) can be visualized.

the ventricular walls being thickened. Hypertrophy of the right ventricle is usually associated with hypertrophy of the right muscular AV valve.

Alterations of the left ventricle are seen less frequently, they may be associated with thickened AV valves indicating valvular damage and insufficiency.[44] The valves are echogenic and easily differentiated; therefore, valvular disease is relatively easy to diagnose. Left ventricular abnormalities are commonly combined with pathologies of the right side of the heart (**Fig. 5**A) and congestion in the pulmonary circulation. Hypertrophy of the right muscular AV valve is usually associated with hypertrophy of the right ventricle.[44]

Signs of congestion (coelomic effusion, hydropericardium, hepatic venous congestion) can as well be easily recognized.[43,44,49]

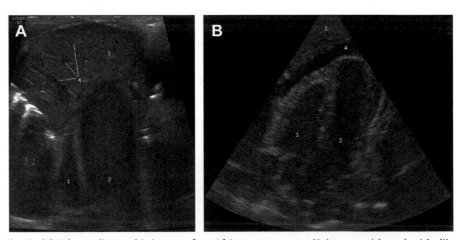

Fig. 5. (B) Echocardiographic image of an African gray parrot (*Psittacus erithacus*) with dilatation of the right ventricle (1) and a normal-sized left ventricle (2) and pericardial effusion (4). In addition, parts of the liver parenchyma (3) can be seen. (A) Echocardiographic image of an African gray parrot (*Psittacus erithacus*) with dilatation of the right (1) and the left ventricle (2) (far less common pathologic finding) and venous congestion of the vessels (4) within the liver (3).

In birds with hydropericardium there is an anechoic region around the heart clearly visible on the sonogram (see **Fig. 5B**). Usually, the pericardium itself is visible as an outer boundary; especially if coelomic effusion is also present. The apex of the heart is movable due to the surrounding fluid, and this can be assessed during the examination. In individual cases, it may be valuable to perform a needle aspirate of the pericardium under ultrasonographic guidance. Furthermore, echocardiography is well suited for determining the degree of success in treating hydropericardium or controlling the contractility of the ventricle once the patient has been administered medication. In cases involving pericarditis, (e. g. infections, gout), the pericardium will be hyperechoic; the assessment is, however, difficult.[14]

Measurements

As mentioned above, subjective assessments of the heart should be combined with measurements (**Table 4**). Interpretation of the results should always be in accordance with each other, as the heart structures are comparably delicate and physiologic differences between individual birds and species occur. It should also be noted, that the technique and method used for the examination may have an influence on the results, as well as the examiners' experience.

The body weight and external palpable length of the sternum may be related to the measurements of the size of the bird. More precise results will be gained using an electrocardiogram additionally so that heart can be investigated in the end-systolic or end-diastolic phase.[50]

The following parameters are important for evaluating the heart's morphology and function: size of the ventricles, thickness of the interventricular septum, contractility of the ventricles Furthermore, the left AV valves, the aortic valves, and the muscular right AV valve can be examined independently of the image quality. The diameter of the aortic root can be assessed, as well as the blood outflow velocity (see later in discussion).

According to Krautwald-Junghanns et al. (1995)[50] measurements in the 2D pictures are performed using the inner edge method. In addition to size, the ventricular contractility (fractional shortening) of the transverse diameter of the left ventricle is a valuable parameter for the assessment of its efficiency.[51] It is calculated using the following formula:

Fractional shortening (%) = (diastolic diameter – systolic diameter) x 100/diastolic value.

Summarizing, with echocardiography, morphologic changes of the epi-, myo-, endo-, and pericardium can be imaged along with valvular dysfunction. Still, reference values of the size and contractility of the heart are available for relatively few avian species.[50,51]

Vessels

The use of echocardiography to image blood vessel walls in birds has not yet been scientifically investigated. Clinical examination of blood vessel walls has shown that the assessment of the aorta close to the heart is possible and that hyperechoic areas indicate the presence of calcification within the vessel wall. However, the examination of vascular disease using echocardiography is very subjective and requires an experienced examiner.

DOPPLER ULTRASONOGRAPHY
Color Doppler

The color Doppler function has been successfully used in different bird species and proved to be a valuable tool in the diagnosis of aneurysms and valve insufficiency.[16,19]

However, the color Doppler function significantly reduces the frame rate; therefore, its applicability in avian echocardiography is demanding. It's use for assessing blood flow in the region of the heart valves is technically possible; but the results strongly depend on the examiners' experience. In the diagnosis of avian cardiovascular diseases, it is primarily used to find a suitable gate for the analysis by means of spectral Doppler.[14,17]

Spectral Doppler

Spectral Doppler ultrasonography is used for assessing the velocity of the blood flow, for this approach the ventromedian coupling side should be used.[44] The spectral Doppler function is used to determine the rate of blood flow (inflow, outflow), which is shown in a 2D curve against time.

In most species, it is possible to visualize the diastolic blood flow at the left and the right AV valves and therefore get values for the inflow in the right and the left ventricles, as well as the systolic outflow in the aorta (**Figure 6**).[52] For these measurements, reference values are available for some psittacine and raptor species.[2,14,52–55]

Again, due to stress-induced bias (increased heart rate and cardiac outflow), the examination is recommended to be conducted under isoflurane anesthesia.[44]

Two methods are available for the spectral Doppler examination:

When examining with the *Pulsed Wave Doppler* (PW Doppler), the speed of sound is limited to 2m/s, but the examiner can select a specific "gate" for the examination.

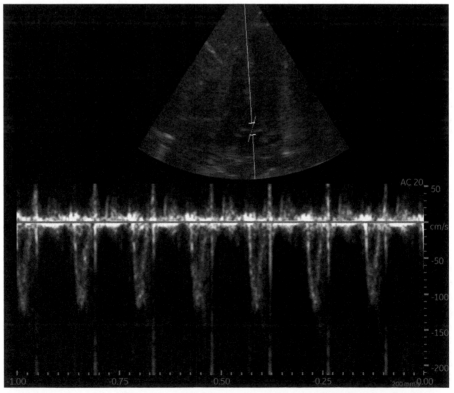

Fig. 6. Measurement of the aortic blood flow velocity of an African gray parrot (*Psittacus erithacus*) using spectral Doppler ultrasonography, with increased outflow rates (>1m/s).

Clinical reports on measurements of diastolic inflow and systolic outflow into the aorta exist,[53,54,56] reference values for psittacine species can be found in **Table 5**. When using *Continuous Wave Doppler* (CW Doppler), it is no longer possible to measure the blood flow velocities from a certain point, which is why there are only single case reports on their use in birds.[49]

In the authors' experience measurement of the blood velocity in the aortic root (see **Table 5**) can provide useful information on possible atherosclerotic changes, as the wall alterations result in smaller vessel diameter and therefore increase the blood flow. Values above 1.5 m/s are often found in birds suspicious of atherosclerotic vessels.[57]

Tissue Doppler Imaging

Recently tissue Doppler imaging was used, to quantify myocardial velocities by measuring the longitudinal peak velocities in the systole and diastole in awake racing pigeons.[58] Still, technical difficulties and individual variabilities seem to be currently a big limitation for the use of this technique to diagnose cardiovascular diseases.[58] However, applying this method in avian medicine provides additional information on the physiology of the heart and may have the opportunity to help diagnose ante-mortem cardiovascular diseases in future.

Computed Tomography and Computed Tomography Angiography

(For further details on computed tomography of the cardiovascular system see article 9. "A Spectral-CT contrast study: demonstration of the avia cardiovascular anatomy and function" in this issue).

Compared with radiography, computed tomography enables better identification of the cardiovascular system without interference from the overlaying structures.[59] Also, CT examination provides an excellent assessment of all major arteries[60]; especially when intravascular contrast media are used.[45,61,62] Likewise, the 4 distinct chambers of the heart can be visualized using intravascular contrast media.[60]

Another great advantage of computed tomography is that the examination time can be kept short with modern devices, reducing the stress on the patient.

The limits to imaging structures are dependent on the spatial resolution of the CT scanners, differences in density between the object of interest, surrounding structures, and size of the object. Further, motion artifacts due to the rapid heart rate of birds, possibly decreasing the accuracy of the diameter measurements have to be taken into count, as well as there are severe limitations for small bird species in the visualization of the smaller arteries (carotid arteries cranially, mesentery carter, branches of the brachial arteries and the abdominal aorta).[61]

For some psittacine species, window dependent protocols for computed tomography angiography (CTA) and reference limits for apparent luminal arterial diameters and ratios are available.[61,63,64] However, more recent studies found disagreements of the luminal arterial diameters when comparing 3 different CTA protocols,[63] limiting the diagnostic power with the existing protocols and current available technical possibilities.

Nevertheless, computed tomographic examinations with or without the use of contrast media can be used to diagnose obvious mineralization of major arteries (**Figure 7**) pericardial effusion (**Figure 8**), cardiomegaly, ventricular dilatation, pulmonary edema, coelomic effusion, and in some cases also ischemic or hemorrhagic infarcts in the brain.[45,65,66]

In future, modern CT technology, contrast agents, and imaging processing software may prove to be invaluable in assessing arterial luminal stenosis, aneurysm, dilatation

Table 5
Reference values on blood flow velocities in the ventricles, and the aortic root of selected pet bird species.

	Amazona Ventralis	Amazona Aestiva	Psittacus Erithacus	Cacatua Galerita	Ara spp.
Diastolic blood flow in the left ventricle (m/s)	0.17 ± 0.02	0.18 ± 0.03	0.39 ± 0.06	0.32 ± 0.15	0.54 ± 0.07
Diastolic blood flow in the right ventricle (m/s)	0.22 ± 0.05	0.22 ± 0.04			
Systolic outflow of the aorta (m/s)	0.84 ± 0.07	0.83 ± 0.08	0.89 ± 0.13	0.78 ± 0.19	0.81 ± 0.16
References	Pees M et al,[52] 2005	Pees M et al,[52] 2005	Carrani F et al,[55] 2003	Carrani F et al,[55] 2003	Carrani F et al,[55] 2003

Examinations were performed under Isoflurane anesthesia. Values are reported as mean ± standard deviation

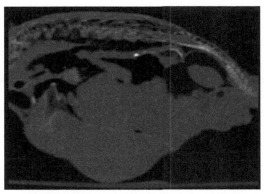

Fig. 7. Sagittal CT of an African gray parrot (*Psittacus erithacus*), in a modified bony window, head points to the left. The ventral wall of the abdominal aorta is mineralized. (*From* Dr. Michaela Gumpenberger, Diagnostic Imaging, Vetmeduni Vienna, with permission).

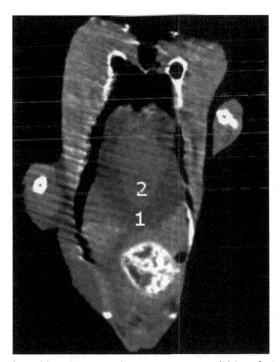

Fig. 8. Coronal CT of a red-lored Amazon (*Amazona autumnalis*) in soft tissue window, head points to the top. A broad hypodense rim (1) is surrounding the heart (2), pushing the liver to caudally and widening the cardio-hepatic waist. The pericardial effusion could be decreased successfully under sonographic control. (*From* Dr. Michaela Gumpenberger, Diagnostic Imaging, Vetmeduni Vienna, with permission).

of the arteries, and calcification of the walls in clinical settings.[45,62] Therefore, further study of CTA and protocols a warranted to become diagnostically useful in cases of cardiovascular diseases.

Magnetic Resonance Imaging

In general, magnetic resonance imaging (MRI) is relatively rarely used in clinical avian medicine, there are 2 main reasons: One is the long scanning time, which is a significant concern for the anesthesiologist who has limited access to the patient. The other reason is the small size of the structures to be imaged and motion artifacts due to rapid respiratory rate and heart rates, which makes it difficult to achieve images of diagnostic quality.

Motion artifacts prevent adequate imaging of the avian heart using MRI and it is also not recommended for the vascular system because of the fast circulation of the contrast media.[45] In addition, there is little empirical data available for avian MRI cardiac image assessment.

Nevertheless, MRI has proven its diagnostic value in cases of cerebral infarction, and hemorrhage secondary to a ruptured midbrain aneurysm, in larger psittacine species (*Ara ararauna, Psittacus erithacus*).[65,66]

Endoscopy

Endoscopy allows direct visualization and detection of gross abnormalities, such as cardiomegaly, pericardial effusion, pericardial thickening, or exudate, arterial discoloration, gross structural changes, neighboring masses, or granulomas.[9] Standard lateral approaches can be used to visualize the abdominal organs and arteries.[67] The more uncommon interclavicular approach[67] allows direct visualization of the great arteries and the base of the heart but is more invasive and may be impaired by fat deposits in overweight birds.[45] Endoscopic examination and guided sampling can be especially valuable in the diagnosis of masses associated with the heart or the major vessels.[68]

CLINICS CARE POINTS

- Frequently described cardiovascular lesions in pet birds are atherosclerosis, pericardial effusions, pericarditis, myocarditis, dilatation or hypertrophy of the ventricles, and valvular endocarditis
- Relative predisposition to cardiovascular diseases, given the species, breed, age, gender, lifestyle, and diet
- Atherosclerosis seems to be most prevalent in female African gray parrots, Amazon parrots, and cockatiels of older age (up to 20 years), on high-fat diets and limited physical activity
- Clinical symptoms are rather unspecific
- Changes in hematology and plasma lipid levels can give a hint on cardiovascular diseases, but won't make a definite diagnosis
- Diagnostic imaging is extremely important when evaluating the avian cardiovascular tract
- Whenever clinical or radiographic examination has revealed a suspicion of heart disease echocardiography should be applied
- Echocardiography allows to evaluate the heart's internal structure and the function
- Advanced imaging methods, especially CT-angiography may be helpful to diagnose arterial luminal stenosis/dilatation, aneurysm, or infarcts; still further improvement on technology and application protocols is warranted
- An overview of diagnostic options is summarized in **Table 6**.

Table 6
Summarizing diagnostic options

Procedure	Described Pathologies	Limitations
Auscultation	Heart murmurs	Due to the rapid heart rate individual beats are not or only hardly differentiable[15]
Pulse palpation	Pulse deficiencies/irregularities	In small and incorporative birds not always applicable
Hematology	Leukocytosis with a left shift, toxic changes of heterophiles – in cases of bacterial endocarditis[7] Leukocytosis, heterophily or lymphopenia in accordance with atherosclerotic lesions[14,19]	No specific diagnostic value in case of cardiovascular diseases
Plasma lipid levels	High total cholesterol and HDL levels can be found in species with higher prevalence of atherosclerosis[9]	Only limited numbers of reference values are available No validated lipoprotein tests for clinical practice[77] Plasma lipid profiles differ throughout the year[78] Until now, no conclusions can be drawn for individual measurements, in individual birds
Blood pressure measurements	May be useful to detect chronic hypertension[29] and therapeutic progress	Strong bias between invasive and noninvasive methods[24,25]; even within noninvasive methods between different cuff placement sides[25] Single measurements of an individual bird should be interpreted with cautions, repeated measurements are more valuable
Electrocardiography	Detection of arrhythmias, conduction disorders[30] Changes in P waves and/or QRS complex can suggest the enlargement of the cardiac chambers[33]	Poor patient compliance, anesthesia in most cases necessary A normal ECG does not rule out cardiac diseases ECG in an awake bird is always comparable to an exercise ECG[34]
Radiography	Changes in heart size, position, shape, and increased radiopacity of the vessels[15] Secondary organ changes (congestion of the liver and/or the lungs, coelomic effusions)[15,43]	Pathologies of the heart or the vessels must be pronounced in other to be visible on radiographs Two-dimensional view only

(continued on next page)

Table 6
(continued)

Procedure	Described Pathologies	Limitations
Angiocardiography	Arterial luminal stenosis, dilatations, and aneurysms[14,17,46]	Advanced imaging modalities must be available, anesthesia always necessary
Echocardiography	Morphologic changes[44] • Dilatation of the ventricles • Thickening of the ventricle walls • Thickening of the interventricular septum • Pathologies of the valves Signs of congestion: hydropericardium; hepatic venous congestion or coelomic effusion[44,49] Doppler ultrasonography: Changes in systolic and diastolic blood flow of the ventricles and the aortic root[14,16,17] Increased aortic systolic blood flow in bird suspicious for atherosclerotic lesions[57]	Not always applicable in small parrot species Anesthesia recommended
CT	Obvious mineralization of major arteries, cardiomegaly, ventricular dilatation, pulmonary edema, coelomic effusion, and in some cases also ischemic or hemorrhagic infarcts in the brain [62,65,66]	Technical limitations on assessing and measuring definitely luminal arterial diameters
MRT	Cerebral infarction and hemorrhage[65,66]	Rarely used (long scanning time, motion artifacts, noisy)
Endoscopy	Detection of gross abnormalities[9] and diagnosis of masses associated with the heart or the major vessels[68]	Invasive technique

DISCLOSURE

The authors have nothing to disclose.

REFERENCES

1. Fitzgerald BC, Dias S, Martorell J. Cardiovascular Drugs in Avian, Small Mammal, and Reptile Medicine. Vet Clin North Am Exot Anim Pract 2018;21(2):399–442.
2. Krautwald-Junghanns M-E, Braun S, Pees M, et al. Research on the Anatomy and Pathology of the Psittacine Heart. J Avian Med Surg 2004;18(1):2–11.
3. Lemon MJ, Pack L, Forzán MJ. Valvular endocarditis and septic thrombosis associated with a radial fracture in a red-tailed hawk (*Buteo jamaicensis*). Can Vet J 2012;53(1):79–82.
4. Huynh M, Carnaccini S, Driggers T, et al. Ulcerative dermatitis and valvular endocarditis associated with Staphylococcus aureus in a hyacinth macaw (*Anadorhynchus hyacinthinus*). Avian Dis 2014;58(2):223–7.
5. Oglesbee BL, Oglesbee MJ. Results of postmortem examination of psittacine birds with cardiac disease: 26 cases (1991-1995). J Am Vet Med Assoc 1998; 212(11):1737–42.
6. Kagohara A, Santos Md, Marinho JPM, et al. Myxomatous degeneration of the left atrioventricular valve in a true parrot (*Amazona aestiva*): a case report. Braz J Vet Med 2020;42(1).
7. Steinagel A, Quesenberry K, Donovan T. Vegetative Endocarditis due to Staphylococcus aureus in an Umbrella Cockatoo (*Cacatua alba*). J Avian Med Surg 2019;33(4):419–26.
8. Carvalho M de, Cunha M, Knöbl T, et al. Cardiac disease in the Spix Macaw (*Cyanopsitta spixii*): two cases. Aust Vet J 2021;0:1–6.
9. Fitzgerald BC, Beaufrère H. Cardiology. In: Speer BL, editor. Current therapy in avian medicine and surgery. 1st edition. Oakley: Elsevier; 2016. p. 252–328.
10. Beaufrère H, Ammersbach M, Reavill DR, et al. Prevalence of and risk factors associated with atherosclerosis in psittacine birds. J Am Vet Med Assoc 2013; 242(12):1696–704.
11. Beaufrère H, Reavill D, Heatley J, et al. Lipid-Related Lesions in Quaker Parrots (*Myiopsitta monachus*). Vet Pathol 2019;56(2):282–8.
12. Gustavsen KA, Stanhope KL, Lin AS, et al. Effects of exercise on the plasma lipid profile in Hispaniolan Amazon Parrots (*Amazona ventralis*) with naturally occurring hypercholesterolemia. J Zoo Wildl Med 2016;47(3):760–9.
13. Johnson JH, Phalen DN, Kondik VH, et al. Atherosclerosis in psittacine birds. Proceedings of the 13th Annual Conference of the association of avian Veterinarians. September 1-5, 1992; New Orleans, Louisiana: p. 87-93.
14. Pees M, Krautwald-Junghanns M-E, Straub J. Evaluating and treating the cardiovascular system. In: Harrison GJ, Lightfood TL, editors. Clinical avian medicine. 1st edition. Palm Beach: Spix Pub; 2006. p. 379–94.
15. Krautwald-Junghanns M-E, Schroff S, Bartels T. Radiographic investigation. In: Krautwald-Junghanns M-E, Pees M, Reese S, et al, editors. Diagnosting imaging of exotic pets. 1st edition. Hannover: Schlütersche; 2011. p. 84–91.
16. Rosenthal K, Miller M, Orosz S, et al. Cardiovascular system. In: Altman RB, Clubb SL, Dorrestein GM, editors. Avian medicine and surgery. 1st edition. Philadelphia: W.B. Saunders Company; 1997. p. 489–500.
17. Krautwald-Junghanns M-E, Kummerfeld N. Erkrankungen des Herzens und der großen Blutgefäße. In: Kaleta EF, Krautwald-Junghanns M-E, editors.

Kompendium der Ziervogelkrankheiten: Papageien - Tauben - Sperlingsvögel. 4th edition. Hannover: Schlütersche; 2011. p. 167–78.

18. Pees M, Krautwald-Junghanns M-E. Cardiovascular physiology and diseases of pet birds. Vet Clin North Am Exot Anim Pract 2009;12(1):81–97.

19. Vink-Nooteboom M, Schoemaker NJ, Kik MJ, et al. Clinical diagnosis of aneurysm of the right coronary artery in a white cockatoo (Cacatua alba). J Small Anim Pract 1998;39(11):533–7.

20. Beaufrère H, Vet M, Cray C, et al. Association of plasma lipid levels with atherosclerosis prevalence in psittaciformes. J Avian Med Surg 2014;28(3):225–31.

21. Beaufrère H, Gardhouse S, Ammersbach M. Lipoprotein characterization in Quaker parrots (Myiopsitta monachus) using gel-permeation high-performance liquid chromatography. Vet Clin Pathol 2020;49(3):417–27.

22. Lichtenberger M. Determination of Indirect Blood Pressure in the Companion Bird. Semin Avian Exot Pet Med 2005;14(2):149–52.

23. Schauer S. Klinische Evaluierung von zwei nichtinvasiven Klinische Evaluierung von zwei nichtinvasiven Methoden zur Blutdruckmessung bei Papageien. [PhD thesis]. München, Germany: Ludwig Maximilian University of Munich; 2015.

24. Acierno MJ, da Cunha A, Smith J, et al. Agreement between direct and indirect blood pressure measurements obtained from anesthetized Hispaniolan Amazon parrots. J Am Vet Med Assoc 2008;233(10):1587–90.

25. Johnston MS, Davidowski LA, Rao S, et al. Precision of repeated, Doppler-derived indirect blood pressure measurements in conscious psittacine birds. J Avian Med Surg 2011;25(2):83–90.

26. Zehnder AM, Hawkins MG, Pascoe PJ, et al. Evaluation of indirect blood pressure monitoring in awake and anesthetized red-tailed hawks (Buteo jamaicensis): effects of cuff size, cuff placement, and monitoring equipment. Vet Anaesth Analg 2009;36(5):464–79.

27. Lichtenberger M, Ko J. Critical care monitoring. Vet Clin North Am Exot Anim Pract 2007;10(2):317–44.

28. Lichtenberger M. Emergency approach to hypotension and acute respiratory distress. Proceedings of the 27th Annual Conference of the Association of Avian Veterinarians. San Antonio, Texas; August 6-10, 2006.

29. Beaufrère H. Avian Atherosclerosis: Parrots and Beyond. J Exot Pet Med 2013;22(4):336–47.

30. Lumeji JT, Ritchie BW. Cardiology. In: Ritchie BW, Harrison GJ, Harrison L, editors. Avian medicine: Principles and application. 1st edition. Florida: Wingers Publishing Inc; 1994. p. 695–722.

31. Pees M, Straub J, Krautwald-Junghanns M-E. Echokardiographische Untersuchungen bei Psittaciformes. Tierarztl Prax Ausg K 2003;31(03):180–7.

32. Hagner D, Prehn H, Krautwald-Junghanns M-E. ECG-leads and trigger pulse generation for echocardiography in unanaesthetized birds. Proceedings of the 3rd Annual Conference of the European Association of Avian Veterinarians, Jerusalem, 1995, p. 189-194.

33. Zandvliet MMJM. Electrocardiography in psittacine birds and ferrets. Semin Avian Exot Pet Med 2005;14(1):34–51.

34. Kummerfeld N. Elektrokardiographie. In: Kaleta EF, Krautwald-Junghanns M-E, editors. Kompendium der Ziervogelkrankheiten: Papageien - Tauben - Sperlingsvögel. 4th edition. Hannover: Schlütersche; 2011. p. 68–70.

35. Papahn AA, Naddaf H, Rezakhani A, et al. Electrocardiogram of Homing Pigeon. J Appl Anim Res 2006;30(2):129–32.

36. Nap AM, Lumeij JT, Stokhof AA. Electrocardiogram of the African grey (*Psittacus erithacus*) and Amazon (*Amazona* spp.) parrot. Avian Pathol 1992;21(1):45–53.
37. Musulin SE, Adin DB. ECG of the Month. Sinus arrhythmia in an African grey parrot. J Am Vet Med Assoc 2006;229(4):505–7.
38. Casares M, Enders F, Montoya JA. Comparative electrocardiography in four species of macaws (genera *Anodorhynchus* and *Ara*). J Vet Med A Physiol Pathol Clin Med 2000;47(5):277–81.
39. Oglesbee BL, Hamlin RL, Klingaman H, et al. Electrocardiographic Reference Values for Macaws (*Ara* species) and Cockatoos (*Cacatua* species). J Avian Med Surg 2001;15(1):17–22.
40. Espino L, Suárez ML, López-Beceiro A, et al. Electrocardiogram reference values for the buzzard in Spain. J Wildl Dis 2001;37(4):680–5.
41. Talavera J, Guzmán MJ, del Palacio MJF, et al. The normal electrocardiogram of four species of conscious raptors. Res Vet Sci 2008;84(1):119–25.
42. Hassanpour H, Moghaddam AKZ, Bashi MC. The normal electrocardiogram of conscious golden eagles (*Aquila chrysaetos*). J Zoo Wildl Med 2010;41(3): 426–31.
43. Krautwald-Junghanns M-E, Pees M, Schroff S. Cardiovascular System. In: Krautwald-Junghanns M-E, Pees M, Reese S, et al, editors. Diagnostic Imaging of exotic pets. Hannover, Germany: Schlütersche Verlagsgesellschaft GmbH & Co.; 2011. p. 84–91.
44. Pees M, Krautwald-Junghanns M E. Avian echocardiography. Semin Avian Exot Pet Med 2005;14(1):14–21.
45. Beaufrère H, Pariaut R, Rodriguez D, et al. Avian vascular imaging: a review. J Avian Med Surg 2010;24(3):174–84.
46. Cowan M, Monks D, Miles S. Diagnosis of cardiac disease in avian species. Proceedings of the 20th AAVAC Annual Conference. Melbourne, Australia. 2012. p. 21-33.
47. Phalen DN, Hays HB, Filippich I J, et al. Heart failure in a macaw with atherosclerosis of the aorta and brachiocephalic arteries. J Am Vet Med Assoc 1996;209(8): 1435–40.
48. Brandão J, Reynolds CA, Beaufrère H, et al. Cardiomyopathy in a Harris hawk (*Parabuteo unicinctus*). J Am Vet Med Assoc 2016;249(2):221–7.
49. Sedacca CD, Campbell TW, Bright JM, et al. Chronic cor pulmonale secondary to pulmonary atherosclerosis in an African Grey parrot. J Am Vet Med Assoc 2009; 234(8):1055–9.
50. Krautwald-Junghanns ME, Schulz M, Hagner D, et al. Transcoelomic two-dimensional echocardiography in the avian patient. J Avian Med Surg 1995;(9): 19–31.
51. Pees M, Straub J, Krautwald-Junghanns M-E. Echocardiographic examinations of 60 African grey parrots and 30 other psittacine birds. Vet Rec 2004; 155(3):73–6.
52. Pees M, Straub J, Schumacher J, et al. [Pilot study for normal color-flow and pulsed-wave spectral Doppler echocardiography in Hispanolian amazons (*Amazona ventralis*) and blue-fronted amazons (*Amazona a. aestiva*)]. Dtsch Tierarztl Wochenschrift 2005;112:39–43.
53. Straub J, Forbes NA, Pees M, et al. Pulsed-wave Doppler-derived velocity of diastolic ventricular inflow and systolic aortic outflow in raptors. Vet Rec 2004;154(5): 145–7.
54. Straub J, Forbes NA, Thielebein J, et al. Pulsed-wave Doppler echocardiography in birds of prey. Vet Rec 2003;153(24):742–6.

55. Carrani F, Gelli D, Salvadori M, Aloisi M., ed. A preliminary echocardiographic initial approach A preliminary echocardiographic initial approach to diastolic and systolic function in medium and large parrots. Proceedings of the Annual Conference of the European Association of Avian Veterinarians; Puerto de la Cruz, Spain; 2003.
56. Straub J, Forbes NA, Thielebein J, et al. The effects of isoflurane anaesthesia on some Doppler-derived cardiac parameters in the common buzzard (*Buteo buteo*). Vet J 2003;166(3):273–6.
57. Schulz Ulrike. *Möglichkeiten der intra vitam Diagnostik und Therapie bei Kongograupapageien (Psittacus erithacus erithacus) mit Verdacht auf Atherosklerose.* [PhD thesis]. Leipzig, Germany: University of Leipzig; 2021.
58. Legler M, Koy L, Kummerfeld N, et al. Diastolic and systolic longitudinal myocardial velocities of healthy racing pigeons (*Columba livia* f. domestica) measured by tissue Doppler imaging. Vet Sci 2021;8(2).
59. Dos Santos GJ, da Silva JP, Hippólito AG, et al. Computed tomographic and radiographic morphometric study of cardiac and coelomic dimensions in captive blue-fronted Amazon parrots (*Amazona aestiva*, Linnaeus, 1758) with varying body condition scores. Anat Histol Embryol 2020;49(2):299–306.
60. Veladiano IA, Banzato T, Bellini L, et al. Normal computed tomographic features and reference values for the coelomic cavity in pet parrots. BMC Vet Res 2016; 12(1):182.
61. Beaufrère H, Rodriguez D, Pariaut R, et al. Estimation of intrathoracic arterial diameter by means of computed tomographic angiography in Hispaniolan Amazon parrots. Am J Vet Res 2011;72(2):210–8.
62. Echols Scott, Krautwald-Junghanns M.-E., Pees M. Computed Tomography: In: Krautwald-Junghanns M-E, Pees M, Reese S, Tully T,editors. Diagnostic Imaging of exotic pets. 2nd ed. Schlütersche Verlagsgesellschaft GmbH & Co.; in print.
63. Yu PH, Lee YL, Chen CL, et al. Comparison of three computed tomographic angiography protocols to assess diameters of major arteries in African grey parrots (*Psittacus erithacus*). Am J Vet Res 2018;79(1):42–53.
64. Lee Y-L, Yu P-H, Chen C-L, et al. Determination of the enhancement effect and diameters of the major arteries of African grey parrots using a dual-head power injector for computed tomographic angiography. Taiwan Vet J 2015;41(03): 165–75.
65. Beaufrère H, Nevarez J, Gaschen L, et al. Diagnosis of presumed acute ischemic stroke and associated seizure management in a Congo African grey parrot. J Am Vet Med Assoc 2011;239(1):122–8.
66. Grosset C, Guzman DS-M, Keating MK, et al. Central vestibular disease in a blue and gold macaw (*Ara ararauna*) with cerebral infarction and hemorrhage. J Avian Med Surg 2014;28(2):132–42.
67. Taylor M. Endoscopic examination and biopsy techniques. In: Ritchie BW, Harrison GR, Harrison LR, editors. Avian medicine principles and application. Lake Worth, Florida: Wingers Publishing Inc; 1994. p. 327–54.
68. Hanley CS, Wilson GH, Latimer KS, et al. Interclavicular Hemangiosarcoma in a Double Yellow-headed Amazon Parrot (A*mazona ochrocephala oratrix*). J J Avian Med Surg 2005;19(2):130–7.
69. Schnellbacher RW, da Cunha AF, Beaufrère H, et al. Effects of dopamine and dobutamine on isoflurane-induced hypotension in Hispaniolan Amazon parrots (*Amazona ventralis*). Am J Vet Res 2012;73(7):952–8.

70. Curro TG, Brunson DB, Paul-Murphy J. Determination of the ED50 of isoflurane and evaluation of the isoflurane-sparing effect of butorphanol in cockatoos (*Cacatua spp.*). Vet Surg 1994;23(5):429–33.

71. Silva JP, Castiglioni MCR, Doiche DP, et al. Radiographic Measurements of the Cardiac Silhouette in Healthy Blue-Fronted Amazon Parrots (Amazona aestiva). J Avian Med Surg 2020;34(1):26–31.

72. Rettmer H, Deb A, Watson R, et al. Radiographic measurement of internal organs in Spix's macaws (*Cyanopsitta spixii*). J Avian Med Surg 2011;25(4):254–8.

73. Straub J, Pees M, Krautwald-Junghanns ME. Measurement of the cardiac silhouette in psittacines. J Am Vet Med Assoc 2002;221(1):76–9.

74. Schnitzer P, Sawmy S, Crosta L. Radiographic Measurements of the Cardiac Silhouette and Comparison with Other Radiographic Landmarks in Wild Galahs (*Eolophus roseicapilla*). Animals (Basel) 2021;11(3).

75. Boskovic M, Krautwald-Junghanns M-E, Failing K, et al. Möglichkeiten und Grenzen echokardiographischer Untersuchungen bei Tag- und Nachtgreifvögeln (Accipitriformes, Falconiformes, Strigiformes). Tierärztliche Praxis 1999;(27):334–41.

76. Schulz M. *Morphologische und funktionelle Messungen am Herzen von Brieftauben (Columba livia forma domestica) mit Hilfe der Schnittbildechokardiographie.* [PhD thesis]. Germany: Gießen; 1995.

77. Reaufrörc H. Clinical lipidology in psittacine birds. Conf Proc Exoticscon virtual 2020;11. 9-3.10.2020.

78. Jahantigh M, Zaeemi M, Razmyar J, et al. Plasma biochemical and lipid panel reference intervals in Common Mynahs (*Acridotheres tristis*). J Avian Med Surg 2019;33(1):15–21.

A Spectral Computed Tomography Contrast Study
Demonstration of the Avian Cardiovascular Anatomy and Function

Rachel Franziska Hein, MedVet[a],*, Ingmar Kiefer, DrMedVet[b],
Michael Pees, ProfDrMedVet[c]

KEYWORDS

- Vascular imaging • CT angiography • Diagnostic imaging • Computer tomography
- Avian • Bolus tracking method • Saline chaser technique

KEY POINTS

- We performed CTA using a spectral CT scanner, which enabled us to improve visualization and characterization of tissues with enhanced image quality.
- We used imaging postprocessing tools after the scan, to visualize the cardiovascular system.
- We used premedication with midazolam and medetomidin and anesthetized with inhalation anesthesia using isoflurane.
- Our CTA protocol involved IV injection of 1 to 2 mL contrast agent per kg followed by a 1 mL saline flush.
- Computed tomographic angiography promises to provide an additional diagnostic possibility for antemortem diagnosis of cardiovascular disease in birds.

INTRODUCTION
Avian Vascular Disease

Cardiovascular diseases are more common in birds than ever expected.[1–6] These diseases are especially prevalent in captive companion avian species, which show increased numbers of vascular changes and cardiac diseases because of physical inactivity, inappropriate diet, and husbandry conditions.[7–10] Retrospective studies

[a] Department for Small Mammal, Reptile and Avian Diseases, University of Veterinary Medicine Hannover, Foundation, Bünteweg 9, Hannover 30559, Germany; [b] Department for Small Animals, Veterinary Teaching Hospital, University of Leipzig, An den Tierkliniken 23, Leipzig 04103, Germany; [c] Department for Small Mammal, Reptile and Avian Diseases, University of Veterinary Medicine Hannover, Foundation, Bünteweg 9, Hannover 30559, Germany
* Corresponding author.
E-mail address: rachel.franziska.hein@tiho-hannover.de

Vet Clin Exot Anim 25 (2022) 435–451
https://doi.org/10.1016/j.cvex.2022.01.008
1094-9194/22/© 2022 Elsevier Inc. All rights reserved.

verify heart diseases as one of the leading causes of death in birds.[1,4,11] More than 36% of the examined birds in a research study by Braun and colleagues[11] (2002) showed macroscopically visible changes in the cardiovascular system, with 99% of all hearts showing histologic alterations.

Among these cardiovascular changes and alterations, atherosclerosis is a common finding in postmortem surveys.[2–5] Atherosclerosis is a chronically inflammatory, degenerative, and progressive vascular disease that is characterized by the accumulation of inflammatory cells, calcium, lipids, carbohydrates, blood and blood products, as well as elastic and collagenous fibers within the intima of affected arteries.[12–14]

Signs for cardiac insufficiency are quite general and include decreased activity, dyspnea, abdominal swelling (ascites), apathy, and unfortunately sudden death.[15] In addition, featherlessness, intermittent limping, and ataxia are described symptoms caused by stenosis of the affected arteries (providing blood and thereby oxygen for the affected area).[16–18]

Factors like age,[9,12,15] gender,[9] species,[19] plasma cholesterol and triglycerides levels,[20,21] inactivity,[22] social stress,[23] inappropriate diet and husbandry conditions,[10,24,25] obesity, and herpesvirus and/or chlamydia infections[26–28] are considered to be predisposing for the development and progression of atherosclerosis.

Atherosclerosis and its associated symptoms, such as coronary heart disease, stroke, and peripheral arterial disease, are among the leading causes of human deaths.[29] Therefore, coronary computed tomographic angiography (CTA) is recommended and in widespread use for the evaluation of (coronary) artery disease in human medicine.[30–32]

Diagnosis of Vascular Disease

The antemortem diagnosis of heart and vascular diseases can be quite challenging due to limited diagnostic methods for evaluating the living bird's heart.[33] The palpation of the pulse, as well as the auscultation of the heart, are part of the routine examination of the cardiac patient in small animals but are not transferable to birds (because of their anatomic specialties/differences such as the keel bone).[34–36]

To aid diagnosis, the following are used: physical examination, biochemistry and hematology, electrocardiography, radiography, echocardiography, angiography, and (as advanced imaging) computed tomography (CT).[37–40]

Ultrasonography is well established for visualization of the heart and the aortic root. However, it has insufficient penetration for the noninvasive imaging of vascular changes.[41–45] Moreover, some pathologic abnormalities cannot be distinguished radiographically due to superposition of anatomic structures.

Computed Tomographic Angiography in Birds

To the authors' knowledge 3 previous studies published in the last 10 years have focused on this topic. The first paper was published by Beaufrère and colleagues[46] (2011). These investigators focused on the establishment of a CTA protocol in 13 healthy amazon parrots and measured the diameter of major arteries; they used a 16-slice CT scanner and recommended the application of 3 mL contrast medium/ kg. All birds were positioned in dorsal recumbency and were anesthetized via a mask using 5% isoflurane in oxygen. To maintain anesthesia, all birds were intubated, and the isoflurane was reduced to 2% to 3%. A heating pad was placed underneath the patient, and a 24- or 26-gauge catheter was placed in the left or the right ulnar vein or the medial tarsal vein. A whole-body scan was followed by a scan in which the area was reduced from the cervical vertebra to the hip joint using the following parameters: 1.25 mm slice thickness, 1.375 pitch, 100 kVp, and 150 mA. Right after a test bolus of 1 mL iohexol/kg over 1 second, the dynamic scan took place using the same technical parameters and 3 mL/kg contrast medium administrated manually over 3 seconds, 3 seconds before CTA initiation. The investigators concluded that CTA was safe and is of diagnostic value in parrots.

The second study, published in 2015 by Lee and colleagues,[47] aimed to establish CTA. Similar to Beaufrère and colleagues (2011),[46] these investigators used a 16-slice CT scanner and examined healthy parrots too. The differences from the prior study were the use of a dual-head power injector and using the bolus tracking method. In addition, they used the contrast material at a dosage of 2 mL and a flow rate of 0.3 mL/s and a 3 mL postflush of saline. The technical parameters were 0.5 mm collimation, 3 mm section width, 0.5 s/rotation scanning speed, 1.0 pitch, 10 mm/s table feed, 120 kVp electric potential, and 50 mA electrical current. The investigators concluded that their method of CTA using a dual-head power injection as well as the bolus tracking method was practical, with a good picture quality that was of diagnostic value.

Yu and colleagues[48] published the most recent study in 2018. The investigators compared 3 different CTA protocols to assess the diameters of major arteries. Similar to the previously mentioned studies, the investigators concentrated on the examination of healthy birds. The first protocol involved a pre-contrast medium infusion - flush and a post - CMI flush of 0.2 Ml saline solution. The intravenous infusion of iopamidol was 2 mL (total volume: 5 mL). Protocol 2 involved a post - CMI (0.4 mL, total volume: 2.4mL) and protocol 3 involved a pre-CMI flush (total volume 4.8mL). All technical parameters (including the 16-slice-CT scanner) were the same as in the prior study. The investigators pronounced protocol 2 as the most reliable but noted that further technique modification is needed.

Therefore, reference values for the CT evaluation of the cardiovascular system in avian species have been established, including in African gray parrots and Hispaniolan amazon parrots. However, no studies have been performed on birds that are clinically suspicious for cardiovascular disease.

Spectral Technology

The IQon Elite Spectral CT (Philips Healthcare, Hamburg, Germany) we used is based on the first detector-based spectral technology and can provide 2 image datasets of the same region and combine conventional CT images with spectral information within the same scan[49]; this is due to the NanoPanel Prism detector, which can capture high and low photon energy at the same time, leading to improved visualization and characterization of tissues with enhanced image quality. In addition to that, every spectral dataset can be analyzed with different diagnostic tools even after the scan. Using these tools one can, for example, adapt the monoenergetic energy levels to isolate the material composition. Furthermore, Z-effective or iodine overlay images can provide additional information and therefore can be helpful for better characterization of pathologic abnormalities.

Approach

The purpose of this study was to establish an angiography protocol for single-source dual-layer CT to visualize the healthy avian cardiovascular system. Ultimately, we hope to improve the positive outcomes in the antemortem diagnosis of cardiovascular disease.

MATERIAL AND METHODS
Animals

A total of 13 birds (3 African gray parrots, 2 amazon parrots, 1 macaw, 2 chicken, 3 pigeons, 1 crow, 1 buzzard) presenting as patients at the Clinic for Birds and Reptiles in Leipzig were included in this study. The ethics committee of the veterinary faculty of the University of Leipzig had approved this study, and informed consent was obtained from every bird's owner before the examination, including education about the risks of general anesthesia.

CTA was performed on these birds as part of the cardiovascular examination and in addition to already established methods.

Clinical Examinations and Blood Analysis

The birds were screened for any disease, especially focusing on cardiovascular disease during the physical examination, radiography, and echocardiography. While performing the physical examination, we were alert to certain signs, such as bluish discoloration of the periorbital skin, abdominal distension, as well as general signs for cardiovascular failure such as dyspnea, tachypnea, cachexia, harsh lung sounds, and peripheral edema.[12,35,37] Blood samples for biochemistry and hematology evaluation were taken and included blood analysis and complete blood cell count.

Radiography and Echocardiography

Standard radiographs were taken in ventrodorsal and laterolateral positions.[35,50] To complete this, we used a particular fixation device to keep the birds in position without having to hold them. The device is made of plexiglass and is equipped with different headpieces, which must be locked in the provided retainer at the top. The hindlimbs can be fixed using shoelaces and the gadgets at the bottom of the device.

The position, size, shape, and in case of a pathologic alteration, enlargement of the cardiac or hepatic silhouette were analyzed, as well as the radiodensity of the large vessels.[50]

Echocardiography was performed while all birds were anesthetized using isoflurane. We placed the scanner on the midline immediately behind the sternum and directed the beam plane craniodorsally. The approach used is called the ventromedian approach. Using this accession, one can obtain 2 longitudinal views of the heart: the vertical view ("two-chamber-view") and the horizontal view ("four-chamber view"). In doing this, we could visualize and measure the heart and the chambers as well as the aortic root. Moreover, we looked for congestion signs like hepatomegaly or ascites and checked not only the frequency of the heart but also the blood flow in the proximal aorta. The function of the atrioventricular valves was also verified.

All measurements were compared with published reference ranges. In this publication, we focused on the patients showing no pathologic abnormalities.

Development of the Computed Tomographic Angiography Protocol

Based on the previously described protocols, we focused on reducing the contrast material volume per kg and the pitch (<1). Injection of a saline solution bolus after applying contrast material allows a 20% reduction of contrast material volume and retaining a related degree of enhancement.[51] Therefore, using this method can save the costs of contrast material. Regarding the pitch, the effective slice thickness increases with a rising pitch, resulting in diminished spatial resolution in the patient's longitudinal direction.[52] Furthermore, typical spiral artifacts on contrast leaps, such as bone edges, increase.[52] By reducing the pitch, we hoped to create more accurate visualizations of the arteries and thus be able to make significantly more accurate measurements in the future. Aside from that, we expected more precise outcomes using a spectral CT instead of a 16-slice CT. All in all, we aimed to shorten the investigation period, extend the volume coverage, and improve the spatial resolution. Furthermore, we used premedication to comfort our patients to provide as nonstressful anesthesia as possible. Considering these deliberations, we ended up performing the CTA according to the following schedule.

Computed Tomographic Angiography

Anesthesia and patient positioning

Each bird was sedated with midazolam (1 mg/kg intramuscularly [IM]) and medetomidin (2 mg/kg IM) 10 to 15 minutes before the CTA procedure. Shortly before the first scan, we placed the bird in dorsal recumbency on the (radiographic) fixation device mentioned earlier and induced anesthesia via face mask with 5% isoflurane in oxygen at an oxygen flow rate of 1 L/min. To maintain anesthesia, we reduced isoflurane down to 2.5% depending on the anesthesia depth of the bird, which was evaluated by corneal reflex, muscle tone, and respiratory frequency. A 24-gauge catheter (VasoVet, B. Braun Melsungen AG, Melsungen, Germany) was placed in the right or left ulnar vein, and an injection plug was placed at the end of the catheter. The catheter was then secured in place with adhesive tape. A tube extension was used to bridge the Y-tubing of the contrast delivery system and the IV line in the patient. To prevent the bird's body temperature to decrease to a health-damaging degree, we placed a pair of surgical gloves filled with warm water on both sides of the body. The heating pad we usually use for surgical procedures would cause irregularities in the CT and result in unusable scans. The catheter was removed after the scan was completed.

Technical Equipment

Computed tomographic scanner

Our CTA examinations were performed with the IQon Elite Spectral CT (Philips Healthcare, Hamburg, Germany). This CT scanner is based on the first detector-based spectral technology that can provide 2 image datasets of the same region while combining conventional CT images with spectral information within the same scan.[49]

Computer Editing Program/software

Cross-sectional images were generated and supplied by the program *IntelliSpace Pacs Radiology*. We created images in different window settings: pulmonary window, mediastinal window, and using IMR. IMR is the abbreviation for Iterative Model Reconstruction and is a reconstruction technique by Philips, promising to provide low-contrast resolution and noise-free images.[53]

Segmentation and volume rendering were performed using *Philips IntelliSpace Portal*.

Contrast Medium

The contrast material we used is called Imeron 300M (Bracco Imaging Deutschland GmbH, Konstanz, Germany). Imeron 300M is a water-soluble (nephrotrop) and low-osmolar injection solution; 1 mL Imeron contains 612.4 mg iomeprol, which is 300 mg iodine.

Contrast Delivery System

The Accutron CT-D double head injector (MEDTRON AG, Saarbrücken, Germany) is a double-syringe contrast delivery system used in CT scans of humans; it is characterized by a preinject function to perform a test injection, as well as the following technical data: injection volume: maximum 200 mL, number of phases: 1 to 6, injection pressure: maximum 21 bar, flow rate: 0.1 to 10 mL/s, and 0 to 255 s injection, phase, and scan delay.[54] One syringe is loaded with contrast material, and the other one with saline solution. Quick handling has been realizable via a wireless touch screen interface. With this interface, we have been able to set delay span, volume, and concentration of the contrast material, as well as flow rate and injection period. We used the following settings for the contrast material: volume, 1 mL/kg; concentration, 100%; flow rate, 0.3 mL/s; and injection period, 4 seconds. The saline solution flush was performed using the following setting: volume, 1 mL; concentration, 0%; flow rate, 0.3 mL/s; and injection period, 4 seconds. In addition, we manually applied the contrast material without needing to be close to the patient by pressing the start key on the interface.

Computed Tomography Angiography Examination

Whole-body scout helical scans were performed before the administration of contrast material in a craniocaudal direction. We used the following scanning parameters: 0.8 mm to 1 mm slice thickness, 0.391 pitch, 0.33 seconds rotation period, 120 kVp, and 30 to 281 mA. The contrast delivery system was vented, and the IV line was preflushed with saline first to ensure that it was unobstructed. While applying the contrast material a dynamic scan was performed using the same parameters and a region of interest in the cephalic artery to monitor the attenuation values. Then we used a real-time bolus tracking method and triggered the scan manually once peak enhancement was reached.

Intravenous contrast media (Imeron 300–300 mg iodine/mL, Bracco Imaging Germany) administration was limited in some cases due to the exceptional low bodyweight of our patients, but we aimed to use 1 mL contrast agent per kg. Generally, we used 1 mL of contrast material at an infusion rate of 0.3 mL/s over an injection period of 4 seconds followed by a 1 mL saline flush at 0.3 mL/s over 4 seconds.

Overall, we performed a series of 2 to 3 scans. The first one captures the first visualization of the arteries and the second one is done to be able to see the venous structures and the perfusion of the organs. (The most delayed scan assessed the whole vascular tree if not seen in the second scan).

RESULTS

CT examination was completed in all birds. There was one extravasation of contrast material or saline solution in one African gray parrot and 2 conspicuous birds (1 amazon parrot and 1 Gy parrot) that did not show an adequate amount of contrast material present in the major arteries.

In the following image series (**Figs. 1 and 2**), one can see the CTA examination of a 21-year-old, male African Gray parrot, which came to the clinic because of chronic and recently hemorrhagic feather plucking. In the radiographic examination, increased radiodensity of the large vessels close to the heart has been diagnosed. The echocardiographic examination did not reveal any pathologic abnormalities.

In the following image series (**Fig. 3**), one can see the progress of a CTA procedure using the example of the CTA examination of the common buzzard starting with a pre-contrast helical scan, followed by the first and second dynamic scan.

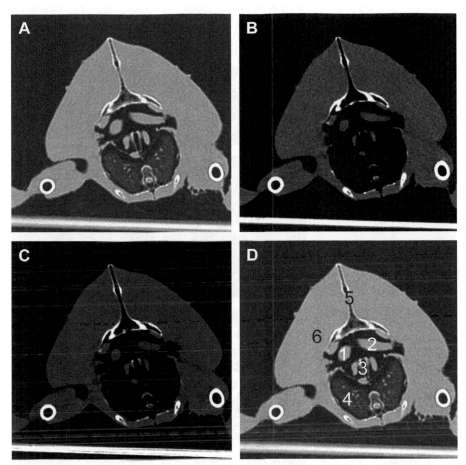

Fig. 1. Computed tomographic angiography of an African gray parrot obtained at the level of the left brachiocephalic trunk before administration of contrast material in a pulmonary window (*A*), in a mediastinal window (*B*), and using IMR (*C*). Using the following settings: 120 kVp, 129 mA, slice location: 187.67 (*D*) the following structures can be identified: (1) right brachiocephalic trunk, (2) left brachiocephalic trunk, (3) syrinx, (4) right lung, (5) carina sterni, (6) right pectoral muscle.

Image Postprocessing (Techniques)

Using segmentation and volume rendering of *Philips IntelliSpace Portal,* we have generated multiple new imaging "sequences" to enhance visualization of selected anatomy. Consequently, we reconstructed the arterial filling and visualized the contrast material-filled cardiovascular system in three dimensions. We focused on the arteries previous studies revealed as the most likely to be affected by atherosclerotic lesions, namely, the beginning of the aorta, the thoracic aorta, both pulmonary arteries, as well as both brachiocephalic trunks.[12,14,16] We tried to follow the route of those vessels as long as possible (**Figs. 4** and **5**).

After the injection of the arteries, we were able to choose just the tissue we injected and remove the overlaying tissue to create these 3D images. With adapting the tissue color, we also created colored images (**Figs. 6–8**).

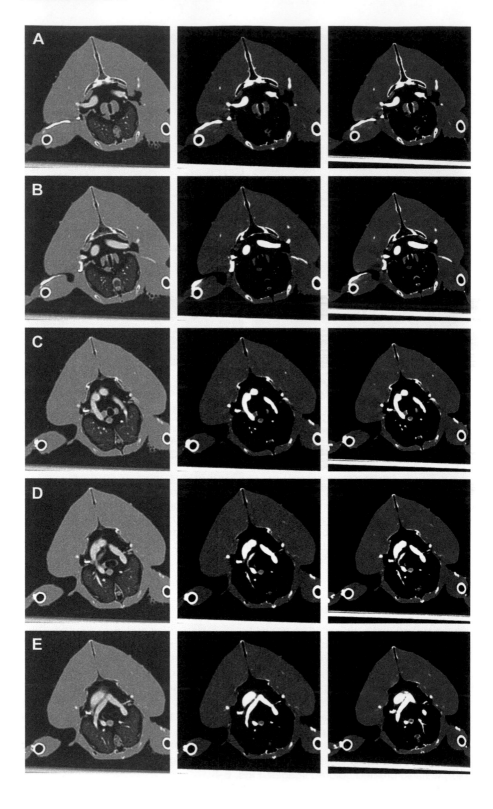

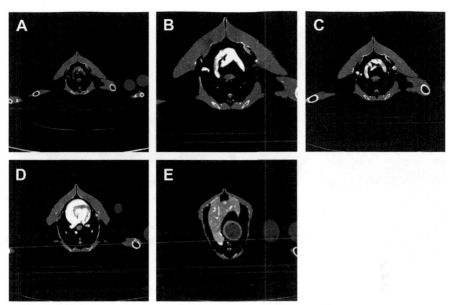

Fig. 3. Precontrast and dynamic scan of the common buzzard. (*A*) Precontrast helical scan at the level of the origin of the aorta and both pulmonary arteries. Settings: 120 kVp, 253 mA, slice location: 246.949, IMR. (*B*) First dynamic scan after the administration of 1 mL contrast material (100% concentration, 0.3 mL/s flow rate, followed by 1 mL saline solution) at the same level. Settings: 120 kVp, 281 mA, IMR. (*C*) Second scan 46 seconds after the first one at the same location. Settings: 120 kVp, 257 mA, IMR. (*D*) The filling of both cardiac ventricles. Settings: 120 kVp, 257 mA, slice location 256.449, IMR. (*E*) Notice the contrast-material-filled hepatic vessels at the second scan. Settings: 120 kVp, 257 mA, slice location: 280.949, IMR.

DISCUSSION

Cardiovascular disease in general and atherosclerosis specifically are some of the leading causes of death in birds. Atherosclerotic lesions such as plaques causing luminal stenosis can be identified using CTA. CTA is a long-established and widely used imaging method to detect those lesions in affected arteries in humans. Therefore, CTA appears to be a promising technique to enable the antemortem diagnosis of atherosclerosis in birds.

Diagnosis of cardiovascular disease from a clinical examination can be difficult. Hence, it is essential to evaluate the signalment and the general and specific medical

Fig. 2. Computed tomographic angiography of the same African gray parrot at the level of the right brachiocephalic trunk (*A*), the left brachiocephalic trunk (*B*), the ascending aorta (*C*), the left pulmonary artery (*D*), and the right pulmonary artery (*E*), after the application of the contrast material (first scan: arterial phase) in different window settings (1, pulmonary window; 2, mediastinal window; 3, IMR). (*A*) Settings: 120 kVp, 145 mA, slice location 185.77. (*B*) Settings: 120 kVp, 146 mA, slice location: 187.37. (*C*) Settings: 120 kVp, 144 mA, slice location 191.77. (*D*) Settings: 120 kVp, 145 mA, slice location 192.97. (*E*) Settings: 120 kVp, 146 mA, slice location 194.17.

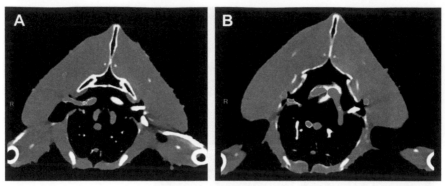

Fig. 4. Illustration of how we "filled" the arteries ((A) right brachiocephalic trunk, (B) left pulmonary artery) using *Philips IntelliSpace Portal* to create a 3D volume-rendered image. The patient was a 9-year-old female African gray parrot presented at the clinic with chronic feather plucking. Radiographic and echocardiographic examinations did not show any abnormalities.

history of every patient. Species, age, husbandry conditions, and food can indicate cardiovascular diseases.[10,12,19,24,25]

We used a single-source dual-layer CT scanner instead of a 16-slice one compared with previously described protocols. According to the SCCT [Society of Cardiovascular Computed Tomography Guidlines commitee] guidelines,[55] a 16-slice scanner is the minimum detector requirement. However, to perform a CTA, a system with at least 32 detector rows is recommended. Consequently, we expected significantly better image quality and more accurate measurements than in previous studies. Furthermore, we could decrease the slice thickness and the pitch to create higher spatial resolution.

Moreover, we used a dual-head power injector to apply the contrast material, in preference to applying it manually while sitting adjacent to the patient. The advantage of this device is not only to allow the contrast material to be followed by a saline solution flush but also to consider, and more importantly, to practice radioprotection; this is a significant advance. Moreover, removing the requirement to load one syringe with contrast material and one with saline solution for each examination is considerably less time consuming.[51]

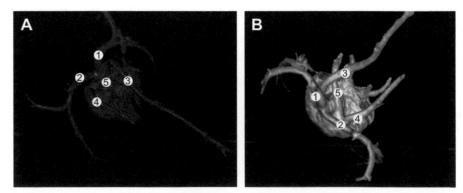

Fig. 5. 3D volume-rendered image of the same African gray parrot as in **Fig. 2**. (1) Right brachiocephalic trunk. (2) Left brachiocephalic trunk. (3) Aorta. (4) Left pulmonary artery. (5) Right pulmonary artery. With (A) and without (B) adapted tissue color.

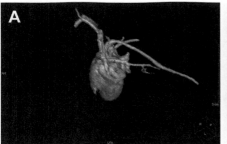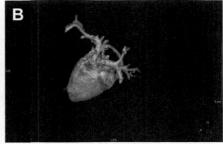

Fig. 6. 3D volume-rendered image of a 3-year-old, male Amazon parrot. Note the origin and the route of (1) the right brachiocephalic trunk, (2) the left brachiocephalic trunk, (3) the aorta, (4) the right pulmonary artery, and the (5) left pulmonary artery. With (*A*) and without (*B*) adapted tissue color.

Based on the previously described protocols by Lee and colleagues[47] (2015) and Yu and colleagues[48] (2018) we performed the CTA using the saline chaser and bolus tracking technique. The benefit of the saline chaser technique is a 20% reduction of contrast material.[51] Benefits are not limited to cost reduction and include clearing the IV catheter for contrast medium, reducing contrast material dilution through mixing with blood, and avoiding contrast material pooling in the wing vein.[51] Concerning the test bolus versus the bolus tracking technique, the advantages of the test bolus technique were a decreased risk of false starts, ensuring adequacy of the IV line, and a chance to observe the patient before the actual scan.[55] However, unlike Beaufrère and colleagues[46] (2011) we focused on the bolus tracking technique, which enabled us to reduce the intravenous applicated volume; this seemed to be more critical when considering the lightweight of our patients.

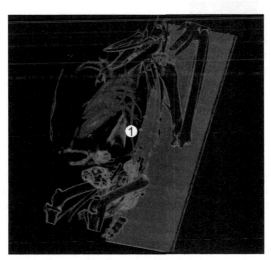

Fig. 7. 3D volume-rendered, bone-masked image of the same African gray parrot as in **Fig. 5**. The bone mask helps demonstrate the localization of the heart and the origin and route of the vessels in situ. Notice the pathway of (1) the aorta, which can be followed down to the hip.

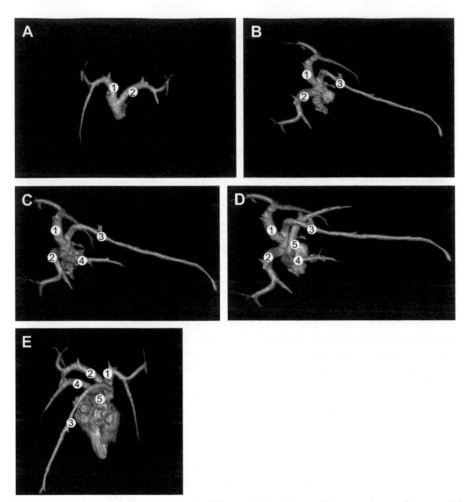

Fig. 8. Series of pictures illustarting the filling and depiction of the vessels step-by-step. (*A*) (1) Right brachiocephalic trunk and (2) left brachiocephalic trunk. (*B*) Additional (3) aorta. (*C*) Additional (4) left pulmonary artery. (*D*) Additional (5) right pulmonary artery. The heart and the great vessels in 3D shown from (*E*) *Facies caudalis.*

Except for the 2 conspicuous birds, that did not show an adequate amount of contrast material present in the major arteries, we could significantly enhance the great arteries using the protocol we created. The African gray parrot suffered an anesthetic accident, whereas the amazon parrot did not show any abnormalities during the CTA procedure, therefore the decreased amount of contrast material was inexplicable. In addition, we visualized the filling process of the cardiovascular system and illustrated this filling in 3-dimensional images. We hope to use these images as a basis for future measurement. However, there are further modifications needed, especially in reducing scanning time and optimizing anesthesia monitoring.

We have been able to create high-quality images with high spatial resolution and 3D images using postprocessing techniques. Therefore, we are optimistic to perform millimeter measurements of the actual vessel lumen (from the inner wall to the opposite inner wall) and at the level of greatest stenosis. We hope that these precise measurements will be of diagnostic value in the future.

All examined birds went through an anesthesia recovery without lasting or clinically shown symptoms or harm. Still, further improvements to the examination procedure to reduce the general risk of anesthesia should be considered.

In addition, Godoy and colleagues[56] (2009) described postprocessing dual-energy CT techniques, suggesting that there are further options available for reconstruction and visualization than those discussed in this article. Consequently, there will be further possibilities to visualize the cardiovascular system and its pathologic chances in birds using dual-energy CT in the future.

SUMMARY

In conclusion, single-source dual-layer CT imaging and the described postprocessing steps is a promising new technique with a potential clinical application in cardiovascular imaging in birds. Nevertheless, further studies are required and further technique modification is needed.

CLINICS CARE POINTS

- Birds with cardiovascular diseases show quite unspecific symptoms.
- Evaluating the patient's signalment, medical history, and husbandry conditions is very important.
- Birds with circulatory problems caused by cardiovascular disease are classified as emergency cases and thus have to be handled as shortly as possible.
- Diagnostic imaging especially radiography, echocardiography, and CT is beneficial when evaluating the cardiovascular system.

ACKNOWLEDGMENTS

The authors would like to thank the staff, especially Stefan Kohl of the Department for Small Animals and Tim Mathes of the Department for Birds and Reptiles of the Veterinary Teaching Hospital of the University of Leipzig, for their medical assistance and collegial support. In addition, we would like to thank Rebecca and Fotios Apokis for linguistic support on an earlier version of this article.

DISCLOSURE

The authors disclose any relationship with a commercial company with a direct financial interest in subject matter or materials discussed in this article or with a company making a competing product.

The authors have nothing to disclose.

REFERENCES

1. Oglesbee BL, Oglesbee MJ. Results of postmortem examination of psittacine birds with cardiac disease: 26 cases (1991-1995). J Am Vet Med Assoc 1998; 212(11):1737–42.
2. Braun S. Pathologische, pathohistologische und mikrobiologische Untersuchungen am Herzen und den großen Blutgefäßen von Vögeln der Ordnung

Psittaciformes. Gießen, Germany: Justus-Liebig-Universität Gießen; 2003. Doctoral Thesis.

3. Krautwald-Junghanns M-E, Braun S, Pees M, et al. Research on the Anatomy and Pathologie of the Psittacine Heart. J Avian Med Surg 2004;18(1):2–11.

4. Kellin N. Auswertung der Sektions- und Laborbefunde von 1780 Vögeln der Ordnung Psittaciformes in einem Zeitraum von vier Jahren (2000 bis 2003). Gießen, Germany: Justus-Liebig-Universität Gießen; 2009. Doctoral Thesis.

5. Nemeth NM, Gonzalez-Astudillo V, Oesterle PT, et al. A 5-Year Retrospective Review of Avian Diseases Diagnosed at the Department of Pathology, University of Georgia. J Comp Pathol 2016;155(2–3):105–20.

6. Gibson DJ, Nemeth NM, Beaufrère H, et al. Captive Psittacine Birds in Ontario, Canada: a 19-Year Retrospective Study of the Causes of Morbidity and Mortality. J Comp Pathol 2019;171:38–52.

7. Dorrestein GM, Zwart P, Borst GH, et al. Ziekte-en doodsoorzaken van vogels. Tijdschrift voor diergeneeskunde 1977;102(7):437–47.

8. Beaufrère H, Nevarez JG, Wakamatsu N, et al. Experimental diet-induced atherosclerosis in Quaker parrots (Myiopsitta monachus). Vet Pathol 2013;50(6): 1116–26.

9. Beaufrère H, Ammersbach M, Reavill DR, et al. Prevalence of and risk factors associated with atherosclerosis in psittacine birds. J Am Vet Med Assoc 2013; 242(12):1696–704.

10. Reichelt C, Wolf P, Cramer K, et al. Situationsanalyse zur derzeitigen Ernährung der am häufigsten gehaltenen Ziervögel in Deutschland. Berliner und Munchener tierarztliche Wochenschrift 2020;(133):159–70.

11. Braun S, Krautwald-Junghanns M-E, Straub J. Zu Art und Häufigkeit von Herzerkrankungen bei in Deutschland in Gefangenschaft gehaltenen Papageienvögeln. DTW Deutsche Tierarztliche Wochenschrift 2002;109(6):255–60.

12. Bavelaar FJ, Beynen AC. Atherosclerosis in parrots. A review. The Vet Q 2004; 26(2):50–60.

13. Fricke C. Atherosklerose bei Graupapageien (Psittacus erithacus) und Amazonen (Amazona spp.). Leipzig, Germany: Veterinary teaching hospital, Department for birds and reptiles, Univeristy of Leipzig; 2006. Doctoral Thesis.

14. Beaufrere H, Nevarez JG, Holder K, et al. Characterization and classification of psittacine atherosclerotic lesions by histopathology, digital image analysis, transmission and scanning electron microscopy. Avian Pathol 2011;40(5):531–44.

15. Beaufrère H. Atherosclerosis: Comparative Pathogenesis, Lipoprotein Metabolism, and Avian and Exotic Companion Mammal Models. J Exot Pet Med 2013;22(4):320–35.

16. Beaufrère H, Holder KA, Bauer R, et al. Intermittent claudication-like syndrome secondary to atherosclerosis in a yellow-naped Amazon parrot (Amazona ochrocephala auropalliata). J Avian Med Surg 2011;25(4):266–76.

17. Grosset C, Guzman DS-M, Keating MK, et al. Central vestibular disease in a blue and gold macaw (Ara ararauna) with cerebral infarction and hemorrhage. J Avian Med Surg 2014;28(2):132–42.

18. Fitzgerald BC, Beaufrere H. Cardiology. In: Speer BL, editor. Current therapy in avian medicine and surgery. First edition. St. Louis, Missouri: Elsevier; 2016. p. 252–328.

19. Fricke C, Schmidt V, Cramer K, et al. Characterization of atherosclerosis by histochemical and immunohistochemical methods in African grey parrots (Psittacus erithacus) and Amazon parrots (Amazona spp.). Avian Dis 2009;53(3):466–72.

20. Finlayson R, Hirchinson V. Experimental atheroma in budgerigars. Nature 1961; 192(4800):369–70.
21. Bavelaar F, Beynen A. Influence of amount and type of dietary fat on plasma cholesterol concentrations in African Grey Parrots. J Appl Es Vet Med 2003;1:1–8.
22. Warnock NH, Clarkson TB, Stevenson R. Effect of exercise on blood coagulation time and atherosclerosis of cholesterol-fed cockerels. Circ Res 1957;5(5):478–80.
23. Ratcliffe HL, Cronin MT. Changing frequency of arteriosclerosis in mammals and birds at the Philadelphia Zoological Garden; review of autopsy records. Circulation 1958;18(1):41–52.
24. Bohorquez F, Stout C. Aortic atherosclerosis in exotic avians. Exp Mol Pathol 1972;17(3):261–73.
25. Harrison GJ, McDonald D. Nutritional Considerations Section 2. In: Lightfoot Harrison. Clin Avian Med 2005;1(1):108–40, 450.
26. Nicholson AC, Hajjar DP. Herpesviruses and thrombosis: Activation of coagulation on the endothelium. Clinica Chim Acta 1999;286(1–2):23–9.
27. Schenker OA, Hoop RK. Chlamydiae and Atherosclerosis: Can Psittacine Cases Support the Link? Avian Dis 2007;51(1):8–13.
28. Pilny AA, Quesenberry KE, Bartick-Sedrish TE, et al. Evaluation of Chlamydophila psittaci infection and other risk factors for atherosclerosis in pet psittacine birds. J Am Vet Med Assoc 2012;240(12):1474–80.
29. Mathers CD, Stein C, Ma Fat D, et al. Global burden of disease 2000: version 2 methods and results. Global Programme on Evidence for health Policy discussion paper No. 50. Geneva, Switzerland: World Health Organization; 2002.
30. Al-Mallah MH, Aljizeeri A, Villines TC, et al. Cardiac computed tomography in current cardiology guidelines. J Cardiovasc computed tomography 2015;9(6): 514–23.
31. Andreini D. Dual Energy Coronary Computed Tomography Angiography for Detection and Quantification of Atherosclerotic Burden: Diagnostic and Prognostic Significance. Rev Esp Cardiol 2016;69(10):885–7.
32. Bartlett ES, Walters TD, Symons SP, et al. Carotid stenosis index revisited with direct CT angiography measurement of carotid arteries to quantify carotid stenosis. Stroke 2007;38(2):286–91.
33. Pees M, Straub J, Krautwald-Junghanns M-E. (2001) Insufficiency of the muscular atrioventricular valve in the heart of a blue-fronted amazon (Amazona aestiva aestiva). The Vet Rec 2001;148(17):540–3.
34. Pees M, Schmidt V, Coles B, et al. Diagnosis and long-term therapy of right-sided heart failure in a yellow-crowned amazon (Amazona ochrocephala). The Vet Rec 2006;158(13):445–7.
35. Pees M, Krautwald-Junghanns M-E. Cardiovascular physiology and diseases of pet birds. The veterinary clinics of North America. Exot Anim Pract 2009;12(1): 81–97.
36. Baumgartner W, Wittek T, Vögel: Pees M. (2018): Allgemeiner klinischer Untersuchungsgang.In: Wittek T, Baumgartner W: Klinische Propädeutik der Haus- und Heimtiere. 9. Aufl.: Enke, p. 50 - 166.
37. DeWit M, Schoemaker NJ. Clinical approach to avian cardiac disease. Semin Avian Exot Pet Med 2005;14(1):6–13.
38. Pees M, Straub J, Krautwald-Junghanns M-E. Echocardiographic examinations of 60 African grey parrots and 30 other psittacine birds. The Vet Rec 2004; 155(3):73–6.
39. Pees M, Straub J, Schumacher J, et al. Pilotstudie zu echokardiographischen Untersuchungen mittels Farb- und pulsed-wave-Spektraldoppler an

Blaukronenamazonen (Amazona ventralis) und Blaustirnamazonen (Amazona a. aestiva). DTW Deutsche Tierarztliche Wochenschrift 2005;112(2):39–40.

40. Johnson-Delaney CA. Practical avian cardiology. Exot DVM 2006;(8):78–85.
41. Krautwald-Junghanns M-E, Pees M, Schütterle N. Echokardiographische Untersuchungen an unsedierten Brieftauben (Columba livia forma domestica) unter besonderer Berücksichtigung des Trainingszustandes. Berliner und Munchener tierarztliche Wochenschrift 2002;115(5–6):221–4.
42. Krautwald-Junghanns M-E, Stahl A, Pees M, et al. Sonographic investigations of the gastrointestinal tract of granivorous birds. Vet Radiol Ultrasound : official J Am Coll Vet Radiol Int Vet Radiol Assoc 2002;43(6):576–82.
43. Pees M, Straub J, Krautwald-Junghanns M-E. Echokardiographische Untersuchung bei Psittaciformes. Teil 2: Sonographisch ermittelte Messwerte zur Herzanatomie und errechnete Parameter der Herzfunktion. Tierärztliche Prax 2003; 31(K):180–7.
44. Pees M, Straub J, Schumacher J, et al. Pilotstudie zu echokardiographischen Untersuchungen mittels Farb- und pulsed-wave-Spektraldoppler an Blaukronenamazonen (Amazona ventralis) und Blaustirnamazonen (Amazona a. aestiva). DTW Deutsche Tierarztliche Wochenschrift 2005;112(2):39–40, 42-43.
45. Beaufrère H, Pariaut R, Nevarez JG, et al. Feasibility of transesophageal echocardiography in birds without cardiac disease. J Am Vet Med Assoc 2010;236(5): 540–7.
46. Beaufrère H, Rodriguez D, Pariaut R, et al. Estimation of intrathoracic arterial diameter by means of computed tomographic angiography in Hispaniolan Amazon parrots. Am J Vet Res 2011;72:210–8.
47. Lee Y-L, Yu P-H, Chen C-L, et al. Determination of the enhancement effect and diameters of the major arteries of african grey parrots using a dual-head power injector for computed tomographic angiography. Taiwan Vet J 2015;41(03): 165–75.
48. Yu PH, Lee YL, Chen CL, et al. Comparison of three computed tomographic angiography protocols to assess diameters of major arteries in African grey parrots (Psittacus erithacus). Am J Vet Res 2018;79(1):42–53.
49. Philips Healthcare. Certainty lives in layers. In: IQon Elite Spectral CT Product Broschure. 2020. Available at: http://www.usa.philips.com/healthcare/product/. Accessed April 07, 2021.
50. Krautwald-Junghanns M-E, Pees M, Reese S, et al. 1st edition. Atlas der bildgebenden Diagnostik bei Heimtieren: Vögel, Kleinsäuger, Reptilien, 2-42. Germany: Schlütersche; 2010. p. 84–91.
51. Haage P, Schmitz-Rode T, Hübner D, et al. Reduction of contrast material dose and artifacts by a saline flush using a double power injector in helical CT of the thorax. AJR Am J roentgenology 2000;174(4):1049–53.
52. Messprinzip F. Bildrekonstruktion, Gerätetypen und Aufnahmetechniken. In: Alkadhi H, Leschka S, Stolzmann P, et al, editors. Wie funktioniert CT? Eine Einführung in Physik, Funktionsweise und klinischeAnwendungen der Computertomographie. Springer; 2011. p. 3–13.
53. Philips Healthcare. Iterative model reconstruction technology. Available at: http://www.usa.philips.com/healthcare/product/HCNCTD449/iterative-model-reconstruction-reconstruction-technology. Accessed July 6, 2021.
54. Medtron AG. Produktkatalog Essential for contrast Version DE 5.0; 10.08. 2020. Available at: https://www.medtron.com/de/computertomographie/. Accessed April 07, 2021.

55. Abbara S, Arbab-Zadeh A, Callister T, et al. SCCT guidelines for performance of coronary computed tomography angiography: A report of the Society of cardio-vascular Computed Tomography Guidelines Committee. J Cardiovasc computed tomography 2009;(3):190–204.
56. Godoy MCB, Naidich DP, Marchiori E, et al. Basic principles and postprocessing techniques of dual-energy CT: illustrated by selected congenital abnormalities of the thorax. J Thorac Imaging 2009;24(2):152–9.

Histopathological Findings in the Cardiovascular System of Psittacidae in Routine Diagnostics

Kathrin Jäger, Dr. med. vet.[a],*,
Argiñe Cerezo-Echevarria, DVM, DipACVP[a], Andres Pohl, Dr. med. vet.[b],
Jens Straub, Dr med vet[c],
Dominik Fischer, Dr. med. vet., DipECZM (Wildlife Population Health)[d],
Heike Aupperle-Lellbach, PD, Dr. med. vet.[a]

KEYWORDS

- Avian • Heart • Aorta • Atherosclerosis • Myocarditis • Lymphoma

KEY POINTS

- 50% of *Psittacus*, *Amazona*, *Agapornis*, and *Ara* birds had cardiac lesions, in contrast to *Melopsittacus* birds, whereby only 6.3% were affected
- Approximately 50% of the cases had epi-, peri-, myo-, and/or endocarditis. These were most often associated with a bacterial septicemic process and, fewer with either viral, fungal, or parasitic infections.
- Cardiac lymphosarcoma was rare in psittacines. Interestingly, other metastatic tumors were not identified.
- One-third of the birds, especially *Psittacus* or *Nymphicus* genera had degenerative vascular lesions, most often located in the large arteries of the heart base.

Histopathology is a key method for the evaluation of cardiac diseases. Nevertheless, history and ancillary testing are crucial for a comprehensive interpretation.

INTRODUCTION

Psittaciformes include over 360 avian species, divided into 2 families; Psittacidae and Cacatuidae.[1,2] This represents enormous species diversity, including small and larger birds with different habitats, diets, and behaviors. Additionally, there are larger

[a] Laboklin GmbH & Co KG, Steubenstr. 3, Bad Kissingen D-97688, Germany; [b] Kleintier- und Vogelpraxis Haldensleben, Papenberg 6, D-39340 Haldensleben; [c] Tierklinik Düsseldorf GmbH, Münsterstraße 359, D-40470 Düsseldorf, Germany; [d] Zoo Wuppertal, Hubertusallee 30, D-42117 Wuppertal, Germany
* Corresponding author.
E-mail address: jaeger@laboklin.com

Vet Clin Exot Anim 25 (2022) 453–467
https://doi.org/10.1016/j.cvex.2022.01.009
1094-9194/22/© 2022 Elsevier Inc. All rights reserved.
vetexotic.theclinics.com

disparities, particularly when comparing companion pets versus free-ranging, wild birds, with potential relevance for longevity, lifestyle, and/or diet.[3] In Germany, in 2019 there were 4 million exotic birds.[4] During 2019 to 2020 in the United States, 5.7 million exotic birds, mostly psittacines and passerines were kept.[5] Due to this, veterinary service is continuously improving, resulting in longer lifespan of the birds under human care. This is leading to increasing cases of chronic or geriatric diseases in exotic birds.

The avian cardiovascular system is highly adapted to the bird's needs, taking into account its activity level, habits, species, and size.[6,7] For the most part, their cardiac anatomy is similar to that of mammals, with 4 chambers (2 atria and 2 ventricles). Interestingly enough, the right-atrioventricular valve, unlike mammals, is a spiral muscular flap devoid of chordae tendineae.[3,7] Histologically, their cardiomyocytes are one-fifth to one-tenth the diameter of mammalian's cardiomyocyte, with no M-band and transverse tubules.[6,7] This adaptation offers a greater surface area, with no need for T-tubules, allowing rapid depolarization[6] and contraction, thus raising the basal heart rate.

Apart from infectious causes and neoplasia, there are various factors that may render the animals prone to cardiovascular diseases. However, there are few studies researching avian cardiovascular disease incidence[8] and, more specifically, in psittacines.[9,10] It is known that psittacines, most specifically *Amazona* spp. and *Psittacus erithacus* are predisposed to atherosclerosis,[6] which becomes more evident with age.[11–13]

The study's aim is to retrospectively characterize the different cardiovascular lesions and incidence in psittacines routinely submitted to LABOKLIN GmbH & Co. KG pathology service.

MATERIAL AND METHODS

There were psittacine organ samples and whole carcasses submitted between 2013 and 2020 to the Pathology Service for routine diagnostics. Samples were fixed in 10% phosphate-buffered formalin. They were trimmed, wax embedded, and cut following laboratory standard procedures. Slides were stained with Hematoxylin–Eosin (HE) and additional stains such as periodic acid-Schiff (PAS), Ziehl–Neelsen, Giemsa, Heidenhain's Azan-trichrome stain, Von Kossa, or Picrosirius red stain were performed on demand.

For retrospective analyses, 363 birds were included. In all cases genus or species, and a final diagnosis were available. In 105 psittacine cases, cardiovascular lesions were re-examined by 2 specialized pathologists for further assessment. Slides were scanned and analyzed through Aperio ImageScope (Leica, Wetzlar, Germany).

Multiple reports have focused on cardiac inflammatory lesion grading.[14–17] In the present study, the distribution (focal, multifocal, diffuse), and severity (mild, moderate, and severe/marked) was noted. The type of inflammation was defined as follows: Fibrinopurulent and purulent inflammation contained heterophils, with/without fibrin. Mixed inflammation additionally had lymphocytes, plasma cells, and histiocytes. Pyogranulomatous and granulomatous inflammation were characterized by a necrotic core, surrounded by lymphocytes, plasma cells, and multinucleated cells, with/without heterophils. Finally, nonpurulent inflammation was an infiltrate with lymphocytes and plasma cells exclusively. Some lesions were further characterized as "fibroblastic," to indicate the presence of granulation tissue, thus giving more of a subacute to chronic timeline to the lesion.

Atherosclerosis was graded according to Beaufrère and colleagues (2011),[18] as type I–VII. These were characterized as follows: Type I: Within the intima, there are macrophages, isolated foam cells, increased extracellular matrix and lipids, and endo-thelial cell vacuolation; Type II: The accumulated macrophages are arranged in sheets with scant extracellular lipid; Type III (Preatheroma): mildly disrupting the artery, there are confluent areas of extracellular lipid and cell remnants; Type IV (Atheroma): dis-rupting the arterial wall, there is a bulging atheromatous lesion with a large lipid core; Type V (Fibroatheroma): Overlying the forementioned lipid core, there is fibro-muscular cap with mild/moderate plaque calcification. Additionally, there is significant luminal stenosis and endothelial defects; Type VI (complicated lesions): similar to type IV–V but with an additional hematoma or fissure; Type VII: Calcifying lesions, osseous metaplasia, large calcium plaques.

Further ancillary testing was initiated on client's request, confirming the presump-tive histopathological diagnosis (see above).

RESULTS

A total of 363 Psittacidae belonging to 37 genera and 54 species were included. The most common genera were *Melopsittacus* (n = 141; 38.8%), *Nymphicus* (n = 45; 12.4%), *Psittacus* (n = 33; 9.1%), *Cyanoramphus* (n = 29; 8.0%), *Amazona* (n = 17; 4.6%), *Agapronis* (n = 17; 4.6%), and *Ara* (n = 10; 2.8%). Age was only provided in 195 out of 363 cases. The cohort was composed of 152 males, 139 females, and 72 individuals of unknown sex. The main lesions were in the gastrointestinal tract (n = 89), liver (n = 80), cardiovascular system (n = 55), and/or respiratory tract (n = 47). Neoplasms were identified in 34 cases (**Fig. 1**).

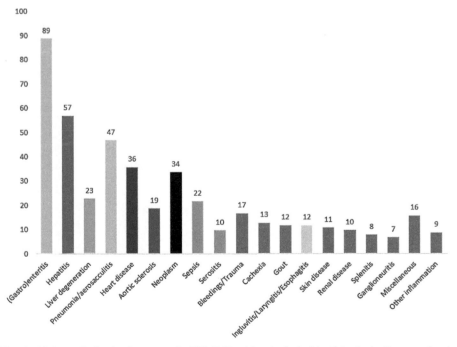

Fig. 1. Main pathologic diagnoses in 363 Psittacidae included in this study. Some animals had several main concomitant diseases.

Although bacteria were the most common infectious cause (n = 66), the majority (n = 43) could not be further characterized; however, Mycobacteria (n = 15) and Chlamydia (n = 8) were confirmed in 23 cases. Mycobacterial infections were seen in Budgerigars (n = 8), Red-crowned parakeets (n = 2), Barred parakeets (n = 1), Cockatiels (n = 1), Lovebirds (n = 1), Parrotlets (n = 1), and Red-winged parrots (n = 1). When identifying fungal agents, the most common organism was *Macrorhabdus ornithogaster* (n = 37), followed by *Aspergillus sp.* (n = 19), yeasts (n = 4), and other nonspecified fungi (n = 5). Parasites, comprised of nematodes (n = 18), *Trichomonas sp.* (n = 3), *Leukocytozoon sp.* (n = 3), *Knemidokoptes pilae* (n = 2), coccidia (n = 1), *Echinuria sp.* (n = 1), trematodes (n = 1), and nonspecified mites (n = 3). When diagnosing viral infections, Avian Borna virus (n = 7), Circovirus (n = 2), and Adenovirus (n = 1) were confirmed using PCR techniques in 10 cases, with other 10 presumed viral infections. On the other hand, noninfectious causes of death included trauma (n = 17), stress (n = 2), intoxication (n = 1), and Vitamin A hypovitaminosis (n = 1), among others.

Cardiovascular lesions were identified in 105 out of 363 cases. Of these, approximately 50% belonged to the genera *Psittacus*, *Amazona*, *Agapornis*, and *Ara*. Furthermore, there were cardiovascular diseases in about 30% of the *Nymphicus* and *Cyanoramphus* genera. In contrast, only 6.3% of *Melopsittacus* were affected (**Fig. 2**). In general, cardiovascular disease was slightly more prevalent in males (n = 47) than females (n = 40). Unfortunately, in 18 cases age was not provided. Most of the 105 Psittacidae had some form of inflammatory (n = 51; 48.5%) or degenerative (n = 15; 14.3%) heart condition, angiosclerosis, mainly in the aorta (n = 28; 26.7%), and/or cardiac lymphoma (n = 5; 4.7%) (**Fig. 3**).

Pericarditis and/or epicarditis were seen in 26 out of 105 birds with cardiovascular lesions. However, in most submitted cardiac samples, the pericardium was not included. Interestingly enough, 5 out of 8 Red-crowned parakeets with cardiovascular lesions had an epi-/pericarditis. These were often associated with other inflammatory conditions, like myocarditis (n = 13), hepatitis (n = 6), pneumonia/aerosacculitis (n = 6), visceral gout (n = 5), sepsis (n = 4), and others. Systemic conditions included

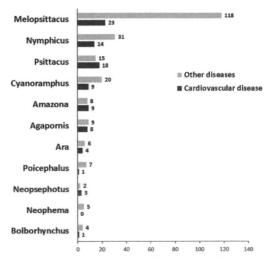

Fig. 2. Occurrence of cardiovascular and noncardiovascular diseases within the most common Psittacidae genera of the study.

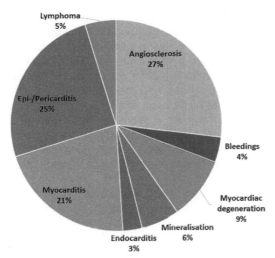

Fig. 3. Main cardiovascular diagnoses in 105 Psittacidae of the study (rounded percentages).

aspergillosis (n = 4), bacterial septicemia (n = 3), chlamydiosis (n = 3), and yeast infections (n = 1).

Grossly, the pericardium was translucent to opaque and variably thickened by an inflammatory exudate (**Fig.** 4A) or nodules (eg, pericardial granulomatous aspergillosis) (**Fig.** 4B). Macroscopically, visceral gout had a white, chalky, opaque pericardial deposition (**Fig.** 4C).

Histologically, 13 cases had mild epi- and/or pericarditis, 6 showed moderate, and 7 severe inflammations. Nonpurulent peri-/epicarditis was mild (n = 7) or moderate (n = 2). One 10-year-old male Cockatiel deceased secondary to trauma, showed a mild lymphoplasmacytic ganglioneuritis, lightly infiltrating the surrounding pericardial fat, epicardium, and myocardium. An underlying viral etiology, such as Avian Borna viruses (eg, Parrot Borna Virus), was suspected but not proven. Similar histologic findings were documented in a juvenile Macaw kept in a flock with intermittent outbreaks of Psittacid Herpes Virus (PsHV-1). Here PsHV-1 was not confirmed, but Avian Borna virus could not be excluded, given the nonpurulent meningoencephalitis, lymphoplasmacytic ganglioneuritis in the heart, (pro-)ventriculus, and abdominal ganglia.

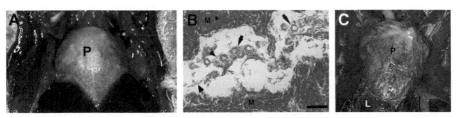

Fig. 4. (A) Purulent pericarditis in a fledgling *Poicephalus gulielmi*: The pericardium (P) is diffusely yellow, turbid, and thickened by pus and fibrin. (B) Pericardial aspergillosis in an *Ara militaris*: Within the marked necrotic material (M) there are numerous fungal hyphae (arrow heads), spores, and coniodophores (fruiting bodies, arrows). (Grocott's methenamine silver stain, bar = 50 μm). (C) Visceral gout in a 4-year-old *Eclectus roratus*: The pericardium (P) and liver surface (L) are covered with abundant whitish crystalline material.

The second most prevalent type of peri-/epicarditis included (pyo)granulomatous inflammation (2x mild, 1x moderate, 5x marked). Marked lesions were associated with visceral gout in three cases, or septic inflammation (2x pneumonia and aerosacculitis, 3x hepatitis). The 9 cases of epi-/pericarditis were classified as purulent/heterophilic (2x mild, 1x moderate), fibrinopurulent (1x mild, 1x moderate), mixed (2x mild, 1x moderate), and fibroblastic (1x severe, associated with visceral gout).

Myocarditis was diagnosed in 21 birds, mainly Budgerigars (n = 9). Seven of these were younger than 6 years; however, 6 years must be regarded as "old" in budgerigars. Unfortunately, only 8 had available age. Most of the samples were grossly unremarkable. Nevertheless, occasionally the myocardium contained patchy, discolorations (**Fig. 5**A). Myocarditis was often associated with hepatitis (n = 5) or other inflammatory lesions (n = 11).

Histologically, myocarditis was mild (11/21), moderate (5/21), or severe (5/21). Eight birds had mild mixed myocarditis, three of which were secondary to *Leucocytozoon*

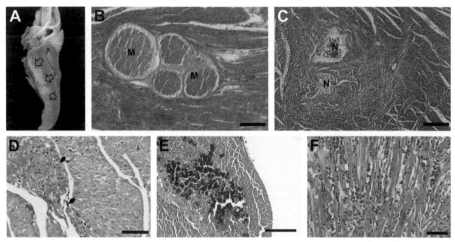

Fig. 5. (*A*) Myocarditis in a *Psittacus erithacus*. Arising from the endocardial surface, there are multifocal to coalescing, irregular, moderately demarcated pale areas in the myocardium. Histologically, these areas correspond with a marked pyogranulomatous myocarditis (arrows). (Formalin-fixed material, longitudinal section left ventricle). (*B*) *Leukocytozoon sp.* in the myocardium of a *Melopsittacus undulatus*: Compressing the adjacent cardiomyocytes, there are multiple, 100 to 200 μm in diameter, protozoal megaloschizonts (M). These are characterized by a granular, basophilic to eosinophilic cytoplasm, with numerous 1 to 2 μm in diameter basophilic, round merozoites. (HE stain, bar = 70 μm). (*C*) Myocardial nematodiasis in a *Triclaria malachitacea*: There are multiple 170 to 400 μm in diameter, cross-sections of degenerated nematode profiles (N) surrounded by a severe mixed inflammation and mild fibrosis. The nematodes are characterized by a thin, smooth, eosinophilic cuticle and a pseudocelom, which often contains cellular debris and degenerated leukocytes. (HE stain, bar = 200 μm). (*D*) Granulomatous myocarditis in *M. undulatus* with intracellular detection of copious acid–fast bacilli, consistent with *Mycobacterium sp.*, that was identified as *M. genavense* by PCR. (Ziehl–Neelsen stain, bar = 60 μm). (*E*) Myocardial mineralization in a *Neopsephotus bourkii*: The affected cardiomyocytes contain intracellular, mineral, granular deposits (black stain), while the surrounding interstitium contains some fibroblasts, fibrosis, few histiocytes, lymphocytes and plasma cells. (Von Kossa stain, bar = 200 μm). (*F*) 26. Myocardial lymphoma in a *Bolborhynchus lineola*. There are multifocal to coalescing aggregates of a monomorphic lymphoid cell population. The cardiomyocytes have signs of degeneration, along with interstitial edema. (HE stain, bar = 50 μm).

sp. infection. The cardiac Leucocytozoonosis were all diagnosed in Budgerigars. Two of these animals were very young. The third one had a history of other 3 very young budgerigars dying within the same enclosure. Histologically, there were 100 to 200 μm diameter, protozoal megaloschizonts, morphologically consistent with *Leukocytozoon* sp within the myocardium, associated with mild lymphoplasmacytic inflammation (**Fig. 5B**).

Nematodes were the causative agents of marked pyogranulomatous myocarditis in a *Triclaria malachitacea*. The bird had a poor body condition and a 1-week long history of gastroenteritis. The bird had received treatment against *M. ornithogaster*. Histologically, within the ventriculus and heart, there were 170 to 400 μm in diameter cross-sections of degenerated nematodes. Within the myocardium, the parasites were surrounded by numerous macrophages, heterophils, and fewer lymphocytes, often associated with fibrosis and edema (**Fig. 5C**). Additionally, there was a moderate subacute granulomatous portal hepatitis, with no etiologic agent on H–E slides.

Myocarditis was characterized as (pyo)granulomatous in 6 hearts (2x mild, 3x moderate, 1x severe). Two Budgerigars had systemic mycobacteriosis with mild/moderate granulomatous myocarditis also affecting liver, spleen, and other organs. Mycobacteriosis was characterized by 1 to 2 μm intrahistiocytic, acid–fast bacilli within areas of myocardial necrosis and inflammation (**Fig. 5D**). In one case, *Mycobacterium genavense* was confirmed using PCR techniques in the National Reference Laboratory for Mycobacteria in Borstel, Germany. Furthermore, a single, 5-year-old Budgerigar had moderate purulent myocarditis and hepatitis, most likely of bacterial origin.

Six hearts contained variable degrees of nonpurulent inflammation (5x mild, 1x moderate). In two birds, the mild nonpurulent myocarditis was considered the main finding, while the other 4 cases had other concomitant inflammatory conditions.

Mild or moderate eosinophilic *myocardial degeneration* (n = 5), moderate or severe fibrosis (n = 3), and/or mild to moderate mineralization (n = 3) were the least common findings. These were often seen in birds older than 10 years, with unremarkable myocardial gross changes.

A 23-year-old female Cockatiel with very poor general condition died despite intensive care. The left intertarsal joint had marked arthritis with associated osteolysis. Interestingly, the myocardium contained areas of *myocardial mineralization* corresponding with a multi-organic disseminated metastatic calcification. Histologically, the cardiomyocytes contained intracellular mineral deposits, often associated with variable amount of fibroplasia and mild interstitial lymphohistiocytic inflammation (**Fig. 5E**).

Lymphoma was diagnosed in 17 cases but only 5 birds had myocardial involvement (**Fig. 5F**) (1 female and 1 male *Bolborhynchus lineola*, 1 male *Cyanoramphus auriceps*, 1 male *Cyanoramphus novaezelandiae*, 1 female *Melopsittacus undulatus*). One of the 2 Barred parakeets was 4.5 years old, while the Red-crowned parakeet and the Budgerigar were both 1 year old. The 2 remaining birds were of unknown age. The history varied among animals, when provided: sudden death, acute dyspnea, reduced body condition, and hepatobiliary disease. In all cases, the heart had mild interstitial infiltration of a few small to intermediate-sized lymphocytes within the myocardium. In all cases, the diagnosis of lymphoma was mainly based on findings in the other affected organs.

Endocarditis was rare (n = 3; 2.8%). One animal, a 9-year-old Cockatiel, had echocardiographic evidence of pericardial effusion and bilateral atrial dilation associated with a severe left atrial fibroblastic inflammation. One 13-year-old *Amazona oratrix* had seizures and marked pyogranulomatous, atrioventricular, valvular endocarditis (**Fig. 6**). And, one *Enicognathus ferrugineus* had a history of sudden death caused

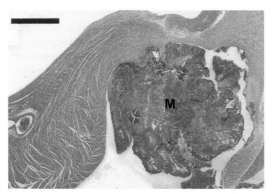

Fig. 6. Valvular endocarditis in an *Enicognathus ferrugineus*: Replacing the atrioventricular leaflet, markedly protruding into the cardiac chamber, there is an irregular inflammatory mass (M) characterized by abundant, liquefactive necrosis admixed with bacterial colonies, leukocytes, fibrin, and mineralization, all rimmed by a thick layer of granulation tissue. (HE stain, bar = 2 mm).

by the septicemic process with marked purulent and thrombotic valvular endocarditis with intralesional bacteria of the right atrioventricular valve.

Degenerative vascular lesions were diagnosed in 28 psittacids (26.6%) without clear sex predisposition (**Table 1**). The age ranged from 6 months to 34 years, (mean: 11.8 years). When assessing the scarce clinical history, sudden death was often reported.

The most prominent changes were identified within large arteries close to the heart base. The vascular lesions were grossly characterized by raised tan plaques most often located at the thoracic aorta's origin in larger birds (**Fig. 7**A). Nevertheless, these lesions may be grossly undiscernible in smaller species.

Histologically, atherosclerotic changes were graded according to Beaufrère and colleagues (2011). They were classified as type I and II (early lesions, n = 5; 17.9%), type III (intermediate lesions, n = 4; 14.3%; **Fig. 7**B), type IV (advanced, n = 6; 21.4%), type V (more advanced, n = 6; 21.4%), type VI (complicated lesions, n = 5; 17.9%), and type VII (calcifying lesions, n = 2; 7.1%; **Fig. 7**C and D).

Table 1
Distribution of age and gender, according to genera, with degenerative vascular lesions of the heart and/or large vessels

Genus	Number	Sex			Mean age (years)
		Male	Female	Unknown	
Psittacus	10	5	4	1	15.25
Nymphicus	6	3	3	0	8.0
Agapornis	4	2	2	0	8.3
Amazona	3	1	0	2	27.0
Melopsittacus	2	1	1	0	unknown
Cacatua	1	1	0	0	unknown
Eolophus	1	0	1	0	unknown
Neopsephotus	1	1	0	0	2.0

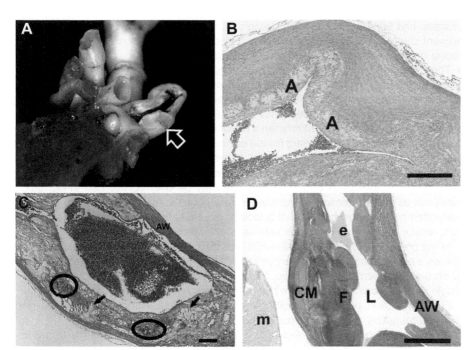

Fig. 7. (A) Aortic atheroma in a *Psittacus erithacus*. There is a tan atherosclerotic plaque within the aortic wall, protruding into the lumen, diminishing it (*arrow*). (B) Aortic atherosclerosis type III (intermediate) in a *P. erithacus*: There is a loss of the subintimal wall structure (A) due to the infiltration of few foamy macrophages, free lipids, and myxoid material. (HE stain, bar = 500 μm). (C) Aortic atherosclerosis type VII in *Amazona versicolor*. The aortic wall (AW) is markedly disrupted within the Tunica media by an accumulation of cholesterol clefts (*arrows*), chondroid and osseous metaplasia and, as well as multifocal mineralization (circles). (HE-stain, bar = 250 μm). (D) Aortic atherosclerosis type VII in a *P.erithacus*, longitudinal section, with partial occlusion of the vascular lumen (L). Different fiber types can be identified: In areas of fibrosis (F), collagen fibers stain red. In the normal aortic wall (AW), elastic fibers stain purple and, in areas of chondroid metaplasia (CM), proteoglycans stain turquoise. Erythrocytes (e) and myocardium (m) stain yellow. (Picrosirius red staining, bar = 2 mm).

Interestingly, there was a 6-month-old Gray parrot with type IV atherosclerosis and concomitant pyogranulomatous pneumonia and aerosacculitis. Furthermore, one lovebird had only splenic atherosclerosis, with multiple foamy macrophages and hemosiderophages. This animal had concomitant severe hepatic lipidosis and 60 g of body weight (physiologic range: 24–48 g).[19] Nevertheless, the heart and associated arteries were unremarkable.

In the present study, there were no cases with cardiac/pericardiac *vasculitis*. Nevertheless, this does not discard subcellular vascular damage during septicemia and/or intoxications.

DISCUSSION

In psittacids, cardiovascular diseases can be either primary or secondary, maybe only contributing (or not) to the clinical signs. Braun and colleagues (2002)[20] demonstrated that, out of 107 psittacines, 36.4% had gross changes on the heart and/or proximal vessels, and 99% of which had histologic abnormalities. This was confirmed by the present study. In contrast, Oglesbee and colleagues (1998)[9] found that after 269 psittacine necropsies, only 9.7% had evident cardiac disease.

The psittacine birds investigated by Oglesbee and Oglesbee (1998)[8] were comparable to our study, including the selection criteria of gross and/or histologic evidence of heart diseases. However, differences between the 2 studies may be due to varying customers' expectations linked with the submission of diagnostic material. For example, in our study, the veterinarian's major concern was the diagnosis of an infectious agent which may be relevant for the enclosure/flock. Therefore, birds from animal husbandry were not so often submitted if there were other known concomitant diseases, old age, or no transmissible diseases suspected. Thus, inflammatory cardiac diseases (both infectious and noninfectious) may be overrepresented in our study. However, although infectious causes were frequently the main concern, further testing was often not pursued because of a lack of available fresh material, the cost of the test, and/or the general diagnosis was satisfying enough for the client.

In the present study, approx. 50% of the birds had some form of cardiac inflammation as a part of a multisystemic process because submitted animals often had acute or chronic septicemia. Furthermore, birds do not have a diaphragm. Thus, within the single coelomic cavity, the heart is similarly affected as the other surrounding organs.

Fungal infection, bacteria—including *Mycobacterium* sp.—and parasites were identified as causative agents in 30 psittacines of this study.

Fungal infection, especially *Aspergillus* sp., is a common finding in the upper and lower respiratory tract of larger psittacines.[21,22] Nevertheless, in the present study, there was only a single, fatal pericardial Aspergillosis in an *Ara militaris*. Although fungal systemic spread can affect the different cardiac structures, there are only few reports describing cardiac *Aspergillus sp.* infection.[23] Therefore, the case in our study aligns nicely with these previously documented results of Carrasco and colleagues (1998).[23]

The different structures of the heart can also be targeted by bacteria such as *Erysipelothrix rhusiopathiae*,[15] *Lactobacillus* spp.,[24] among others[15,16,24,25] resulting in peri-, epi-, myo-, or endocarditis.[6,15,17,24,26] Mycobacteriosis can often cause fatal chronic diseases in single birds[27] and flocks.[28] This is a raising concern, given its zoonotic potential.[29,30]

In this study, 15 birds had systemic mycobacteriosis, the majority of which were Budgerigars (n = 8). Palmieri and colleagues (2013) identified *Mycobacterium genavense* as the most common form of Mycobacteriosis in selected psittacines including Budgerigars.[31] However, the most affected species were Amazon parrot and Gray cheeked parakeet, accounting for 26% and 18.7% of the total mycobacterial infections, respectively.[31] In our study, further PCR mycobacterial characterization was performed in only one Budgerigar, identifying *M. genavense*. This further corresponds to the aforementioned results of Palmieri and colleagues (2013).[31] Two Budgerigars of our study had cardiac mycobacteriosis. This may represent the first description of cardiac mycobacteriosis in Budgerigars, although this has been previously documented in few other psittacines (*Callocephalon fimbriatum*,[32] *Eclectus roratus, Amazona oratrix,* and *Pionites melanocephala*[27]).

Parasitic myocarditis was rare, including *Leucocytozoon* sp. infection in 3 Budgerigars and detection of myocardial nematode larvae in a Blue bellied parrot. Although gastrointestinal parasitic infestations are commonly seen in psittacines,[33,34] there are few reports about myocardial parasites, of for example, *Sarcocystis sp.*[35] or filariasis in the aorta and brachiocephalic trunks of Ramphastids.[36] Toxoplasma infection probably related to granulomatous myocarditis was documented in a flock of parrots and Mynahs.[37]

Leukocytozoon sp. in blood smears, liver, spleen, and lungs have been documented Budgerigars,[38] Barakeets,[38] a Gray headed parrot[39,40] and other birds.[38] However, to the best of authors' knowledge, the cases in this study seem to be the first ones identifying fatal myocardial leukocytozoonosis in Budgerigars.

In the present study, there was a suspicion of Parrot Borna virus causing cardiac lymphoplasmacytic epicardial ganglioneuritis in a Cockatiel and in a Macaw, but could not be further proven. Nevertheless, this seems most likely given the characteristic histologic appearance of this entity in psittacines with frequent involvement of the heart.[14,41]

Noninfectious peri- and/or epicarditis was associated with gout, which is common in captive psittacines.[42] Noninfectious causes for myocarditis and/or peri-/epicarditis include, for example, gout, lipidosis, or hemosiderosis,[42] but the two latter were not found in this study.

Endocarditis was the least common form of inflammation in this study (n = 3), although this is well known in psittacines.[24,25,43,44] In our study, the birds had died suddenly or had acute dyspnea. Nevertheless, the literature indicates that trauma (eg, feather damage, self-mutilation, pododermatitis, or owner's tough manipulation) with bacterial infection—especially *Staphylococcus aureus*—or chronic infections of the salpinx, liver, or skin can result in inflammatory heart damage.[13,17,44]

Cardiomyocyte eosinophilic degeneration, fibrosis, and/or mineralization were uncommon findings in this study and clear etiologic specificity could not be evaluated. General causes for myocardial degeneration include vitamin E and/or selenium deficiency, vascular abnormalities, or cardiomyocyte toxicity, including avocado or chronic endotoxemia.[13,17] In our study, a Cockatiel had multifocal cardiac mineralization with multiorgan involvement, suggesting a metastatic calcification. Other possible causes include renal and/or parathyroid hormonal dysfunction[45] due to old age (23 years) or marked hypercalcemia secondary to calcium sensitizers' ingestion or Vitamin D3 hypervitaminosis.[46] Interestingly, no myocardial degeneration or underlying necrosis was seen histologically in this cockatiel (eg, due to vitamin E and/or selenium deficiency), that would have predisposed it to dystrophic mineralizations.[17]

Lymphosarcoma is a very common diagnosis in psittacines and passerines.[47] There are different types described, often with multicentric involvement.[48–52] In psittacines, unlike other birds, it has not been linked to any underlying viral disease[52 53]. In the current study, 17 animals were diagnosed with lymphoma, 5 of them with concurrent cardiac metastasis. This ratio is similar to dogs, whereby 7/13 cases had cardiac metastasis, and unlike cats, whereby only 2/13 had cardiac involvement.[54] To the best research of the authors, this study includes the first description of 5 cases with cardiac lymphoma metastases in psittacines.

Atherosclerosis is considered one of the most common lesions in large parrots, more so populations of over 20 to 30 years of age. Interestingly, Amazon parrots, and especially in *Amazona aestiva, Psittacus erithacus, Nymphicus* sp., Cockatoos, and Macaws are particularly prone to it.[11,12] This species distribution was comparable to the present study. Regarding the age of the species affected by degenerative vascular lesions in this study, the mean age of Lovebirds was 8.3 years and 27 years in Amazons. Unfortunately, there are only very few larger studies in literature focusing on psittacids' average lifespan.[55] When compared with the reported average life expectancy, the cases of our study included young-adult to mid-aged animals suffering from atherosclerosis. Interestingly enough, within our collection there was a 6-month-old Gray parrot with moderate aortic atherosclerosis grade IV.[18] Although this has been previously reported in such a young animal,[56] this was considered exceptionally rare.

Vasculitis was not seen in our study; however, noninfectious cardiac vasculitis in psittacines may be secondary to toxic cardiomyopathy, especially lead poisoning.[57,58]

One limitation of this retrospective study was that the animal's species, history, and age were not always available. Moreover, often only a selected panel of organs was submitted, thus not evaluating all organs and truly determining if the cardiac lesion may be the primary lesion or just secondary to a disseminated inflammatory condition. This, along with the lack of history and/or the reported "sudden death," makes it challenging to assess the true clinical relevance of the cardiac disease and its contributing role to the cause of death.

In conclusion, when evaluating cardiac disease in a diagnostic setting, the entire case has to be considered as a whole (history, clinical examinations, gross examination, histopathology, and further diagnostics). Histopathology is a key tool for the evaluation of cardiac diseases, but the interpretation is hindered if not supported by appropriate signalment, history, clinical data, and complete set of organs. When sending organ samples, a representative section must be submitted to evaluate not only cardiac but also systemic disease and fresh material should be refrigerated for possible further testing. This allows a global view of the cardiac changes and ponder its clinical significance. Additionally, if there are several animals within the enclosure with similar clinical signs, sending more than one deceased animal may aid to interpret if the changes are representative or not of the entire population. These advances in diagnostics and especially in the development of sensible housing and management protocols (including husbandry, diet, social and functional needs of birds) are key for successful therapy and—even more desirable—prevention of psittacine cardiac disease.

In summary, this study on 363 psittacides identified cardiovascular lesions in about one-third of the cases submitted. Inflammatory lesions were often secondary to systemic infections while degenerative vascular lesions mainly affected larger arteries and aorta. Furthermore, this study included the first description of cardiac metastases of lymphoma in five psittacines, of cardiac mycobacteriosis in 2 Budgerigars as well as of fatal myocardial leukocytosis in 3 Budgerigars.

ACKNOWLEDGMENTS

The authors would like to thank the veterinary staff of the Clinic for Birds, Reptiles, Amphibians and Fish of Justus Liebig University Giessen, Germany, of the Veterinary Practice for Small Animals and Birds in Haldensleben, Germany and of the Animal Clinic Dusseldorf, Germany for assistance and support of clinical veterinary diagnostics, laboratory analysis, and part of the gross examinations.

DISCLOSURE

The authors K. Jäger, A. Cerezo-Echevarria, and H. Aupperle-Lellbach are employed by Laboklin GmbH &Co KG, Bad Kissingen, Germany, a veterinary diagnostic laboratory.

REFERENCES

1. psittaciform | Definition & Characteristics. Encyclopedia Britannica. Available at: https://www.britannica.com/animal/psittaciform. Accessed June 15, 2021.

2. The IUCN Red List of Threatened Species. IUCN Red List of Threatened Species. Available at: https://www.iucnredlist.org/en. Accessed June 30, 2021.

3. Kubale V, Miller G, Merry K, et al. Avian Cardiovascular Disease Characteristics, Causes and Genomics. 2018. https://www.intechopen.com/books/application-of-genetics-and-genomics-in-poultry-science/avian-cardiovascular-disease-characteristics-causes-and-genomics. Accessed February 11, 2021.
4. Pets: number by type Germany 2019. Statista. Available at: https://www.statista.com/statistics/552971/pets-number-by-type-germany/. Accessed June 16, 2021.
5. Pet Industry Market Size, Trends & Ownership Statistics. American Pet Products Association. Available at: https://www.americanpetproducts.org/. Accessed June 16, 2021.
6. Strunk A, Wilson GH. Avian cardiology. Vet Clin Exot Anim Pract 2003;6(1):1–28.
7. Cardiovascular system. In: pathology of pet and aviary birds. John Wiley & Sons, Ltd; 2015. p. 1–19. https://doi.org/10.1002/9781118828007.ch1.
8. Olkowski AA, Classen HL. High incidence of cardiac arrhythmias in broiler chickens. Zentralbl Veterinarmed A 1998;45(2):83–91.
9. Oglesbee BL, Oglesbee MJ. Results of postmortem examination of psittacine birds with cardiac disease: 26 cases (1991-1995). J Am Vet Med Assoc 1998; 212(11):1737–42.
10. Juan-Sallés C, Soto S, Garner MM, et al. Congestive Heart Failure in 6 African Grey Parrots (Psittacus e erithacus). Vet Pathol 2011;48(3):691–7.
11. Beaufrere H, Ammersbach M, Reavill D, et al. Prevalence and risk factors in psittacine atherosclerosis: a multicenter case-control study. J Am Vet Med Assoc 2013;242(12):1696–704.
12. Beaufrère H, Ammersbach M, Reavill DR, et al. Prevalence of and risk factors associated with atherosclerosis in psittacine birds. J Am Vet Med Assoc 2013; 242(12):1696–704.
13. Schmidt RE, Reavill DR, Phalen DN. Pathology of pet and aviary birds, 2. Wiley; 2015.
14. Vice CA. Myocarditis as a component of psittacine proventricular dilatation syndrome in a Patagonian conure. Avian Dis 1992;36(4):1117–9.
15. Galindo-Cardiel I, Opriessnig T, Molina L, et al. Outbreak of Mortality in Psittacine Birds in a Mixed-Species Aviary Associated With *Erysipelothrix rhusiopathiae* Infection. Vet Pathol 2012;49(3):498–502.
16. Vapniarsky N, Barr BC, Murphy B. Systemic Coxiella-like infection with myocarditis and hepatitis in an eclectus parrot (Eclectus roratus). Vet Pathol 2012; 49(4):717–22.
17. WitDVMaNico Martinede, Schoemaker J. Clinical approach to avian cardiac disease. Semin Avian Exot Pet Med 2005;14:6–13. No 1 (January).
18. Beaufrère H, Nevarez JG, Holder K, et al. Characterization and classification of psittacine atherosclerotic lesions by histopathology, digital image analysis, transmission and scanning electron microscopy. Avian Pathol J WVPA 2011;40(5): 531–44.
19. Wellensittich - zootier-lexikon.org. Available at: https://www.zootier-lexikon.org/index.php?option=com_k2&view=item&id=2573:wellensittich-melopsittacus-undulatus&Itemid=667. Accessed June 30, 2021.
20. Braun S, Krautwald-Junghanns ME, Straub J. [About type and incidence of heart disease in psittacines kept in captivity in Germany]. DTW Dtsch Tierarztl Wochenschr 2002;109(6):255–60.
21. Kaplan W, Arnstein P, Ajello L, et al. Fatal aspergillosis in imported parrots. Mycopathologia 1975;56(1):25–9.
22. Hauck R, Cray C, França M. Spotlight on avian pathology: aspergillosis. Avian Pathol 2020;49(2):115–8.

23. Carrasco L, Gómez-Villamandos JC, Jensen HE. Systemic candidosis and concomitant aspergillosis and zygomycosis in two Amazon parakeets (*Amazona aestiva*). Mycoses 1998;41(7–8):297–301.
24. Foldenauer U, Rusch M, Simova-Curd S, et al. Endocarditis due to Lactobacillus jensenii in a Salvin's Amazon parrot (Amazona autumnalis salvini). Avian Pathol 2009;38(1):55–8.
25. Isaza R, Buergelt C, Kollias GV. Bacteremia and Vegetative Endocarditis Associated with a Heart Murmur in a Blue-and-Gold Macaw. Avian Dis 1992;36(4): 1112–6.
26. Kellin N. Auswertung der Sektions- und Laborbefunde von 1780 Vögeln der Ordnung Psittaciformes in einem Zeitraum von vier Jahren (2000 bis 2003). GEB-IDN/ 6957. Available at: http://geb.uni-giessen.de/geb/volltexte/2009/6957/. Accessed February 11, 2021.
27. McRee AE, Higbie CT, Nevarez JG, et al. Mycobacteriosis in Captive Psittacines: A Brief Review and Case Series in Common Companion Species (Eclectus roratus, Amazona oratrix, and Pionites melanocephala). J Zoo Wildl Med 2017; 48(3):851–8.
28. Schmitz A, Korbel R, Thiel S, et al. High prevalence of Mycobacterium genavense within flocks of pet birds. Vet Microbiol 2018;218:40–4.
29. Schmidt V, Schneider S, Schlömer J, et al. Transmission of tuberculosis between men and pet birds: a case report. Avian Pathol 2008;37(6):589–92.
30. Boseret G, Losson B, Mainil JG, et al. Zoonoses in pet birds: review and perspectives. Vet Res 2013;44(1):36.
31. Palmieri C, Roy P, Dhillon AS, et al. Avian Mycobacteriosis in Psittacines: A Retrospective Study of 123 Cases. J Comp Pathol 2013;148(2):126–38.
32. Gelis S, Gill JH, Oldfield T, et al. Mycobacteriosis in Gang Gang Cockatoos (Callocephalon fimbriatum). Vet Clin North Am Exot Anim Pract 2006;9(3):487–94.
33. Tsai SS, Hirai K, Itakura C. Histopathological survey of protozoa, helminths and acarids of imported and local psittacine and passerine birds in Japan. Jpn J Vet Res 1992;40(4):161–74.
34. Papini R, Girivetto M, Marangi M, et al. Endoparasite Infections in Pet and Zoo Birds in Italy. Sci World J 2012;2012:1–9.
35. Latimer KS, Perry RW, Mo IP, et al. Myocardial sarcocystosis in a grand eclectus parrot (Eclectus roratus) and a Moluccan cockatoo (Cacatua moluccensis). Avian Dis 1990;34(2):501–5.
36. Sanchez-Godoy FD, Juarez-Murguia A, Hernandez-Castro R, et al. Characterization of aortic and brachiocephalic filariasis by Filarioidea sp (Nematoda:Spirurida:Filarioidea) in Mexican ramphastids. Int J Parasitol Parasites Wildl 2020;11: 282–6.
37. Dhillon AS, Thacker HL, Winterfield RW. Toxoplasmosis in mynahs. Avian Dis 1982;26(2):445–9.
38. Simpson V. Leucocytozoon-like infection in parakeets, budgerigars and a common buzzard. Vet Rec 1991;129(2):30–2.
39. Galosi L, Scaglione FE, Magi GE, et al. Fatal Leucocytozoon Infection in a Captive Grey-headed Parrot (Poicephalus robustus suahelicus). J Avian Med Surg 2019; 33(2):179.
40. García-del-Río M, Sancho R, Martínez J, et al. Blood Parasite Infections in Strigiformes and Psittaciformes Species in Captivity with a New Record of Potential Fatal Blood Parasite Transmission to Parrots. J Zoo Wildl Med 2021;51(4).
41. Leal de Araujo J, Hameed SS, Tizard I, et al. Cardiac Lesions of Natural and Experimental Infection by Parrot Bornaviruses. J Comp Pathol 2020;174:104–12.

42. Nemeth NM, Gonzalez-Astudillo V, Oesterle PT, et al. A 5-Year Retrospective Review of Avian Diseases Diagnosed at the Department of Pathology, University of Georgia. J Comp Pathol 2016;155(2–3):105–20.
43. Huynh M, Carnaccini S, Driggers T, et al. Ulcerative Dermatitis and Valvular Endocarditis Associated with *Staphylococcus aureus* in a Hyacinth Macaw (*Anadorhynchus hyacinthinus*). Avian Dis 2014;58(2):223–7.
44. Steinagel A, Quesenberry K, Donovan T. Vegetative Endocarditis due to Staphylococcus aureus in an Umbrella Cockatoo (Cacatua alba). J Avian Med Surg 2019;33(4):419.
45. Urist MR. Avian Parathyroid Physiology: Including a Special Comment on Calcitonin. Am Zool 1967;7(4):883–95.
46. Olds JE, Burrough E, Madson D, et al. Clinical Investigation into Feed-Related Hypervitaminosis D in a Captive Flock of Budgerigars (Melopsittacus undulatus): Morbidity, Mortalities, and Pathologic Lesions. J Zoo Wildl Med 2015;46(1):9–17.
47. Coleman CW. Lymphoid Neoplasia in Pet Birds: A Review. J Avian Med Surg 1995;9(1):3–7.
48. Burgos-Rodríguez AG, Garner M, Ritzman TK, et al. Cutaneous Lymphosarcoma in a Double Yellow-headed Amazon Parrot (Amazona ochrocephala oratrix). J Avian Med Surg 2007;21(4):283–9.
49. Souza MJ, Newman SJ, Greenacre CB, et al. Diffuse Intestinal T-cell Lymphosarcoma in a Yellow-Naped Amazon Parrot (*Amazona Ochrocephala Auropalliata*). J Vet Diagn Invest 2008;20(5):656–60.
50. Nevarez JG, Doo-Youn C, Tully TN. What Is Your Diagnosis? J Avian Med Surg 2011;25(3):231–3.
51. Lennox A, Clubb S, Romagnano A, et al. Monoclonal Hyperglobulinemia in Lymphosarcoma in a Cockatiel (*Nymphicus hollandicus*) and a Blue and Gold Macaw (*Ara ararauna*). Avian Dis 2014;58(2):326–9.
52. Gibson DJ, Nemeth NM, Beaufrère H, et al. Lymphoma in Psittacine Birds: A Histological and Immunohistochemical Assessment. Vet Pathol 2021. https://doi.org/10.1177/03009858211002180. 03009858211002180.
53. Harrison GJ, Lightfoot TL. Clinical Avian Medicine. :14.
54. Aupperle H, März I, Ellenberger C, et al. Primary and Secondary Heart Tumours in Dogs and Cats. J Comp Pathol 2007;136(1):18–26.
55. Miesle JJ. The Geriatric Psittacine | IVIS. Published January 13. 2017. Available at: https://www.ivis.org/library/reviews-veterinary-medicine/geriatric-psittacine. Accessed June 13, 2021.
56. Fricke C, Schmidt V, Cramer K, et al. Characterization of Atherosclerosis by Histochemical and Immunohistochemical Methods in African Grey Parrots (Psittacus erithacus) and Amazon Parrots (Amazona spp.). Avian Dis 2009;53(3):466–72.
57. Oglesbee BL. Case Reports. Vet Clin North Am Small Anim Pract 1991;21(6):1299–306.
58. Denver MC, Tell LA, Galey FD, et al. Comparison of two heavy metal chelators for treatment of lead toxicosis in cockatiels. Am J Vet Res 2000;61(8):935–40.

Cardiovascular Diseases in Pet Birds
Therapeutic Options and Challenges

Brenna Colleen Fitzgerald, DVM, Diplomate ABVP (avian practice)[a,b,*]

KEYWORDS

- Cardiovascular • Avian • Heart failure • Arrhythmia • Pericardial effusion
- Atherosclerosis • Hypertension • Treatment

KEY POINTS

- Cardiovascular disease, including congestive heart failure (CHF), pericardial disease and effusion, and atherosclerosis, is becoming increasingly better recognized in companion birds.
- Birds with cardiac disease often present with signs of CHF. The mainstays for treatment of CHF in small animal medicine, namely diuretics, vasodilators, and positive inotropes, can also be applied to treatment of the condition in birds. Negative inotropic drugs and lifestyle changes can also have merit.
- CHF may be accompanied by disease processes, such as hypertrophic cardiomyopathy, systemic and/or pulmonary hypertension, and arrhythmias, which need to be addressed accordingly.
- Treatment of pericardial effusion and cardiac tamponade should initially focus on fluid removal, followed by treatment of the underlying cause.
- Atherosclerosis is a disease that predominantly affects psittacine birds; treatment of this condition involves both controlling risk factors and managing sequelae, including peripheral hypoperfusion, ischemic stroke, and CHF.

INTRODUCTION

Cardiovascular disease has traditionally been thought to be a rare occurrence in companion birds, but a growing body of evidence collected over the last few decades indicates otherwise. It is frequently encountered in practice, predominantly in psittacine birds, and poses a serious threat to the quality of life and longevity of these and many other avian species. Successful intervention requires a foundational understanding of

[a] Avian Exclusive Veterinary Consultation (AEVC), Englewood, Colorado; [b] Homestead Animal Hospital, Centennial, Colorado
* Homestead Animal Hospital. 6900 S Holly Circle, Centennial, Colorado 80112
E-mail address: fitzgeralddvm@gmail.com

Vet Clin Exot Anim 25 (2022) 469–501
https://doi.org/10.1016/j.cvex.2022.01.005
1094-9194/22/© 2022 Elsevier Inc. All rights reserved.
vetexotic.theclinics.com

relevant anatomy and physiology, heightened awareness of risk factors and clinical disease states, accurate and timely diagnosis, and innovative treatment approaches.

At the present time, therapeutic interventions for cardiovascular disease in birds are largely empirical and extrapolated, where possible, from small animal and human medicine. Case reports of cardiovascular disease in which treatment was attempted are relatively few, but include cases of vascular disease (eg, atherosclerosis and associated pathologic conditions such as stroke and intermittent claudication), pericardial disease (eg, pericardial effusion), cardiac disease to include endocarditis, myocarditis, and end-stage disease (ie, congestive heart failure [CHF]), and cardiac arrhythmias.[1–24] There is a paucity of pharmacokinetic and pharmacodynamic data and no clinical trials in avian species for cardiovascular therapeutic agents. At present, the wide array of causative conditions, affected species, therapeutic interventions proposed or attempted, and outcomes precludes any conclusive association between therapeutic protocols and survival time.

The long-term prognosis for most cardiovascular diseases is considered guarded to poor, given that treatment is limited to management for a finite period, rather than resolution of disease in most cases. Prognosis is partly contingent on timely diagnosis, which proves challenging given the absence or subtlety of clinical signs and the limited sensitivity of available diagnostic modalities before disease has become advanced. Primary goals are to identify and control risk factors, where possible, and following diagnosis of cardiovascular disease, to maintain quality of life and extend survival time. The following sections review treatment options that show promise for management of recognized disease states, including CHF and related conditions, pericardial disease/effusion, and clinical atherosclerotic disease in birds. Medications that have been used empirically, and those for which pharmacokinetic and pharmacodynamic data are available, are presented in **Table 1**.

CONGESTIVE HEART FAILURE AND RELATED CONDITIONS

CHF occurs when the heart is unable to empty the venous reservoirs, manifested by vascular congestion and transudation of fluid within tissues and body cavities (congestive signs).[25,52–55] In the case of right-sided CHF, peripheral venous congestion, hepatic congestion, ascites, and pericardial effusion are often present. Pulmonary edema and congestion of the pulmonary veins occur with left-sided CHF, and a combination of signs may be seen with biventricular failure.[25,26,52,55] Heart failure (HF) can further be characterized as systolic (inadequate ventricular ejection), diastolic (inadequate ventricular filling), or a combination of the two. In either scenario, stroke volume and cardiac output decrease.[53,54]

CHF is not a primary disease in itself, but an ultimate consequence of structural or functional abnormalities of the cardiovascular or pulmonary systems (**Box 1**), compounded by the chronic effects of compensatory mechanisms. Not all cardiovascular disease necessarily leads to CHF, but it is a frequent clinical endpoint encountered in avian species. HF can result from primary myocardial failure (eg, dilated cardiomyopathy [DCM]), ventricular pressure overload (eg, outflow obstruction, systemic or pulmonary hypertension [PH]) or volume overload (eg, valvular insufficiency), conduction disturbances, or diastolic dysfunction (eg, myocardial hypertrophy, cardiac tamponade). For more details, please see Ref.[53,54,56]

Successful medical management is partly contingent on the earliest possible detection of disease. This can be enabled by teaching the companion bird owner to identify clinical signs, even if subtle, by regular physical examinations on an annual or semiannual basis, by considering the option of baseline diagnostic imaging for at-risk

Table 1
Selected agents for treatment of cardiovascular disease in birds

Drug	Species	Dose/Frequency	Basis	Reference
Diuretics				
Furosemide	Parrots, raptors, mynah birds, African penguins (*Spheniscus demersus*)	0.1–2.2 mg/kg IM, IV, SC, po q6–24h	EU	4,5,14,15,21,22,25,26,46,47
	Parrots	1–11 mg/kg IM q2–12h (acute treatment)	EU	Fitzgerald
		1–70 mg/kg po q6–12h (maintenance)	EU	Fitzgerald
	Chickens (*Gallus gallus domesticus*)	2.5 mg/kg IM	PD	28
		5 mg/kg po	PD	28
Spironolactone	Chickens	1 mg/kg po	PD	28
	Gray parrot (*Psittacus erithacus*)	1 mg/kg po q12h	EU	4
	Parrots	1–13 mg/kg po q8–12h	EU	Fitzgerald
Vasodilators				
Isoxsuprine	Yellow-naped Amazon parrot (*Amazona auropalliata*)	10 mg/kg po q24h	EU	20
	Parrots	10–15 mg/kg po q12h	EU	Fitzgerald
	Golden eagle (*Aquila chrysaetos*)	10 mg/kg po q24h	EU	11
	Bengal eagle owl (*Bubo bubo bengalensis*), lanner falcon (*Falco biarmicus*)	5–10 mg/kg po q24h	EU	44
Enalapril	Pigeons (*Columba livia*)	1.25 mg/kg po q8–12h	PK	29
	Amazon parrots	1.25 mg/kg po q8–12h	PK	29
	Parrots	1–5 mg/kg po q12–24h	EU	7,8,46
	Parrots	1.25–11 mg/kg pc q8–12h	EU	Fitzgerald
	African penguin	0.8 mg/kg po q12h	EU	21
	African penguin	0.25 mg/kg po q24h	EU	22
Benazepril	Gray parrot	0.5 mg/kg po q24h	EU	4
Sildenafil	Parrots	1–11 mg/kg po q8–12h	EU	Fitzgerald
	Mealy Amazon parrot (*A farinosa*)	2.5–3 mg/kg po q8h	EU	16
	African penguin	1 mg/kg po q12h	EU	21
Positive Inotropes				

(continued on next page)

Table 1
(continued)

Drug	Species	Dose/Frequency	Basis	Reference
Digoxin	Parrots, raptors, passerines	0.01–0.02 mg/kg po q12h	EU	46
	Budgerigars (*Melopsittacus undulatus*)	0.02 mg/kg po q24h	PK	48
	Quaker parrots (*Myiopsitta monachus*)	0.05 mg/kg po q24h	PK	49
	Sparrows	0.02 mg/kg po q24h	PK	48
	Indian ringneck parakeet (*Psittacula krameri*)	0.025 mg/kg po q24h	EU	5
	Indian hill mynah (*Gracula religiosa*)	0.01 mg/kg po q24h	EU	14
	Chickens	0.01 mg/kg po q24h	EU	50
	Chickens	0.33 mg/kg IV	PK	51
	Ducks (*Anas platyrhynchos domesticus*), turkeys (*Meleagris gallopavo*)	0.066 mg/kg IV	PK	51
Pimobendan	Hispaniolan Amazon parrots (*A ventralis*)	10 mg/kg po q12h	PK	30
	Parrots	6–20 mg/kg po q8–12h	EU	Fitzgerald 4,17,31
	Parrots	0.25 mg/kg po q12h	EU	15
	Harris hawk (*Parabuteo unicinctus*)	0.25 mg/kg po q12h	PK, EU	11
	Golden eagle	0.25 mg/kg po q12h	EU	21
	African penguin	6 mg/kg po q12h	EU	22
	African penguin	0.25 mg/kg po q12h	EU	
Dobutamine	Hispaniolan Amazon parrots	5–15 µg/kg/min (CRI)	PD	39
Dopamine	Hispaniolan Amazon parrots	5–10 µg/kg/min (CRI)	PD	39
Negative Inotropes				
Carvedilol	Turkeys[a]	1–20[b] mg/kg po q24h	PD	27
	Parrots	1–9 mg/kg po q12–24h	EU	Fitzgerald
Propranolol	Turkeys[a]	10 mg/kg po q8h	PD	32
	Turkeys[a]	10–30 mg/kg po q8h	PD	33
Atenolol	Most species	0.2 mg/kg IM, 0.04 mg/kg IV	EU	26
	Golden eagle	0.5 mg/kg po q12h	EU	11
	Turkeys[a]	10–30 mg/kg po q24h	PD	33

Carteolol	Turkeys[a]	0.01–10 mg/kg po q12h	PD	34
Sotalol	Golden eagle	1–2[c] mg/kg po q12h	EU	11
Amlodipine	Parrots	0.1–0.5 mg/kg po q12–24h	EU	12
Nifedipine	Turkeys[a]	10–50 mg/kg po q8h	PD	33
Diltiazem	Most species	1–2 mg/kg po q8–12h	EU	35
	Chickens	15 mg/kg po q12h	PD	36
Verapamil	Chickens	5 mg/kg po q12h	PD	37
Parasympatholytics				
Atropine	Most species	0.01–0.2 mg/kg IM, IV, IO	EU	25,46
	Moluccan cockatoo (*Cacatua moluccensis*)	0.05 mg/kg IM	EU	17
Glycopyrrolate	Most species	0.01–0.02 mg/kg IM	EU[a]	43
Other Antiarrhythmics				
Lidocaine (preservative-free)	Hispaniolan Amazon parrots	2.5 mg/kg IV	PK, PD	41
	Chickens	6 mg/kg IV	PD	42
	Chickens	2.5 mg/kg IV	PK, PD	40
Propantheline	Moluccan cockatoo	0.3 mg/kg po q8h	EU	17
Miscellaneous				
Pentoxifylline	Parrots	15–25 mg/kg po q8–12h	EU	Fitzgerald
	Most species	15 mg/kg po q8–12h	EU	38
	Gray-headed parrot (*Poicephalus fuscicollis suahelicus*)	25 mg/kg po q12h	EU	45

Abbreviations: CRI, continuous rate infusion; EU, empirical use; IO, intraosseous infusion; IV, intravenously; PD, pharmacodynamic study; PK, pharmacokinetic study; SC, subcutaneously.
[a] Broad-breasted white turkey poults.
[b] Some birds receiving carvedilol at 20 mg/kg had significantly decreased heart rate and BP for up to 8 h.
[c] The higher dose of 2 mg/kg caused significant bradycardia in this eagle.

Box 1
Documented causes of congestive heart failure in domestic and companion birds[56]
Dilated cardiomyopathy
Hypertrophic cardiomyopathy
Atherosclerosis
Systemic hypertension
Pulmonary hypertension
Pulmonary fibrosis/mycosis
Arrhythmias
Cardiac infection
Nutritional causes
Iron storage disease
Toxic causes
Valvular insufficiency
Valvular stenosis
Septal defects
Pericardial effusion

individuals to screen for subclinical cardiovascular disease, and by heightened awareness in the clinical setting.

In a patient presenting with acute or decompensated HF, initial treatment aims to stabilize the patient, followed by design of a longer-term management strategy. In the author's experience, this has met with highly variable success, but some birds have been maintained in stable condition for up to 9 years. Survival time for selected clinical cases of CHF in birds is shown in **Table 2**.

The mainstays of treatment of CHF in small animal medicine, namely diuretics, vasodilators (including angiotensin-converting enzyme inhibitors [ACEI]), and positive inotropes, can be applied to treatment of the condition in birds.[1,3–5,8,14,15,21,22,25,56,59,60] Beta-blockers (BBs), considered part of standard treatment in humans, may also have potential application.[27,61–65] In addition, known or hypothesized underlying cause or causes should be addressed, if possible. Some causes, including bacterial and fungal infections, parasitic disease, and certain toxic insults, carry a better prognosis for recovery.

Diuretics

Marked reduction of excessive circulating plasma volume (hypervolemia), edema, and effusion is an immediate treatment priority in any avian patient with CHF. Alleviation of this relative fluid overload can be accomplished through the use of diuretics, principally furosemide. Diuretics should not be used alone long term, as they further activate the renin-angiotensin-aldosterone system (RAAS).[66] Of the various diuretics available, furosemide is most commonly used in companion birds.

Furosemide

Furosemide is a potent loop diuretic that inhibits the sodium, potassium, and chloride cotransporter in the ascending limb of the loop of Henle, thereby promoting diuresis

Table 2
Survival time after diagnosis and treatment for selected cases of congestive heart failure in birds[a]

Species	Ultimate Diagnosis	CHF	Treatment	Survival Time	Reference
Gray parrot (*P erithacus*)	Atherosclerosis Right AV valve insufficiency Cor pulmonale Myocardial fibrosis	Right	Coelomocentesis Furosemide Spironolactone Benazepril Pimobendan	35 d	Sedacca et al,[4] 2009
Gray parrot (*P erithacus*)	Valve regurgitations, hyperechoic aorta	Biventricular	Furosemide Imidapril Pimobendan	30 d	Beaufrere et al,[31] 2007
Indian ringneck parakeet (*Psittacula krameri*)	Left and right AV valve insufficiency (myxomatous degeneration of left AV valve and hypertrophy of right AV valve) Myocardial degeneration and necrosis	Biventricular	Furosemide Digoxin	10 mo	Oglesbee and Lehmkuhl,[5] 2001
Blue-fronted Amazon parrot (*Amazona aestiva*)	Right AV valve insufficiency (congenital defect)	Right	Supportive Furosemide Digoxin	8 d	Pees et al,[13] 2001
Yellow-crowned Amazon parrot (*Amazona ochrocephala*)	Cause undetermined	Right	Supportive Furosemide Enalapril	27 mo	Pees et al,[8] 2006
Severe macaw (*Ara severa*)	Atherosclerosis Diffuse fatty infiltration of the right ventricular myocardium	Biventricular	Furosemide	70 d	Phalen et al,[3] 1996
Gray-cheeked parakeet (*Brotogeris pyrrhopterus*)	Atherosclerosis Left and right AV valve	Biventricular	Supportive	3 d	Mans and Brown,[57] 2007

(continued on next page)

Table 2
(continued)

Species	Ultimate Diagnosis	CHF	Treatment	Survival Time	Reference
Umbrella cockatoo (*Cacatua alba*)	insufficiency Myocardial degeneration and fibrosis				
Umbrella cockatoo (*Cacatua alba*)	Atherosclerosis Aneurysm of right coronary artery Myocardial fibrosis	Right	Supportive Furosemide	Euthanized at diagnosis	Vink-Nooteboom et al,[58] 1998
Umbrella cockatoo (*C alba*)	Atherosclerosis Left AV valve insufficiency (myxomatous degeneration and mineralization)	Left	Unspecified	Euthanized within 1 d of diagnosis	Baine,[23] 2012
Pukeko (*Porphyrio melanotus*)	Atherosclerosis Left AV valve insufficiency (endocardiosis) Left atrial thrombus Atrial fibrillation Myocardial degeneration	Biventricular	Supportive Digoxin	49 d	Beehler et al,[24] 1980
Red-tailed hawk (*Buteo jamaicensis*)	Dilated cardiomyopathy	Right	Supportive Furosemide	Euthanized 2 d after presentation	Knafo et al,[1] 2011
Indian hill mynah (*Gracula religiosa*)	Left AV valve insufficiency	Biventricular	Supportive Coelomocentesis Furosemide Digoxin	10 mo	Rosenthal and Stamoulis,[14] 1993
Greater hill mynah (*G religiosa intermidia*)	Coronary mineralization	Right	Coelomocentesis	12 d	Ensley et al,[2] 1979
Mallard hybrid duck (*Anas* spp)	Congenital left AV valve stenosis and subvalvular aortic stenosis	Biventricular	Supportive Coelomocentesis Furosemide	29 d	Mitchell et al,[6] 2008

Species	Diagnosis		Treatment	Duration	Reference
African penguin (*Spheniscus demersus*)	Right AV valve insufficiency (endocardiosis)	Right	Supportive, Coelomocentesis, Furosemide, Enalapril, Pimobendan, Sildenafil	124 d	Cusack et al,[21] 2016
African penguin (*S demersus*)	Right AV valve insufficiency (congenital valvular dysplasia and myxomatous degeneration), Myocardial fibrosis	Right	Supportive, Furosemide, Enalapril, Pimobendan	10 d	McNaughton et al,[22] 2014
Harris hawk (*Parabuteo unicinctus*)	Cardiomyopathy	Biventricular	Furosemide, Pimobendan	6 mo	Brandao et al,[15] 2016
*Yellow-naped Amazon parrot (*A auropalliata*)[b]	Atherosclerosis	Biventricular	Supportive, Coelomocentesis, Furosemide, Spironolactone, Enalapril, Sildenafil, Pimobendan, Carvedilol	8 mo	Author
*Gray parrot (*P erithacus*)	Dilated cardiomyopathy, Atherosclerosis	Right	Supportive, Furosemide, Spironolactone, Enalapril	30 d	Author
*Gray parrot (*P erithacus*)	Atherosclerosis	Biventricular	Supportive, Furosemide, Spironolactone, Enalapril, Pimobendan	14 mo	Author

(continued on next page)

Table 2
(continued)

Species	Ultimate Diagnosis	CHF	Treatment	Survival Time	Reference
*Gray parrot (P erithacus)	Open	Right	Supportive Furosemide Enalapril Sildenafil Pimobendan Omega-3 fatty acid supplementation	108 mo to present	Author
*Gray parrot (P erithacus)	Left AV valve insufficiency Atherosclerosis	Biventricular	Supportive Furosemide Spironolactone Enalapril Sildenafil Pimobendan	17 mo	Author
*Gray parrot (P erithacus)	Open	Left	Supportive Furosemide Enalapril Pimobendan	73 mo to present	Author
*Gray parrot (P erithacus)	Atherosclerosis Endocardiosis (left AV valve) Right ventricular hypertrophy Thickened pericardium Diffuse hepatopathy	Right	Supportive Furosemide Spironolactone Enalapril Sildenafil Isoxsuprine Pimobendan	16 mo	Author
*Sun conure (Aratinga solstitialis)	Mycobacteriosis	Right	Supportive Antimicrobials Furosemide Spironolactone	6 m to present	Author

Species	Pathology	Heart failure	Treatment	Follow-up	Source
			Enalapril Pimobendan		
*Orange-winged Amazon parrot (Amazona amazonica)	Open	Biventricular	Supportive Furosemide Enalapril Isoxsuprine Pimobendan	41 mo to present	Author
*Goffin's cockatoo (Cacatua goffiniana)	Right ventricular hypertrophy Markedly thickened right AV valve	Right	Supportive Furosemide Enalapril Sildenafil Pimobendan	6 mo to present	Author
*Indian ringneck parakeet (P krameri)	Atherosclerosis Ovarian neoplasia with local metastasis	Biventricular	Supportive Coelomocentesis Pericardiocentesis Furosemide Spironolactone Enalapril Carvedilol Pimobendan	7 mo	Author
*Indian hill mynah (G religiosa)	Open	Biventricular	Furosemide Spironolactone Enalapril Pimobendan	19 mo	Author

a Cases managed by the author and colleagues (B. C. Fitzgerald, unpublished data) are indicated with an asterisk.
b Case discussed in the text under hypertrophic cardiomyopathy.

and excretion of sodium and chloride.[66-68] Parenteral administration of furosemide is an essential step in management of the acute crisis in avian patients, as this route allows for a rapid onset of action. A relatively high initial dose is often required. Following stabilization of the patient, a maintenance dose of furosemide can be used to enable the long-term management of chronic CHF.[66,67,69]

Furosemide has been found to be efficacious with a rapid onset of action in birds, despite the presence of only 10% to 30% of looped nephrons in the avian kidney.[70] It has been used successfully for the treatment of pericardial effusion, CHF, pulmonary edema, and ascites.[8,13,25,26,56] Route of administration may significantly influence bioavailability, as suggested by a study in chickens (adult laying hens) showing significantly increased urine output following parenteral administration, but no such increase following oral administration, even at twice the parenteral dose (see **Table 1**).[28]

Doses that have been used vary widely (see **Table 1**). The dose and administration interval are best determined by clinical response (namely normalization of respiratory rate and effort) balanced with maintenance of acceptable hydration. The degree of clinical response can be of diagnostic and prognostic value; a positive response supports the working diagnosis of CHF and suggests a more favorable prognosis. Alternatively, a poor response warrants reevaluation of the working diagnosis or, if the diagnosis is sound, suggests a poorer prognosis. In the author's experience, a dose range of 1 to 5 mg/kg intramuscularly (IM) has been efficacious when stabilizing most psittacine patients. An initial frequency of 2 hours is usually followed by a shift to 6- to 12-hour intervals. There have been isolated cases with severely decompensated disease in which higher doses (7–11 mg/kg IM every 12 hours) were required to gain control of congestive signs. In patients whose disease is less severe and advanced, a lower initial dose and frequency (1–5 mg/kg IM every 12 hours) may be adequate. Once the patient has been stabilized, furosemide can be administered orally, with the dose increased at least 2-fold (presuming oral bioavailability is 60%–75% as in humans[68]) given every 8 to 12 hours. Ultimately, the goal for long-term management is to identify the lowest dose and frequency that controls congestive signs; adjustments will be needed over time, as the disease condition changes or progresses. Patients with more severe, advanced disease may require a higher dose and frequency (30–70 mg/kg per os [po] every 6–12 hours) to maintain control of congestive signs.

Adverse effects of loop diuretics include dehydration, hypotension, (prerenal) azotemia, and depletion of electrolytes, especially chloride, potassium, and magnesium.[60,66,68] With chronic use, renal functional status (blood uric acid) and electrolytes should therefore be monitored carefully.[25] In addition, caution and lower doses are warranted when using this drug in patients with renal disease, as well as in lories and lorikeets (subfamily Loriinae), which have been reported to be extremely susceptible to adverse effects of furosemide.[26]

Other diuretics

Spironolactone, an aldosterone antagonist that is classified as a potassium-sparing diuretic, may have merit as part of the treatment regime in cases where congestive signs cannot be controlled with furosemide and an ACEI alone.[71] Its combined use with furosemide may also be considered to offset potassium loss.[4,67,71] Aside from its diuretic effects, spironolactone is thought to prevent or decrease myocardial fibrosis in humans[66] and counteract the myriad deleterious effects of aldosterone in CHF.[72] Reports on its use or efficacy in avian species are scarce. In the author's experience, doses between 1 and 13 mg/kg by mouth every 8 to 12 hours have been well tolerated in numerous patients with CHF.

Vasodilators

ACE inhibitors

ACEI are typically combined with diuretics and positive or negative inotropes and comprise an essential component of long-term medical management of CHF by blunting the effects of the RAAS. By interfering with angiotensin II (AII) formation and limiting aldosterone production, ACEI promote vasodilation and reduce sodium and water retention, thereby decreasing total peripheral resistance and pulmonary vascular resistance (afterload) and circulating volume (preload), allowing an increase in cardiac output.[25,29,73,74] Enalapril is thought to attenuate myocardial remodeling in humans and dogs.[75] In both species,[76,77] ACEI have been found beneficial to increase survival times.

Enalapril has been the most commonly used ACEI in birds, with empirical evidence suggesting it is both safe and efficacious.[29] Enalapril has been used, both alone and in combination with furosemide, to treat CHF with reduction in pericardial effusion, ascites, and hepatic congestion documented by echocardiography, and reportedly increased quality of life and longevity in birds with severe cardiac pathologic condition.[8,29,56] The author has found that when edema and effusion are mild, they can in some cases be resolved with enalapril alone without concurrent use of a diuretic. Pharmacokinetic data support a dose of at least 1.25 mg/kg by mouth every 8 to 12 hours in pigeons and Amazon parrots, although the half-life was shorter, and lower maximum plasma concentrations were reached in the latter species.[29] The author has used higher doses (4–11 mg/kg by mouth every 8–12 hours) in psittacine birds with appreciable symptomatic benefit and no apparent adverse effects.

Potential adverse effects of ACEI include hypotension, renal dysfunction, and hyperkalemia.[74] Dehydration has been reported with long-term, higher-dose therapy (5 mg/kg daily) in birds, although the drug generally appears well tolerated.[29] The risk of hyperkalemia is likely diminished by concurrent use of furosemide, but may be relatively greater if spironolactone is used as well.[73] When using ACEI, it is reasonable to consider similar biochemical and hematologic monitoring as for furosemide, but no significant changes in these parameters were found in pigeons receiving 10 mg/kg enalapril once daily for 3 weeks.[29]

Other vasodilators

Sildenafil is a selective pulmonary vasodilator that reduces pulmonary vascular resistance and right ventricular afterload.[78–80] Compared with mammals, birds are thought to have a greater propensity for developing PH and right-sided, rather than left-sided CHF.[55,81] The inclusion of sildenafil should be considered in treatment of patients with CHF with cor pulmonale. The author has used sildenafil for this indication in psittacine birds at a dose and frequency of 1 to 11 mg/kg by mouth every 8 to 12 hours.

Positive Inotropes

Positive inotropes, such as digoxin and pimobendan, have been used or proposed for treatment of HF in avian species, but pharmacodynamic data are lacking, and pharmacokinetic data and information as to their efficacy and margin of safety are extremely limited.[7,25,29,30] Both drugs are used to enhance myocardial contractility and are appropriate for treatment of HF because of systolic dysfunction. They are contraindicated in cases of hypertrophic cardiomyopathy (HCM; where diastolic dysfunction is the primary problem), and of outflow obstruction (eg, aortic stenosis).[25,67,82] Likewise, it should be questioned whether their use is appropriate in birds with HF secondary to atherosclerotic disease and luminal stenosis of major arteries. In those cases with severe systolic dysfunction, however, it is fair to consider their inclusion in the treatment regime in an effort to stabilize the patient, if not also to manage CHF over the long term. Once the patient has been stabilized, the clinician can also consider either alternative or concurrent use of a BB (see the following section). Digoxin may have value in certain HF cases, particularly when supraventricular tachyarrhythmia is a feature.[26] For more information on digoxin and its application in the treatment of CHF, please see Refs.[56,83]

Pimobendan

Pimobendan, a calcium sensitizer and phosphodiesterase inhibitor, is a positive inotrope and vasodilator (inodilator), as well as a positive lusitrope. It enhances myocardial contractility, primarily through calcium sensitization of cardiac myofibrils and by phosphodiesterase III inhibition, without increasing myocardial oxygen consumption.[30,84] Inhibition of phosphodiesterase III and V promotes systemic and pulmonary arterial and venous dilation, thereby reducing afterload and preload, respectively.[30] Pimobendan is commonly used in small animal cardiology and has been shown to increase both survival time and quality of life in dogs with DCM and HF secondary to mitral valve disease.[85]

There are 2 reported cases where pimobendan (0.25–0.6 mg/kg every 12 hours) was used in conjunction with a diuretic and an ACEI to treat CHF in psittacines, with mixed results.[4,31] The apparent limited clinical effect may be explained by underdosing. A pharmacokinetic study in Hispaniolan Amazon parrots (*Amazona ventralis*) demonstrated that a single oral dose of 10 mg/kg is required to achieve a peak plasma concentration of 8.26 ng/mL, comparable to levels considered therapeutic in dogs and humans.[30] Extrapolation of the dose used in this study to other species groups should be done with caution. Plasma concentrations in a Harris hawk (*Parabuteo unicinctus*) with CHF receiving 10 mg/kg pimobendan by mouth peaked at 25,196 ng/mL. However, there was no indication of toxicosis.[15]

Bioavailability of pimobendan can be affected by pharmacologic composition. An oral suspension formulated from commercially available tablets (crushed and combined with a suspending vehicle) produced 6 times greater plasma concentrations than a suspension made from the bulk chemical (powder). The investigators proposed that the difference might be attributed to the citric acid excipient present in the commercially available tablets, which facilitated oral absorption.[30]

Adverse effects have not been recognized in birds, but the safety and efficacy of this drug in avian species have not been established. The author has incorporated pimobendan (6–20 mg/kg by mouth every 8–12 hours) into the treatment regime for management of CHF in many companion birds.

Negative Inotropes

Negative inotropes, including BBs and calcium channel blockers (CCBs), may have merit as adjunctive treatment for CHF, particularly when ventricular hypertrophy and tachyarrhythmia are contributing factors.

Beta-blockers

BBs are sympatholytic agents that block the binding of endogenous catecholamines to β-adrenoreceptors. They are negative inotropes, chronotropes, and lusitropes that also slow atrioventricular (AV) nodal conduction:

- First-generation, nonselective BBs (eg, propanolol, carteolol, sotalol) block both β_1- and β_2-adrenoreceptors.
- Second-generation BBs (eg, atenolol, metoprolol) are relatively β_1-selective.

- Carvedilol, a third-generation BB, is both a nonselective β-adrenoreceptor antagonist and a selective $α_1$-adrenoreceptor antagonist, such that it also has vasodilatory action to reduce afterload.[62,86–90]

BBs are part of core therapy for HF in humans, in both early and advanced stages.[61,63,64] They counter the increased sympathetic tone and RAAS activation characteristic of the neuroendocrine system that is central to the pathogenesis and progression of CHF.[65,67] By retarding its deleterious effects, β-blockade ultimately improves systolic function despite the attendant negative inotropic effect. Longer-term actions of BBs include regression of myocardial hypertrophy, reversal of remodeling, and normalization of ventricular geometry. The antioxidant properties of some BBs, including carvedilol, may also contribute to their beneficial effects. In human cardiovascular medicine, second- and third-generation BBs are used in combination with diuretics and ACEI for treatment of chronic, stable CHF related to left ventricular systolic dysfunction (including DCM).[61,63,65,67]

In dogs, these drugs have also garnered interest as adjunctive treatment for CHF, although their efficacy has not yet been established.[62,67,88] BBs and ACEI are also used in humans to prevent HF in cases with structural cardiac abnormalities (eg, left ventricular hypertrophy, valvular disease) and systolic dysfunction that are as yet asymptomatic.[61] Similarly, BBs have been suggested as part of treatment for preclinical chronic degenerative AV valve disease (CVD) and preclinical DCM in dogs, as they might delay progression to HF.[62]

The beneficial effects of BBs have been documented in avian models of HF.[27,32–34] The author suggests that BBs may have application in avian cardiology as adjunctive treatment of CHF, provided the condition is first stabilized using conventional management strategies. The author has used carvedilol, in conjunction with diuretics and an ACEI, as part of treatment for CHF in psittacines, specifically when concentric ventricular hypertrophy, tachycardia, and diastolic dysfunction were features. Concurrent administration of a positive inotrope (eg, pimobendan) during the period of BB uptitration may allow patients to tolerate initiation of treatment.

For detailed information on the avian pharmacologic data, potential indications, goals and guidelines for use, and contraindications and adverse effects of BB, please see Refs.[56,83]

Calcium channel blockers

CCBs, including nifedipine, verapamil, diltiazem, and amlodipine, inhibit influx of extracellular calcium ions across cardiomyocyte and vascular smooth muscle cell membranes, thereby inhibiting contraction. Effects are negative inotropy and chronotropy, slowing of the sinus rate and AV nodal conduction, and vasodilation. CCBs are classified by their relative selectivity for the vasculature or for the myocardium; those that predominately promote peripheral vasodilation and reduce total peripheral resistance (eg, nifedipine and amlodipine) are indicated primarily for treatment of hypertension, and those that influence conduction (eg, verapamil and diltiazem) are indicated for treatment of supraventricular tachyarrhythmias.[12,35,91–93] Adverse effects of CCBs include bradycardia, hypotension and reflex tachycardia, and AV block.[35,91–93] Contraindications include sinoatrial (SA) nodal dysfunction, second- or third-degree AV block, and decompensated HF.[35,92,93]

In human patients with HF with systolic dysfunction, CCBs confer no survival benefit and may exacerbate the condition.[61] Nevertheless, CCBs warrant mention because their cardioprotective effects have been investigated in avian models of HF and found to rival those of BBs.[33,36,37,94] Both nifedipine and verapamil are cardioprotective (nifedipine > verapamil), but the mechanisms by which these drugs confer their benefits are unknown.[33,94] There is one case series of 5 psittacine birds treated with amlodipine for presumed systemic hypertension (see the following section).[12]

Treatment of Related Conditions

CHF may be accompanied by disease processes such as HCM, systemic and/or PH, and arrhythmias.

Hypertrophic cardiomyopathy

HCM comprises hyperplasia or thickening of individual muscle fibers of the heart. HCM in pet birds is usually secondary to pressure overload states (cardiomyopathy of overload), including arterial luminal stenosis owing to advanced atherosclerosis, and PH.[3,25,55,59,95,96] As in mammals, the affected ventricle or ventricles ultimately undergo concentric hypertrophy, in which the ventricular wall thickens with a corresponding decrease in chamber volume. Eventual ischemia of the hypertrophied myocardium results in fibrosis and increased collagen content, impairing both systolic and diastolic function.[53,54] Analogous conditions in human and small animal medicine are ventricular outflow obstructions, such as subvalvular aortic stenosis and primary HCM to include the obstructive type characterized by systolic anterior motion of the mitral valve. BBs are used in treatment of these conditions; their potential benefit is based on reduction of heart rate and myocardial oxygen consumption, as well as improved diastolic filling and coronary artery flow.[62,97] However, in cats, evidence of their efficacy is scarce, with little to no indication that they improve survival in patients with CHF.[62,98]

Anecdotally, BBs can have merit for treatment of HCM in birds. The author has used carvedilol, with or without an ACEI inhibitor, in a small number of psittacines with suspected atherosclerotic disease and concentric ventricular hypertrophy that had not yet progressed to failure. In each of these cases, there has been symptomatic improvement in the form of increased energy and activity level, appetite, and body weight. In the case of a 34-year-old, female yellow-naped Amazon parrot (see **Table 2**), there was marked concentric hypertrophy of both ventricles, diastolic dysfunction, and sinus tachycardia. Following initial management with standard therapy, clinical status deteriorated, and carvedilol was added to the treatment regime; pimobendan was discontinued. Following these changes, rapid and marked clinical improvement was seen, and the patient remained stable for an additional 7 months.

Systemic hypertension

Systemic hypertension occurs in poultry species and can result in severe ventricular hypertrophy and CHF.[99] Although not defined in psittacines, systemic hypertension is likely also a disease entity in this group.[12,100,101] In human and small animal medicine, BBs are often used in conjunction with ACEI, CCBs, and/or diuretics to reduce arterial blood pressure (BP).[61,62,102] In humans, such treatment markedly reduces the risk of developing HF, and combined therapy with a BB and ACEI is recommended in cases of diastolic HF with concurrent hypertension.[61] In cats, the CCB amlodipine is the treatment of choice for systemic hypertension; it has been shown to significantly reduce BP, and in one study, resolved secondary ventricular hypertrophy in 50% of subjects.[12,102]

In companion birds, application of BBs, CCBs, or other antihypertensive drugs for treatment of systemic hypertension is complicated by the fact that there is no practical means to obtain accurate and repeatable arterial BP measurements in the clinical setting and no established definition of hypertension exists.[12,103–105] Direct BP measurement, although accurate, requires invasive techniques; indirect BP measurements do not seem to correlate well with direct arterial BPs in birds.[12,103,104] However, if in select cases, BP measurements are obtained and support a diagnosis of hypertension (direct systolic BP > 240 mm Hg; indirect systolic BP consistently ≥270 mm Hg),[12,100,106] combined treatment of an ACEI with a BB or a CCB may be considered.

Recently, Fink and Mans[12] published a case series of 5 companion psittacine birds treated with amlodipine for presumed systemic hypertension (see **Table 1**). Clinical signs and physical examination abnormalities included lethargy, ataxia, seizures, lameness, blindness, heart murmur, tachycardia, and bradycardia. Hypertension was diagnosed on the basis of indirect BP measurements (taken under sedation) exceeding 200 mm Hg. Amlodipine was used together with enalapril in 2 cases. There were owner-reported clinical improvements for all cases, and indirect BP measurements decreased by 10% to 43%. It should be noted that the methodology used for indirect BP measurement (cuff size, placement, and location) were not always consistent between visits, which could account to some degree for the variability of values obtained.[12,105]

Pulmonary hypertension

Compared with mammals, birds are thought to have a greater propensity for developing PH and right-sided, rather than left-sided CHF owing to the morphology of the right AV valve, less deformable nucleated erythrocytes, and the rigid, nondistensible lungs, which limit the ability of the blood capillaries to expand and accommodate greater blood flow.[55,81] PH can result from pulmonary vascular disease (to include atherosclerosis), chronic pulmonary disease and/or hypoxia, congenital left-to-right shunts, or left-sided heart disease and failure.[3,16,25,55,59,78,70,05,90] Secondary polycythemia, which develops as a consequence of chronic hypoxemia, can be a complicating factor in many disease conditions, including PH. Increased blood viscosity and larger and less deformable erythrocytes result in increased resistance to blood flow in the lung and other tissues.[16,36,37,95,96,107–109]

The known or hypothesized underlying cause or causes of PH should be addressed, if possible, but pulmonary vasodilators (sildenafil), CCBs, pentoxifylline, and periodic phlebotomy may have symptomatic benefit in birds with a presumptive or definitive diagnosis of PH.[16] Similarly, the inclusion of these drugs should be considered in the treatment of patients with CHF with cor pulmonale.

Pulmonary Vasodilators

Sildenafil is a selective pulmonary vasodilator that acts by specifically inhibiting phosphodiesterase V, an enzyme that degrades cyclic guanosine monophosphate (cGMP) in pulmonary vascular smooth muscle cells. The resulting increase in cGMP enhances nitric oxide–mediated pulmonary vasodilation, thereby reducing pulmonary vascular resistance and right ventricular afterload. The drug does not typically lower systemic arterial BP or alter heart rate.[78–80,110,111] Its hypotensive effects may be increased upon concurrent use of α-adrenoceptor blockers, amlodipine, or other hypotensive drugs. In addition, its metabolism may be reduced by administration of azole antifungals.[80] In humans and dogs, sildenafil is an effective treatment for PH[78–80,110,111] and has been shown to improve quality of life and mitigate secondary polycythemia in dogs.[78,80,110]

Prolonged (>15 months) use of sildenafil (2.5–3 mg/kg by mouth every 8 hours), in addition to therapeutic phlebotomy and supplemental oxygen, resolved clinical signs (lethargy, anorexia, ataxia, tachypnea/dyspnea, and oxygen dependence) in a 25-year-old, male mealy Amazon parrot (*Amazona farinosa*) with suspected PH and secondary, absolute polycythemia.[16] The author has treated an unknown-age, female rose-breasted cockatoo (*Eolophus roseicapilla*) with suspected PH, in which clinical signs (lethargy and exercise intolerance) rapidly resolved with administration of sildenafil (2 mg/kg by mouth every 12 hours) and enalapril (3 mg/kg by mouth every 12 hours). Over a period of 1 year, doses of both drugs were gradually increased to 5 mg/kg by mouth every 12 hours. Right ventricular hypertrophy decreased 6 months into treatment.

Other Treatment Options

Patients with suspected PH may also benefit from an ACEI,[74,112–114] pimobendan,[30,79,84] CCBs,[36,37] pentoxifylline, and therapeutic phlebotomy.[16,97] Pentoxifylline, a methylxanthine derivative, increases flexibility and deformability of erythrocytes and leukocytes and decreases blood viscosity in mammals. It thereby promotes blood flow through damaged or occluded microvasculature[38,115,116] and thus may have merit in avian patients with PH and secondary polycythemia and hyperviscosity syndrome. For more on these therapeutic options, please see Ref.[83]

Arrhythmias

Cardiac arrhythmias range from clinically insignificant to life-threatening, and/or terminal events.[11,17,26,39,91,117–123] Clinical signs may be absent or include weakness, syncope, or sudden death. Arrhythmias rarely constitute a primary disease process; they can develop secondary to cardiac chamber dilatation, myocarditis, or cardiomyopathy of any cause, as well as toxicoses, nutritional deficiencies, electrolyte imbalances, and various anesthetic agents.[11,26,91,118,119] They can be potentiated by catecholamine release as occurs with handling stress and painful conditions.[26,120,121] Clinically significant cardiac arrhythmias likely represent the minority, but those that are symptomatic, causing hemodynamic instability, and complicating or precipitating HF warrant characterization and appropriate treatment.[61,91] To date, reports of antiarrhythmic therapy in birds are extremely few.

Treatment of Tachyarrhythmias

Aside from digoxin, BBs and CCBs are used in small animal cardiology for treatment of supraventricular tachyarrhythmias, including atrial fibrillation, in order to slow the ventricular response rate.[91] Their use is generally contraindicated in patients with acute or decompensated CHF unless the arrhythmia is contributing to the condition such that conventional treatment alone has failed to stabilize the patient.[35,91–93] Even in this scenario, these drugs must be used with great caution, beginning at low dosages, with the aim of decreasing ventricular rate only marginally.[91]

Sotalol was used to control supraventricular tachycardia in a 19-year-old golden eagle (see **Table 1**) with marked left atrial and ventricular dilatation, marked left ventricular systolic dysfunction, and stenosis of the right brachiocephalic trunk (most consistent with an atherosclerotic lesion). Sotalol was used in conjunction with isoxsuprine and pimobendan, resulting in resolution of the arrhythmia and restoration of normal chamber sizes and systolic function.[11]

Lidocaine is a parenteral antiarrhythmic agent used to control life-threatening ventricular tachyarrhythmias.[91] At usual doses, there is minimal effect on the cardiac conduction system or on myocardial contractility.[91,124] To the author's knowledge, there are no reports describing its use for treatment of tachyarrhythmias in avian species, but its pharmacokinetics and cardiovascular effects have been evaluated during experimental studies.[40–42]

Treatment of Bradyarrhythmias

Bradyarrhythmias, and in particular, second- and third-degree AV block, have been noted in birds with cardiac disease.[17,26,119] Escape beats and escape rhythms may be seen with severe bradyarrhythmias; they are of ectopic origin and perform an essential salvage function by preventing asystole at low heart rates. QRS morphology of ventricular escape beats may be abnormal (wide and bizarre), but these should not be confused with premature beats (additional beats added to already normal or rapid heart rate), because in the case of escape beats, antiarrhythmic therapy is contraindicated.[91,119]

Antimuscarinic agents, including atropine and glycopyrrolate, can be used for both the diagnosis and the treatment of bradycardias related to increased vagal tone, including SA arrest and first- and second-degree AV block.[25,43,59,125] They are also used as antidotes for organophosphate and carbamate intoxication.[43,125] These drugs are contraindicated in patients with tachycardia or tachyarrhythmias and must be used cautiously in patients with HF. Because the activity of atropine and glycopyrrolate is short lived, they are mainly used during treatment of bradycardia during anesthesia. For long-term use, propantheline, an oral antimuscarinic agent, has been used to normalize heart rate and rhythm in a 30-year-old Moluccan cockatoo (*Cacatua moluccensis*) with second-degree AV block (Mobitz type 2).[17]

Supportive Care and Husbandry Considerations

Along with medical management of CHF, it is often necessary to address concurrent problems and meet specific supportive needs. Patients may be presented in a severely debilitated state, with cachexia, dehydration, secondary renal dysfunction, and injuries. In addition to rest and judicious, limited handling and restraint to minimize stress, inpatient supportive care measures may include oxygen supplementation, nutritional support, fluid therapy (although parenteral fluid administration must be carefully questioned), and analgesia. Once the patient has been stabilized and discharged, longer-term management strategies should also incorporate exercise restriction, housing modifications, and dietary and lifestyle changes.

Supportive care

Avian patients with HF are typically dyspneic because of pulmonary edema, intracoelomic air sac compression by ascitic fluid, and/or pericardial effusion. Oxygen supplementation is indicated for patients with pulmonary edema, whereas physical fluid removal is more efficacious to stabilize those with air sac compression and cardiac tamponade.

Coelomocentesis will rapidly relieve air sac compression in the case of ascites. It is justified as a short-term stabilization strategy in patients with severe respiratory compromise. When large fluid volumes are present, the procedure can be performed relatively safely with (ideally) or without ultrasound guidance. Small fluid volumes will usually resolve with medical management alone without the need for physical fluid removal. Although coelomocentesis can be performed periodically over the long term, it should not be substituted for pharmacologic management.

Fluid therapy challenges

Maintaining the delicate balance between management of hypervolemia and concurrent dehydration and renal dysfunction is a profound clinical challenge, requiring close monitoring for changes in clinical status and adjustment of the treatment plan accordingly. Fluid therapy is generally not indicated in the treatment of CHF, where a primary, immediate goal is reduction of fluid overload. Initial treatment of acute and decompensated CHF frequently results in some degree of dehydration and prerenal azotemia, but these abnormalities can resolve over a few days without fluid therapy once food and water intake have normalized.

In cases with persistent, severe azotemia, it may be necessary to administer small volumes of parenteral fluids, but patients for which hemodynamic stability cannot be achieved without severe renal compromise have a poor prognosis. Subcutaneous fluid absorption may fail in cases of right-sided CHF.

Exercise restriction and housing
Weakness and ataxia may limit patient mobility and access to food and water and predispose to falls. This necessitates housing modifications designed to limit exertion and allow easy, immediate access to food and water. As even debilitated birds will often persist in trying to climb or perch, enclosures that prevent or limit this activity are ideal. Incubators, aquarium setups, or plastic or acrylic bins with a soft substrate serve this purpose well and permit visual monitoring. Depending on patient strength and stability, a low, secure, and stable perch can be provided. Once the patient regains strength and exercise tolerance, housing can be adjusted to allow greater activity (eg, small cage or crate, furnished with low perches and readily accessible dishes); some patients will ultimately be able to return to a traditional cage with no specific exercise restrictions.

Diet and lifestyle
Longer-term husbandry considerations, including dietary changes (to include optimum nutrition and sodium restriction) and lifestyle changes, mirror those discussed for atherosclerosis. Dietary changes should not be made until the patient is well stabilized.

Other
Considering that most patients will require long-term (if not life-long) medical management, operant learning methods and food vehicles should be used to facilitate low-stress medication administration.[126]

Inpatient Versus Outpatient Care and Follow-Up Considerations
Patients with acute and decompensated CHF should be hospitalized for initial treatment. Inpatient care should be continued until the patient has been stabilized to the extent that appetite and water intake are acceptable, hypervolemia is adequately controlled and hydration is adequate, oxygen supplementation is no longer needed, and parenteral medications are withdrawn.

Following discharge, effective long-term management requires close monitoring and regular follow-up in order to reevaluate patient status and make adjustments to the treatment regime accordingly. Follow-up should include physical examination, repeat radiographic and/or ultrasonographic imaging, and biochemical and hematologic monitoring. Most patients with CHF should have their first follow-up visit 1 week after discharge. Depending on patient progress and stability, the frequency of recheck visits can be progressively reduced to 3- or 6-month intervals. Treatment success is dependent in large part on owner compliance, so thorough client education and regular communication are essential.

Prognostic Considerations and Setting Client Expectations
The prognostic picture must be critically assessed on a case-by-case basis. The long-term prognosis is guarded to poor in most cases given that the condition is often incurable and can only be managed for a finite period of time. The therapeutic objectives

---

Box 2
Client discussion points regarding prognostic picture, treatment goals, and expectations

- Owners should be made aware, from the outset, that successful treatment will almost always require intensive, inpatient care initially and close monitoring, regular communication, and follow-up once the patient is discharged
  - In most situations, treatment represents a significant financial investment, both initially and over the long term
  - In most cases the patient will require ongoing medical treatment lifelong; some of the required medications may be costly
  - Regular reassessment and adjustment of the treatment plan will be needed as the patient condition changes and progresses
  - Dietary and husbandry changes may be recommended in accordance with patient stability and the specific aspects of their condition
- Owners must understand that individual response to treatment is highly variable and difficult to predict
  - Some patients cannot be stabilized even with appropriate intensive treatment
  - Some patients may stabilize initially, but their stability cannot be maintained
  - Patients responding favorably to treatment may remain stable for only a matter of weeks to as long as several years

---

are to maintain quality of life and extend survival time, with the understanding that most patients will ultimately become refractory to treatment. Patients that exhibit a fair-poor response to initial intensive therapy or fail to maintain stability once treatment is transitioned to an (oral) maintenance strategy have a poorer prognosis. Furthermore, if hemodynamic stability cannot be achieved without severe renal compromise, the prognosis should be considered grave. As soon as CHF is diagnosed, the prognostic picture should be openly discussed with the pet bird owner and treatment goals explained (**Box 2**).

PERICARDIAL EFFUSION/CARDIAC TAMPONADE

Pericardial effusion is characterized by an inappropriate accumulation of fluid within the pericardial sac. Possible causes are listed in **Box 3**, although in some cases an underlying cause cannot be identified, and the condition is ruled idiopathic. Severe pericardial effusion or restrictive pericarditis can compress the heart, resulting in impaired ventricular filling (diastolic dysfunction), and subsequent decreases in stroke volume and cardiac output. This condition (cardiac tamponade) can become life-

---

Box 3
Causes of pericardial effusion in birds[18,56]

Infectious pericarditis

Noninfectious pericarditis (visceral gout)

Right-sided CHF

Hemopericardium (trauma, aneurismal rupture, coagulopathy)

Cardiac or pericardial neoplasia

Metabolic derangements (eg, hypoproteinemia)

Toxic causes

threatening. Because the intramural pressure of the thinner-walled right ventricle is overcome more rapidly than that of the left, cardiac tamponade results more quickly in right-sided CHF than in left-sided failure.[26,127]

Treatment for pericardial effusion and cardiac tamponade is based first on removal of the fluid, and second on treatment of the underlying cause of fluid accumulation.[25,26,127,128] Fluid removal can be accomplished either by ultrasound-guided[7,18,25,29] or endoscopic pericardiocentesis or by endoscopic or surgical fenestration of the pericardium.[26,59,128,129]

Although diuretics are generally contraindicated in cardiac tamponade because they decrease the preload necessary to maintain ventricular filling pressure and cardiac output, furosemide with or without an ACEI may be useful to reduce pericardial fluid of low volume related to CHF in birds.[8,13,25,26,29]

ATHEROSCLEROTIC DISEASE

Atherosclerosis is a chronic inflammatory and degenerative disease of the arterial wall wherein the lumen narrows by progressive accumulation of fibrofatty atheromatous plaques within the intima. Advanced lesions are characterized by severe arterial stenosis and occlusion, and by calcification and osseous metaplasia. Atherosclerosis is likely an underlying factor in most noninfectious cardiovascular diseases in pet birds. Prevalence is highest in gray parrots (Psittacus spp), Amazon parrots (Amazona spp), and cockatiels (Nymphicus hollandicus). Other risk factors include increasing age, female sex and female reproductive activity, high-calorie, fat, and cholesterol diets, dyslipidemia (eg, hypercholesterolemia, hypertriglyceridemia), and limited physical activity.[101,130–137]

Clinical signs are attributed to advanced lesions, whereas early and intermediate lesions are generally silent and subclinical. Unlike humans, recognizable clinical disease is primarily the product of progressive, flow-limiting arterial stenosis rather than thromboembolism and acute arterial obstruction.[101,130,131,133] Clinical signs vary depending on the vessels affected, severity of atherosclerotic lesions, and presence of concurrent disease, including cardiac disease and CHF.[101,132] Patients often present for falling or collapse, frequently accompanied by transient or persistent weakness and dysfunction of one or more limbs. Exercise-induced intermittent weakness and pain in the pelvic limbs, resolving with rest, is termed intermittent claudication.[10,20,95,138,139] There may be persistent neurologic abnormalities identified on physical examination, including reduced mentation, blindness, anisocoria, seizures, vestibular signs, paresis of one or both pelvic limbs, and ataxia. These signs are considered most consistent with stroke, but rarely is this confirmed diagnostically.[9,101]

Treatment of atherosclerosis involves both controlling risk factors and managing sequelae, including peripheral hypoperfusion, intermittent claudication, ischemic stroke, and CHF.[11,101] Atherosclerotic lesions cannot be resolved, but diet, husbandry, and lifestyle changes may help to prevent, slow progression, or decrease the size of lesions.[101,133–135] Medical management focuses primarily on improving peripheral perfusion. Peripheral vasodilators, used either singly or in combination, may have symptomatic benefit by decreasing vascular resistance and reducing afterload.

Vasodilation

Isoxsuprine
Isoxsuprine is a peripheral vasodilator that causes vascular smooth muscle relaxation predominately through α-adrenoceptor blockade.[140,141] To a much lesser degree, it is

a β-adrenoreceptor agonist and as such may have positive chronotropic and inotropic effects (via β-1 adrenoreceptors) and further vasodilatory effects (via β-2 adrenoreceptors).[140–142] Isoxsuprine is known to increase erythrocyte deformability in humans.[143] In veterinary medicine, isoxsuprine is used to increase peripheral blood flow in horses with vascular disorders of the lower limb and to address trauma-induced wingtip edema in raptors.[20,44] In a published report (see **Table 1**), a 35-year-old yellow-naped Amazon parrot with presumptive atherosclerosis was treated with isoxsuprine. Clinical signs of lethargy, weakness, hyporexia, weak grip, and ataxia resolved with treatment, recurred when the drug was discontinued, and again resolved once it was reinstituted.[20] The author has observed similar, apparent symptomatic improvement when using isoxsuprine (10–15 mg/kg by mouth every 12 hours) in numerous cases of clinical, presumed atherosclerosis (some of which were later confirmed at necropsy and by histopathology). Many of these patients have been treated and followed for several months to several years, over which time frequency and severity of stroke-like events, intermittent claudication episodes, and other clinical signs appeared to decrease.

Angiotensin-converting enzyme inhibitors
ACEI, including enalapril, result in vasodilation by blocking the formation of AII.[73,74] AII promotes vasoconstriction and venoconstriction by mediating release of catecholamines, which act on the vascular smooth muscle via α-adrenergic receptors.[144] By blocking formation of AII, ACEI reduce both total peripheral resistance and pulmonary vascular resistance.[74] Although the relative vasodilatory effect of an ACEI compared with isoxsuprine in birds is not known, it is conceivable that the 2 used in combination would have synergistic effects: an ACEI by limiting α-adrenoreceptor stimulation and isoxsuprine by α-adrenoreceptor antagonism. The author has treated patients with clinical (presumed) atherosclerotic disease using enalapril at a dose and frequency of 1.25 to 5 mg/kg by mouth every 8 to 12 hours. In more severe cases, this is paired with isoxsuprine.

Sildenafil
Sildenafil has predominantly been used for the treatment of PH in humans and dogs.[78–80,110,111] In birds, the drug may have merit in cases with suspected atherosclerosis of the pulmonary arteries, potentially in combination with other vasodilators.

Other Medical Managements

Pentoxifylline
In human medicine, pentoxifylline has been used for treatment of peripheral vascular and cerebrovascular disease by improving microcirculatory blood flow.[38,115,116] In small mammal models, the drug was found to increase tissue perfusion, mitigate inflammation, and attenuate atherosclerotic plaque formation.[38,115] Thus, pentoxifylline may have value in improving peripheral perfusion in birds with atherosclerotic disease, including those with concurrent polycythemia.[38,45,115] The author has used it for these indications in numerous psittacine patients (15–25 mg/kg by mouth every 8–12 hours).

Statins
Statins are a group of lipid-lowering drugs used extensively in human medicine for their antiatherosclerotic effects through inhibition of cholesterol synthesis and other mechanisms. Several products are commercially available for human use, including atorvastatin (Lipitor) and rosuvastatin (Crestor).[145] Statins have been used empirically in psittacine birds, but their use is controversial because target lipid levels that would

reduce atherosclerosis risk are unestablished,[136] and because their efficacy is not supported by available pharmacodynamic and pharmacokinetic data.[146,147] Consequently, the author does not recommend use of statins in psittacines considered either to have or to be at risk for atherosclerotic disease. Instead, vasodilatory therapy (for symptomatic patients) and dietary and lifestyle changes to prevent and address dyslipidemia are more appropriate.

Supportive Care and Husbandry Considerations

Supportive care

Patients with signs of stroke may have marked neurologic deficits to include reduced mentation, limb paresis, and ataxia that prevent normal eating and drinking and impair mobility. They may experience seizures or suffer injuries from falls. Supportive care measures to consider for these patients include fluid and nutritional support, analgesia, anticonvulsant therapy when needed, and management of secondary conditions, such as trauma and aspiration pneumonia. The benzodiazepines diazepam (0.5–2 mg/kg IM) or midazolam (1–2 mg/kg IM) can be used for emergency control of seizures.[57] Options for longer-term anticonvulsant therapy are levetiracetam (50–150 mg/kg by mouth every 8–12 hours), zonisamide (20 mg/kg by mouth every 8–12 hours), and gabapentin (15–20 mg/kg by mouth every 8–12 hours).[9,148–153] The author has used levetiracetam alone or in combination with zonisamide and gabapentin to control seizure activity in psittacine birds with severe atherosclerotic disease.

Exercise restriction versus promotion of exercise

For patients with advanced, clinical atherosclerotic disease, exercise restriction should be part of the longer-term treatment plan, as well as appropriate housing modifications to accommodate and protect birds with persistent deficits. In contrast, increasing opportunities for exercise (especially flight) from early in life may have preventative value.[101,154]

Dietary management

Dietary management to avoid dyslipidemia may have both therapeutic and preventative value, particularly for at-risk species. Such measures include the following[101,133–135,155]:

- Moderation of dietary calories and fat and prevention and resolution of obesity
- Provision of formulated (rather than seed-based) diets, supplemented with fresh vegetables and fruits
- Avoidance of dietary sources of cholesterol (animal-based products)
- Supplementation with omega-3 fatty acids, particularly α-linolenic acid (found in flaxseed oil), has been shown to improve lipid metabolism, reduce inflammation, and minimize development (or slow progression) of atherosclerosis in several avian species[156–159]

Other

Along with dietary changes, control of female reproductive activity may help prevent atherosclerotic disease.[56,134]

DISCLOSURE

The author has nothing to disclose.

REFERENCES

1. Knafo SE, Rapoport G, Williams J, et al. Cardiomyopathy and right-sided congestive heart failure in a red-tailed hawk (*Buteo jamaicensis*). J Avian Med Surg 2011;25(1):32–9.
2. Ensley PK, Hatkin J, Silverman S. Congestive heart failure in a greater hill mynah. J Am Vet Med Assoc 1979;175(9):1010–3.
3. Phalen DN, Hays HB, Filippich LJ, et al. Heart failure in a macaw with atherosclerosis of the aorta and brachiocephalic arteries. J Am Vet Med Assoc 1996;209:1435–40.
4. Sedacca CD, Campbell TW, Bright JM, et al. Chronic cor pulmonale secondary to pulmonary atherosclerosis in an African grey parrot. J Am Vet Med Assoc 2009;234(8):1055–9.
5. Oglesbee BL, Lehmkuhl L. Congestive heart failure associated with myxomatous degeneration of the left atrioventricular valve in a parakeet. J Am Vet Med Assoc 2001;218(3):376–80, 360.
6. Mitchell EB, Hawkins MG, Orvalho JS, et al. Congenital mitral stenosis, subvalvular aortic stenosis, and congestive heart failure in a duck. J Vet Cardiol 2008; 10(1):67–73.
7. Straub J, Pees M, Enders F, et al. Pericardiocentesis and the use of enalapril in a Fischer's lovebird (*Agapornis fischeri*). Vet Rec 2003;152:24–6.
8. Pees M, Schmidt V, Coles B, et al. Diagnosis and long-term therapy of right-sided heart failure in a yellow-crowned Amazon (*Amazona ochrocephala*). Vet Rec 2006;158(13):445–7
9. Beaufrere H, Nevarez J, Gaschen L, et al. Diagnosis of presumed acute ischemic stroke and associated seizure management in a Congo African grey parrot. J Am Vet Med Assoc 2011;239(1):122–8.
10. Beaufrere H, Holder KA, Bauer R, et al. Intermittent claudication-like syndrome secondary to atherosclerosis in a yellow naped Amazon parrot (*Amazona ochrocephala auropalliata*). J Avian Med Surg 2011;25(4):266–76.
11. Oster SC, Jung SW, Moon R. Resolution of supraventricular arrhythmia using sotalol in an adult golden eagle (*Aquila chrysaetos*) with presumed atherosclerosis. J Exot Pet Med 2019;29:136–41.
12. Fink DM, Mans C. Use of amlodipine in psittacine birds: 5 cases (2010-2018). J Avian Med Surg 2021;35(2):155–60.
13. Pees M, Straub J, Krautwald-Junghanns ME. Insufficiency of the muscular atrioventricular valve in the heart of a blue-fronted Amazon (*Amazona aestiva aestiva*). Vet Rec 2001;148:540–3.
14. Rosenthal K, Stamoulis M. Diagnosis of congestive heart failure in an Indian hill mynah bird (*Gracula religiosa*). J Assoc Avian Vet 1993;7(1):27–30.
15. Brandao J, Reynolds CA, Beaufrere H, et al. Cardiomyopathy in a Harris hawk (*Parabuteo unicinctus*). J Am Vet Med Assoc 2016;249:221–7.
16. Brady SM, Burgdorf-Moisuk A, Silverman S, et al. Successful treatment of suspected pulmonary arterial hypertension in a mealy Amazon parrot (*Amazona farinosa*). J Avian Med Surg 2016;30:368–73.
17. Van Zeeland Y, Schoemaker N, Lumeij J. Syncopes associated with second degree atrioventricular block in a cockatoo. In: Proc Annu Conf Assoc Avian Vet. 2010:345–346.
18. McCleery B, Jones MP, Manasse J, et al. Pericardial mesothelioma in a yellow-naped Amazon parrot (*Amazona auropalliata*). J Avian Med Surg 2015;29: 55–62.

19. Grosset C, Guzman DS, Keating MK, et al. Central vestibular disease in a blue and gold macaw (*Ara ararauna*) with cerebral infarction and hemorrhage. J Avian Med Surg 2014;28:132–42.

20. Simone-Freilicher E. Use of isoxsuprine for treatment of clinical signs associated with presumptive atherosclerosis in a yellow-naped Amazon parrot (*Amazona ochrocephala auropalliata*). J Avian Med Surg 2007;21(3):215–9.

21. Cusack L, Field C, McDermott A, et al. Right heart failure in an African penguin (*Spheniscus demersus*). J Avian Med Surg 2016;30:243–9.

22. McNaughton A, Frasa S Jr, Mishra N, et al. Valvular dysplasia and congestive heart failure in a juvenile African penguin (*Spheniscus demersus*). J Zoo Wildl Med 2014;45:987–90.

23. Baine K. Atypical heart disease in an umbrella cockatoo. In: Proc Annu Conf Assoc Avian Vet. 2012:285.

24. Beehler B, Montali R, Bush M. Mitral valve insufficiency with congestive heart failure in a pukeko. J Am Vet Med Assoc 1980;177:934–7.

25. Pees M, Krautwald-Junghanns ME, Straub J. Evaluating and treating the cardiovascular system. In: Harrison GJ, Lightfoot TL, editors. Clinical avian medicine, Vol 1. Palm Beach (FL): Spix Publishing; 2006. p. 379–94.

26. Lumeij J, Ritchie B. Cardiology. In: Ritchie BW, Harrison GJ, Harrison LR, editors. Avian medicine: principles and applications. Lake Worth (FL): Wingers Publishing; 1994. p. 695–722.

27. Okafor CC, Perreault-Micale C, Hajjar RJ, et al. Chronic treatment with carvedilol improves ventricular function and reduces myocyte apoptosis in an animal model of heart failure. BMC Physiol 2003;3:6.

28. Esfandiary A, Rajaian H, Asasi K, et al. Diuretic effects of several chemical and herbal compounds in adult laying hens. Int J Poult Sci 2010;9(3):247–53.

29. Pees M, Kuhring K, Demiraij F, et al. Bioavailability and compatibility of enalapril in birds. In: Proc Annu Assoc Avian Med. 2006:7–11.

30. Guzman DS, Beaufrere H, KuKanich B, et al. Pharmacokinetics of single oral dose of pimobendan in Hispaniolan Amazon parrots (*Amazona ventralis*). J Avian Med Surg 2014;28(2):95–101.

31. Beaufrere H, Aertsens A, Fouquet J. Un cas d'insuffisance cardiaque congestive chez un perroquet gris. L'Hebdo Vet 2007;200:8–10.

32. Gwathmey JK. Morphological changes associated with furazolidone-induced cardiomyopathy: effects of digoxin and propranolol. J Comp Path 1991;104:33–45.

33. Glass MG, Fuleihan F, Liao R, et al. Differences in cardioprotective efficacy of adrenergic receptor antagonists and Ca^{2+} channel antagonists in an animal model of dilated cardiomyopathy. Circ Res 1993;73(6):1077–89.

34. Gwathmey JK, Kim CS, Hajjar RJ, et al. Cellular and molecular remodeling in a heart failure model treated with the β-blocker carteolol. Am J Phys 1999;276:H1678–90.

35. Plumb DC. Diltiazem HCl. In: Plumb DC, editor. Plumb's veterinary drug handbook. 9th edition. Stockholm (WI): John Wiley & Sons; 2018. p. 518–21.

36. Yang Y, Gao M, Guo Y, et al. Calcium antagonists, diltiazem and nifedipine, protect broilers against low temperature-induced pulmonary hypertension and pulmonary vascular remodeling. Anim Sci J 2010;81:494–500.

37. Yang Y, Qiao J, Wang H, et al. Calcium antagonist verapamil prevented pulmonary arterial hypertension in broilers with ascites by arresting pulmonary vascular remodeling. Eur J Pharmacol 2007;561:137–43.

38. Wellehan JFX. Frostbite in birds: pathophysioloy and treatment. Compend Contin Educ practicing veterinarian 2003;25:776–81.

39. Schnellbacher RW, da Cunha AF, Beaufrère H, et al. Effects of dopamine and dobutamine on isoflurane-induced hypotension in Hispaniolan Amazon parrots (*Amazona ventralis*). Am J Vet Res 2012;73(7):952–8.

40. da Cunha AF, et al. Pharmacokinetics/pharmacodynamics of bupivacaine and lidocaine in chickens. In Proc Annu Conf Assoc Avian Vet. 2011; p. 313.

41. da Cunha AF, et al. Pharmacokinetics and pharmacodynamics of lidocaine in Hispaniolan Amazon parrots (Amazona ventralis). In: Proc Annu Conf Assoc Avian Vet. 2012:313.

42. Brandao J, da Cunha AF, Pypendop B, et al. Cardiovascular tolerance of intravenous lidocaine in broiler chickens (*Gallus gallus domesticus*) anesthetized with isoflurane. Vet Anaesth Analg 2014;42(4):442–8.

43. Plumb DC. Glycopyrrolate. In: Plumb DC, editor. Plumb's veterinary drug handbook. 9th edition. Stockholm (WI): John Wiley & Sons; 2018. p. 765–8.

44. Lewis JC, Storm J, Greenwood AG. Treatment of wing tip oedema in raptors. Vet Rec 1993;133(13):328.

45. Martel-Arquette A, Mans C, Sladky K. Management of severe frostbite in a grey headed parrot (*Poicephalus fuscicollis suahelicus*). J Avian Med Surg 2016;30:39–45.

46. Hawkins MG, Guzman DSM, Beaufere H, et al. Birds. In: Carpenter J, Marion C, editors. Exotic animal formulary. 5th edition. St. Louis (MO): Elsevier; 2018. p. 198–398.

47. Ritchie BW, Harrison GJ. Formulary. In: Ritchie BW, Harrison GJ, Harrison LR, editors. Avian medicine: principles and application. Lake Worth (FL): Wingers Publishing, Inc; 1994. p. 457–78.

48. Hamlin R, Stalnaker P. Basis for use of digoxin in small birds. J Vet Pharmacol Ther 1987;10(4):354–6.

49. Wilson R, Zenoble R, Horton C, et al. Single dose digoxin pharmacokinetics in the Quaker conure (*Myiopsitta monachus*). J Zoo Wildl Med 1989;20(4):432–4.

50. Alvarez Maldonado MVZ. Reporte preeliminar: digitalizacion en pollos de engorda como metodo preventivo en el syndrome ascitico. Proc 35th West. Poult Dis Conf 1986.

51. Pedersoli WM, Ravis WR, Lee HS, et al. Pharmacokinetics of single doses of digoxin administered intravenously to ducks, roosters, and turkeys. Am J Vet Res 1990;51(11):1751–5.

52. Krautwald-Junghanns ME, Braun S, Pees M, et al. Research on the anatomy and pathology of the psittacine heart. J Avian Med Surg 2004;18:2–11.

53. de Morais HA, Schwartz DS. Pathophysiology of heart failure. In: Ettinger SJ, Feldman EC, editors. Textbook of veterinary internal medicine. 6th edition. St. Louis (MO): Elsevier Saunders; 2005. p. 914–40.

54. Sisson DD. Pathophysiology of heart failure. In: Ettinger SJ, Feldman EC, editors. Textbook of veterinary internal medicine. 7th edition. St. Louis (MO): Elsevier Saunders; 2010. p. 1143–58.

55. Oglesbee BL, Oglesbee MJ. Results of postmortem examination of psittacine birds with cardiac disease: 26 cases (1991-1995). J Am Vet Med Assoc 1998;212:1737–42.

56. Fitzgerald BC, Beaufrere H. Cardiology. In: Speer BL, editor. Current therapy in avian medicine and surgery. St. Louis (MO): Elsevier; 2016. p. 252–328.

57. Mans C, Brown CJ. Radiographic evidence of atherosclerosis of the descending aorta in a grey-cheeked parakeet (*Brotogeris pyrrhopterus*). J Avian Med Surg 2007;21(1):56–62.
58. Vink-Nooteboom M, Schoemaker N, Kik M, et al. Clinical diagnosis of aneurysm of the right coronary artery in a white cockatoo (*Cacatua alba*). J Small Anim Pr 1998;39(11):533–7.
59. de Wit M, Schoemaker NJ. Clinical approach to avian cardiac disease. Semin Avian Exot Pet Med 2005;14:6–13.
60. Bonagura JD, Keene BW. Drugs for treatment of heart failure in dogs. In: Bonagura JD, Twedt DC, editors. Kirk's current veterinary therapy XV. St. Louis (MO): Elsevier Saunders; 2014. p. 762–72.
61. Yancy CW, Jessup M, Bozkurt B, et al. 2013 ACCF/AHA guideline for the management of heart failure: a report of the American College of Cardiology Foundation/American Heart Association Task Force on Practice Guidelines. Circulation 2013;128:e240–327.
62. Gordon SG. Beta blocking agents. In: Ettinger SJ, Feldman EC, editors. Textbook of veterinary internal medicine. 7th edition. St. Louis (MO): Elsevier Saunders; 2010. p. 1207–11.
63. Gibbs CR, Davies MK, Lip GYH. ABC of heart failure. Management: digoxin and other inotropes, β blockers, and antiarrhythmic and antithrombotic treatment. BMJ 2000;320(7233):495–8.
64. Klapholz M. Beta-blocker use for the stages of heart failure. Mayo Clin Proc 2009;84(8):718–29.
65. Mann D, Bristow M. Mechanisms and models in heart failure: the biomechanical model and beyond. Circulation 2005;111:2837–49.
66. Schroeder N. Diuretics. In: Ettinger SJ, Feldman EC, editors. Textbook of veterinary internal medicine. 7th edition. St. Louis (MO): Elsevier Saunders; 2010. p. 1212–4.
67. Bulmer BJ, Sisson DD. Therapy of heart failure. In: Ettinger SJ, Feldman EC, editors. Textbook of veterinary internal medicine. 6th edition. St. Louis (MO): Elsevier Saunders; 2005. p. 948–72.
68. Plumb DC. Furosemide. In: Plumb DC, editor. Plumb's veterinary drug handbook. 9th edition. Stockholm (WI): John Wiley & Sons; 2018. p. 726–31.
69. Cote E. Clinical veterinary advisor: dogs and cats. St. Louis (MO): Mosby Inc.; 2007.
70. Goldstein D, Skadhauge E. Renal and extrarenal regulation of body fluid composition. In: Whittow G, editor. Sturkie's avian physiology. 5th edition. San Diego (CA): Academic Press; 2000. p. 265–97.
71. Plumb DC. Spironolactone. In: Plumb DC, editor. Plumb's veterinary drug handbook. 9th edition. Stockholm (WI): John Wiley & Sons; 2018. p. 1510–3.
72. Swift S. Aldosterone inhibitors. In: Ettinger SJ, Feldman EC, editors. Textbook of veterinary internal medicine. 7th edition. St. Louis (MO): Elsevier Saunders; 2010. p. 1223–5.
73. Bulmer B. Angiotensin converting enzyme inhibitors and vasodilators. In: Ettinger SJ, Feldman EC, editors. Textbook of veterinary internal medicine. 7th edition. St Louis (MO): Elsevier Saunders; 2010. p. 1216–23.
74. Plumb DC. Enalapril maleate. In: Plumb DC, editor. Plumb's veterinary drug handbook. 9th edition. Stockholm (WI): John Wiley & Sons; 2018. p. 581–5.
75. Cohn JN. Structural basis for heart failure. Circulation 1995;91:2504–7.
76. BENCH (BENazepril in Canine Heart disease) Study Group. The effect of benazepril on survival times and clinical signs of dogs with congestive heart failure:

results of a multicenter, prospective, randomized, double-blinded, placebo-controlled, long-term clinical trial. J Vet Cardiol 1999;1(1):7–18.

77. Solvd Investigators. Effect of enalapril on survival in patients with reduced left ventricular ejection fractions and congestive heart failure. N Engl J Med 1991; 325:293–302.

78. Kellihan HB. Pulmonary hypertension and pulmonary thromboembolism. In: Ettinger SJ, Feldman EC, editors. Textbook of veterinary internal medicine. 7th edition. St. Louis (MO): Elsevier Saunders; 2010. p. 1138–41.

79. Powers LV. Pulmonary arterial hypertension in companion birds. Proc Annu Assoc Avian Med 2014;295–9.

80. Plumb DC. Sildenafil citrate. In: Plumb DC, editor. Plumb's veterinary drug handbook. 9th edition. Stockholm (WI): John Wiley & Sons; 2018. p. 1485–7.

81. Julian RJ. Ascites in poultry. Avian Pathol 1993;22(3):419–54.

82. Plumb DC. Pimobendan. In: Plumb DC, editor. Plumb's veterinary drug handbook. 9th edition. Stockholm (WI): John Wiley & Sons; 2018. p. 1318–22.

83. Fitzgerald BC, Dias S, Martorell J. Cardiovascular drugs in avian, small mammal, and reptile medicine. Veterinary Clin North Am Exot Anim Pract 2018;21(2):399–442.

84. Fuentes VL. Inotropes: inodilators. In: Ettinger SJ, Feldman EC, editors. Textbook of veterinary internal medicine. 7th edition. St. Louis (MO): Elsevier Saunders; 2010. p. 1202–7.

85. Summerfield NJ, Boswood A, O'Grady MR, et al. Efficacy of pimobendan in the prevention of congestive heart failure or sudden death in Doberman pinschers with preclinical dilated cardiomyopathy. J Vet Intern Med 2012;26(6):1337–49.

86. Plumb DC. Propanolol HCl. In: Plumb DC, editor. Plumb's veterinary drug handbook. 9th edition. Stockholm (WI): John Wiley & Sons; 2018. p. 1396–9.

87. Plumb DC. Atenolol. In: Plumb DC, editor. Plumb's veterinary drug handbook. 9th edition. Stockholm (WI): John Wiley & Sons; 2018. p. 133–6.

88. Plumb DC. Carvedilol. In: Plumb DC, editor. Plumb's veterinary drug handbook. 9th edition. Stockholm (WI): John Wiley & Sons; 2018. p. 266–9.

89. Plumb DC. Metoprolol. In: Plumb DC, editor. Plumb's veterinary drug handbook. 9th edition. Stockholm (WI): John Wiley & Sons; 2018. p. 1098–101.

90. Plumb DC. Sotalol HCl. In: Plumb DC, editor. Plumb's veterinary drug handbook. 9th edition. Stockholm (WI): John Wiley & Sons; 2018. p. 1503–5.

91. Cote E, Ettinger SJ. Electrocardiography and cardiac arrhythmias. In: Ettinger SJ, Feldman EC, editors. Textbook of veterinary internal medicine. 6th edition. Saint Louis (MO): Elsevier Saunders; 2005. p. 1040–76.

92. Plumb DC. Verapamil HCl. In: Plumb DC, editor. Plumb's veterinary drug handbook. 9th edition. Stockholm (WI): John Wiley & Sons; 2018. p. 1670–4.

93. Plumb DC. Amlodipine besylate. In: Plumb DC, editor. Plumb's veterinary drug handbook. 9th edition. Stockholm (WI): John Wiley & Sons; 2018. p. 81–3.

94. Liao R, Carles M, Gwathmey JK. Animal models of cardiovascular disease for pharmacologic drug development and testing: appropriateness of comparison to the human disease state and pharmacotherapeutics. Am J Ther 1997;4: 149–58.

95. Fricke C, Schmidt V, Cramer K, et al. Characterization of atherosclerosis by histochemical and immunohistochemical methods in African grey parrots (*Psittacus erithacus*) and Amazon parrots (*Amazona* spp.). Avian Dis 2009;53:466–72.

96. Zandvliet MMJM, Dorrestein GM, van der Hage M. Chronic pulmonary interstitial fibrosis in Amazon parrots. Avian Pathol 2001;30:517–24.

97. Oyama MA, Sisson DD, Thomas WP, et al. Congenital heart disease. In: Ettinger SJ, Feldman EC, editors. Textbook of veterinary internal medicine. 7th edition. St. Louis (MO): Elsevier Saunders; 2010. p. 1250–98.

98. MacDonald K. Myocardial disease, feline. In: Ettinger SJ, Feldman EC, editors. Textbook of veterinary internal medicine. 7th edition. St. Louis (MO): Elsevier Saunders; 2010. p. 1328–41.

99. Crespo R, Shivaprasad H. Developmental, metabolic, and other noninfectious disorders. In: Saif Y, Fadly A, Glisson J, et al, editors. Diseases of poultry. 12th edition. Ames (IA): Blackwell Publishing; 2008. p. 1149–95.

100. Lichtenberger M. Determination of indirect blood pressure in the companion bird. Semin Avian Exot Pet Med 2005;14(2):149–52.

101. Beaufrere H. Avian atherosclerosis: parrots and beyond. J Exot Pet Med 2013; 22(4):336–47.

102. Snyder PS, Cooke KL. Management of hypertension. In: Ettinger SJ, Feldman EC, editors. Textbook of veterinary internal medicine. 6th edition. St. Louis (MO): Elsevier Saunders; 2005. p. 477–9.

103. Acierno MJ, de Cunha A, Smith J, et al. Agreement between direct and indirect blood pressure measurements obtained from anesthetized Hispaniolan Amazon parrots. J Am Vet Med Assoc 2008;233:1587–90.

104. Zehnder AM, Hawkins MG, Pascoe PJ, et al. Evaluation of indirect blood pressure monitoring in awake and anesthetized red-tailed hawks (Buteo jamaicensis): effects of cuff size, cuff placement, and monitoring equipment. V Anesth Analg 2009;36(5):464–79.

105. Johnston MS, Davidowski LA, Rao S, et al. Precision of repeated, Doppler-derived indirect blood pressure measurements in conscious psittacine birds. J Avian Med Surg 2011;25(2):83–90.

106. Schnellbacher R, da Cunha A, Olson EE, et al. Arterial catheterization, interpretation, and treatment of arterial blood pressures and blood gases in birds. J Exot Pet Med 2014;23:129–41.

107. Assi TB, Baz E. Current applications of therapeutic phlebotomy. Blood Transfus 2014;12:s75–83.

108. Fudge AM, Reavill DR. Pulmonary artery aneurysm and polycythaemia with respiratory hypersensitivity in a blue and gold macaw (Ara ararauna). Proc Europ Conf Avian Med Surg. 1993:382-387.

109. Taylor M. Polycythemia in the blue and gold macaw: a report of three cases. In: Proc 1st Int Conf Zoo Avian Med 1987:95-104.

110. Brown AJ, Davison E, Sleeper MM. Clinical efficacy of sildenafil in treatment of pulmonary arterial hypertension in dogs. J Vet Intern Med 2010;24:850–4.

111. Michelakis E, Tymchak W, Lien D, et al. Oral sildenafil is an effective and specific pulmonary vasodilator in patients with pulmonary arterial hypertension: comparison with inhaled nitric oxide. Circulation 2002;105:2398–403.

112. Fathi M, Haydari M, Tanha T. Effects of enalapril on growth performance, ascites mortality, antioxidant status and blood parameters in broiler chickens under cold-induced ascites. Poult Sci J 2015;3:121–7.

113. Hao XQ, Zhang SY, Cheng XC, et al. Imidapril inhibits right ventricular remodeling induced by low ambient temperature in broiler chickens. Poult Sci 2013;92: 1492–7.

114. Hao XQ, Zhang SY, Li M, et al. Imidapril provides a protective effect on pulmonary hypertension induced by low ambient temperature in broiler chickens. J Renin Angiotensin Aldosterone Syst 2014;15:162–9.

115. Scagnelli A. Therapeutic review: pentoxifylline. J Exot Pet Med 2017;26:238–40.

116. Plumb DC. Pentoxifylline. In: Plumb DC, editor. Plumb's veterinary drug handbook. 9th edition. Stockholm (WI): John Wiley & Sons; 2018. p. 1284–7.

117. Martinez L, Jeffrey J, Odom T. Electrocardiographic diagnosis of cardiomyopathies in Aves. Poul Av Biol Rev 1997;8(1):9–20.

118. Sturkie PD. Heart: contraction, conduction, and electrocardiography. In: Sturkie PD, editor. Avian physiology. 4th edition. New York: Springer-Verlag; 1986. p. 130–66.

119. Zandvliet MMJM. Electrocardiography in psittacine birds and ferrets. J Exot Pet Med 2005;14(1):34–51.

120. Rembert MS, Smith JA, Strickland KN, et al. Intermittent bradyarrhythmia in a Hispaniolan Amazon parrot (*Amazona ventralis*). J Avian Med Surg 2008; 22(1):31–40.

121. Nap AM, Lumeij JT, Stokhof AA. Electrocardiogram of the African grey (*Psittacus erithacus*) and Amazon (*Amazona* spp.) parrot. Avian Pathol 1992;21(1):45–53.

122. Kushner LI. ECG of the month. Atrioventricular block in a Muscovy duck. J Am Vet Med Assoc 1999;214(1):33–6.

123. Mukai S, Noboru M, Nishimura M, et al. Electrocardiographic observation on spontaneously occurring arrhythmias in chickens. J Vet Med Sci 1996;58(10): 953–61.

124. Plumb DC. Lidocaine HCl (intravenous; systemic). In: Plumb DC, editor. Plumb's veterinary drug handbook. 9th edition. Stockholm (WI): John Wiley & Sons; 2018. p. 951–8.

125. Plumb DC. Atropine sulfate. In: Plumb DC, editor. Plumb's veterinary drug handbook. 9th edition. Stockholm (WI): John Wiley & Sons; 2018. p. 144–9.

126. Speer BL, Hennigh M, Muntz B, et al. Low-stress medication techniques in birds and small mammals. Vet Clin North Am Exot Anim Pract 2018;21(2):261–85.

127. Tobias AH. Pericardial disorders. In: Ettinger SJ, Feldman EC, editors. Textbook of veterinary internal medicine. 6th edition. St. Louis (MO): Elsevier Saunders; 2005. p. 1104–18.

128. Echols S. Collecting diagnostic samples in avian patients. Vet Clin North Am Exot Anim Pract 1999;2:621–49.

129. Hernandez-Divers SJ, McBride M, Hanley C. Minimally invasive endosurgery of the psittacine cranial coelom. Exot DVM 2004;6:33–7.

130. Beaufrere H, Nevarez JG, Holder K, et al. Characterization and classification of psittacine atherosclerotic lesions by histopathology, digital image analysis, transmission and scanning electron microscopy. Avian Pathol 2011;40(5): 531–44.

131. Beaufrere H, Ammersbach M, Reavill DR, et al. Prevalence of and risk factors associated with atherosclerosis in psittacine birds. J Am Vet Med Assoc 2013; 242(12):1696–704.

132. Walsh AL, Shivaprasad HL. Unusual lesions of atherosclerosis in psittacines. J Exot Pet Med 2013;22(4):366–74.

133. Beaufrere H. Atherosclerosis: comparative pathogenesis, lipoprotein metabolism, and avian and exotic companion mammal models. J Exot Pet Med 2013;22(4):320–35.

134. Beaufere H. Clinical lipidology in psittacine birds. In: Proc Am Board Vet Pract Symposium. 2019:42-44.

135. Beaufere H. Clinical lipidology in psittacine birds. Proc Annu Conf Assoc Avian Vet 2020;120–31.

136. Beaufrere H, Gardhouse S, Ammersbach M. Lipoprotein characterization in Quaker parrots (*Myiopsitta monachus*) using gel-permeation high-performance liquid chromatography. Vet Clin Pathol 2020;49(3):417–27.

137. Beaufrere H, Gardhouse SM, Wood RD, et al. The plasma lipidome of the Quaker parrot (*Myiopsitta monachus*). PLoS One 2020;15(12):e0240449.

138. Johnson JH, Phalen DN, Kondik VH, et al. Atherosclerosis in psittacine birds. Proc Annu Conf Assoc Avian Vet 1992;87–93.

139. Bennett RA. Neurology. In: Ritchie BW, Harrison GJ, Harrison LR, editors. Avian medicine: principles and applications. Lake Worth (FL): Wingers Publishing; 1994. p. 723–47.

140. Elliott J, Soydan J. Characterisation of beta-adrenoceptors in equine digital veins: implications of the modes of vasodilatory action of isoxsuprine. Equine Vet J Suppl 1995;0(19):101–7.

141. Belloli C, Carcano R, Arioli F, et al. Affinity of isoxsuprine for adrenoreceptors in equine digital artery and implications for vasodilatory action. Equine Vet J 2000; 32(2):119–24.

142. Plumb DC. Isoxsuprine HCl. In: Plumb DC, editor. Plumb's veterinary drug handbook. 9th edition. Stockholm (WI): John Wiley & Sons; 2018. p. 888–9.

143. Aarts PA, Banga JD, van Houwelingen HC, et al. Increased red blood cell deformability due to isoxsuprine administration decreases platelet adherence in a perfusion chamber: a double-blind cross-over study in patients with intermittent claudication. Blood 1986;67:1474–81.

144. Smith FM, West NH, Jones DR. The cardiovascular system. In: Whittow GC, editor. Sturkie's avian physiology. 5th edition. San Diego (CA): Academic Press; 2000. p. 141–231.

145. Paoletti R, Bolego C, Cignerella A. Lipid and non-lipid effects of statins. In: von Eckarstein A, editor. Atherosclerosis: diet and drugs. Berlin (Germany): Springer Verlag; 2005. p. 365–88.

146. Beaufrere H, Papich MG, Brandao J, et al. Plasma drug concentrations of orally administered rosuvastatin Hispaniolan Amazon parrots (*Amazona ventralis*). J Avian Med Surg 2015;29:18–24.

147. Robertson JA, Guzman DSM, Graham JL, et al. Evaluation of orally administered atorvastatin on plasma lipid and biochemistry profiles in hypercholesterolemic Hispaniolan Amazon parrots (*Amazona ventralis*). J Avian Med Surg 2020; 34(1):32–40.

148. Powers LV, Papich MG. Pharmacokinetics of orally administered phenobarbital in African grey parrots (*Psittacus erithacus erithacus*). J Vet Pharmcol Ther 2011;34(6):615–7.

149. Keller KA, Guzman DSM, Boothe DM, et al. Pharmacokinetics and safety of zonisamide after oral administration of single and multiple doses to Hispaniolan Amazon parrots (*Amazona ventralis*). Am J Vet Res 2019;80(2):195–200.

150. Schnellbacher R, Beaufrere H, Arnold RD, et al. Pharmacokinetics of levetiracetam in healthy Hispaniolan Amazon parrots (*Amazona ventralis*) after oral administration of a single dose. J Avian Med Surg 2014;28(3):193–200.

151. Kabakchiev C, Laniesse D, James F, et al. Diagnosis and long-term management of post-traumatic seizures in a white-crowned pionus (*Pionus senilis*). J Am Vet Med Assoc 2020;256(10):1145–52.

152. Visser M, Boothe DM. Population pharmacokinetics of levetiracetam and zonisamide in the African grey parrot (Psittacus erithacus). In: Proc Annu Conf Assoc Avian Vet. 2015:7-10.

153. Guzman DSM. Advances in avian clinical therapeutics. J Exot Pet Med 2014; 23:6–20.
154. Gustavsen KA, Stanhope KL, Lin AS, et al. Effects of exercise on the plasma lipid profile in Hispaniolan Amazon parrots (*Amazona ventralis*) with naturally occurring hypercholesterolemia. J Zoo Wildl Med 2016;47(3):760–9.
155. Belcher C, Heatley JJ, Petzinger C, et al. Evaluation of plasma cholesterol, triglyceride, and lipid density profiles in captive monk parakeets (*Myiopsitta monachus*). J Exot Pet Med 2014;23(1):71–8.
156. Bavelaar FJ, Beynen AC. Severity of atherosclerosis in parrots in relation to the intake of alpha-linolenic acid. Avian Dis 2003;47(3):566–77.
157. Petzinger C, Heatley JJ, Cornejo J, et al. Dietary modification of omega-3 fatty acids for birds with atherosclerosis. J Am Vet Med Assoc 2010;236(5):523–8.
158. Bavelaar FJ, Beynen AC. Atherosclerosis in parrots. A review. Vet Q 2004;26(2): 50–60.
159. Echols MS. Using nutritional supplements in birds. Proc Wild West Vet Conf 2016.

Cardiology in Rodents, Rabbits, and Small Exotic Mammals—Diagnostic Workup

Vladimir Jekl, MVDr, PhD., DiplECZM (Small Mammal)[a,b,*],
Carlos F. Agudelo, MVDr, PhD[c], Karel Hauptman, MVDr, PhD[a]

KEYWORDS

- Rabbit • Guinea pig • Chinchilla • Rat • Electrocardiography • Radiography
- Cardiac disease • Echocardiography

KEY POINTS

- Cardiac diseases start to have a higher incidence, especially in older rabbits and rodents; however, the true incidence in these exotic companion mammals is still unknown because of the lack of information in the literature.
- Diagnostics of the exact cardiopathy is necessary for proper cardiac disease therapy and management.
- Thoracic radiographs can be challenging to evaluate; however, radiography should precede echocardiography or electrocardiography.
- Echocardiography or electrocardiography are golden standards in the evaluation of the heart structure and its function.

BACKGROUND

The incidence of cardiac diseases in pet rabbits and rodents increased over the past decade because these exotic companion mammal species live longer in captivity. Moreover, diagnostics methods and techniques developed quickly, are more precise, and can imagine/diagnose the heart disease even in small-sized animals. Despite their frequent use as laboratory animals, spontaneous cardiac diseases are still reported in the literature as sporadic or clinical findings[1–4] are not supported by further diagnostics of the exact disorder, for example, using echocardiography and electrocardiography (ECG).

[a] Jekl and Hauptman Veterinary Clinic – Focused on Exotic Companion Mammal Care, Mojmirovo Namesti 3105/6a, Brno 61200, Czech Republic; [b] Department of Pharmacology and Pharmacy, Faculty of Veterinary Medicine, VETUNI Brno, Palackeho Tr. 1946/1, Brno 61242, Czech Republic; [c] Dogs and Cat Clinic, Faculty of Veterinary Medicine, VETUNI Brno, Palackeho Tr. 1946/1, Brno 61242, Czech Republic
* Corresponding author. Jekl and Hauptman Veterinary Clinic – Focused on Exotic Companion Mammal Care, Mojmirovo Namesti 3105/6a, Brno 61200, Czech Republic.
E-mail address: VladimirJekl@gmail.com

Vet Clin Exot Anim 25 (2022) 503–524
https://doi.org/10.1016/j.cvex.2022.01.010
1094-9194/22/© 2022 Published by Elsevier Inc.

vetexotic.theclinics.com

Published prevalence of confirmed cardiac diseases by ECG and echocardiography in pet guinea pigs comprised 1.2% of affected individuals from the retrospective study in 1000 animals.[2] Prevalence of heart murmurs is in chinchillas very high (23%, 59 chinchillas from 260 animals); however, only 15 animals were examined using echocardiography.[1] In a health survey of 167 pet rabbits and 375 pet rats, cardiac disease was not reported to be present.[5,6] Based on the author's experience, many cardiac disorders are not detected as auscultation of the heart, and detection of abnormal heart sounds can be challenging, especially for unexperienced practitioners or practitioners working predominantly with dogs and cats. Further cardiac disease diagnostics may be also a question of increased costs. Nevertheless, more and more animal owners are willing to increase the wellbeing of their pets, so exact diagnostics of many diseases, cardiac disease included, and also their potential prevalence, is increasing.

ANATOMY AND TOPOGRAPHIC ANATOMY
Topographic Anatomy

The heart is a conical, elongated organ and has a pointed apex and is of similar function in other mammalian species.

In rabbits, guinea pigs, chinchillas, and rats, the heart occupies a large space in the thoracic cavity as these species possess a narrow thoracic cavity. It extends from the sternum to the vertebral column and leaves only a narrow space for lungs on each side. In rabbits and rats, despite the heart being the largest organ in the thoracic cavity, the heart weight/body weight ratio of pet rabbits is, in comparison with wild hares, 4 times smaller.[7] Also, the heart weight/body weight ratio of pet rats is about 50% smaller than that of wild rats.[7]

The heart is located in the midline with slightly left orientation at the level of second to fourth intercostal space with the apex directed caudoventrally. In rabbits, it is located little bit more caudally between second (third) and fifth (sixth) intercostal space (**Fig. 1**).

All the species listed above have both left and right cranial vena cava, which can be used for blood sampling, especially in rodents.[8,9]

Selected Cardiac Anatomic and Functional Variations

Rabbits
A unique feature of the cardiovascular system of the rabbit is that the right atrioventricular valve has only 2 cusps, rather than 3 as in many other mammals. The sinoatrial node is less complex than in other species, a feature that facilitates precise determination of the location of the pacemaker. The aortic nerve subserves no known

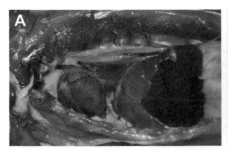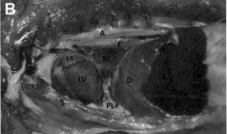

Fig. 1. Topographic anatomy of a rabbit thorax (*A, B*)—lateral view after thoracic wall and left lung excision. D, diaphragm; E, esophagus; L, liver; LA, left atrium; LV, left ventricle; PL, phrenicopericardial ligament; RL, right lung; S, sternum. (*Courtesy of* Vladimir Jekl.)

chemoreceptors and responds to baroreceptors only, whereas the nerve to the carotid sinus subserves both.[10] Rabbit has limited vascularization of the myocardium, which makes them prone to ischemia.[11]

The normal respiratory rate is 30 to 60 breaths per minute. The resting heart rate of conscious healthy rabbits varies from 180 bpm to 250 bpm.

In the adult rabbit, the thymus persists and consists of a right ventral lobe, dorsal thoracic lobe, and left thoracic lobe. The thymus extends into the thoracic inlet.[12]

Guinea pigs and chinchillas

Guinea pigs are noted for the spectacular collateralization of their coronary arteries, making them unlikely to develop myocardial infarction.[11] Guinea pigs have lower basal and peak coronary blood flow than the rat, however.[13]

The right coronary artery is absent in chinchillas.

The normal respiratory rate in guinea pigs is 40 to 120 breaths per minute. The resting heart rate of conscious healthy guinea pigs varies from 300 bpm to 500 bpm.[14] The normal respiratory rate in chinchillas is 40 to 80 breaths per minute and the resting heart rate of healthy chinchillas is 200 to 300 bpm.[15]

Rats

Of the rodents, rats have the thinnest pulmonary artery and the thickest pulmonary vein. Cardiac striated muscle in the rat extends to lung tissue, which makes these species particularly susceptible to infectious agents spread between the heart, pulmonary veins, and lungs. Blood supply to the heart of the rat differs from other mammals and is largely extracoronary from branches of the internal mammary and subclavian arteries.

The normal respiratory rate is 71 to 146 breaths per minute. The resting heart rate of conscious healthy guinea pigs varies from 300 to 500 bpm.[16]

Please note that respiratory and heart rates can increase significantly in all animals in stress because of increased sympathetic tone.

HISTORY AND CLINICAL EXAMINATION
History

Animals with cardiac diseases may be present with nonspecific signs of general weakness, loss of activity, weight loss, and dyspnea. Practitioners need to distinguish other diseases, which can cause dyspnea in particular animal species, for example, primary respiratory disease, lymphoproliferative disorders, or other systemic diseases. Respiratory disorders can be also associated with cardiac disease, especially in cases of congestive heart failure (CHF) and lung edema. Complete history, previous medication included, should be part of the first approach to the patient. In case of emergency cases, a short history should be obtained first, and additional history should be taken after patient stabilization.

Clinical Examination

All the animals should be handled gently and in a quiet examination room, as stress from the strange environment can increase respiratory and heart rates, and can even worsen clinical signs of the disease. If necessary, rabbits, guinea pigs, chinchillas, and rats can be sedated with midazolam, preferably intramuscularly. The recommended midazolam dosage is published within the range of 0.5 to 1 mg/kg[17]; however, authors (VJ, KH) recommend lower dosages of 0.2 to 0.5 mg/kg, as especially rabbits and chinchillas can be heavily sedated with higher dosages.

Thorough clinical examination is mandatory in all animal species. Animals with suspected cardiac disease, assessment of body condition, respiration, mucosal color evaluation, capillary refill time (CRT) estimation, thoracic auscultation, and pulse wave symmetry (femoral artery in rabbits, central ear artery in larger rabbits) are important parts of the examination. In the case of healthy rabbits, guinea pigs, chinchillas, and rats, breathing can be seen as periodic thoracic movement with minimal involvement of the diaphragm. Mucosal color is best evaluated on conjunctiva and gingiva at the area of the incisors, where CRT can be also measured.

Thoracic auscultation should be performed using preferably a neonatal stethoscope. The thorax of these animals is minute, and the smallest chest piece is necessary to obtain the best possible quality of information from the auscultation. Even the neonatal chest pieces can be too large compared with the size of the thorax to be able to auscultate separately different lung and heart structures.[18] Heart should be auscultated from several sides, lateral part of the chest and also close to the sternum of the thoracic cavity, as some mild abnormal heart sounds (eg, heart murmurs in chinchillas) can be evident from only one side. Two heart sounds consist normally of the standard two sounds of "lub" (louder, S1) and "dub" (softer, S2). In guinea pigs, the S1 may be normally preceded by a fourth heart sound corresponding to atrial contraction.[19]

Rectal temperature is preferably measured by the authors at the end of clinical examination, as it is one of the most stressful procedures. Hyperthermia is associated with tachycardia and hypothermia with bradycardia.[20] Hypothermic rabbits have a 3 times higher risk of mortality than normothermic rabbits, so treatment of these rabbits should be started immediately.[21]

Cardiac disease may be considered if any of the following are known from the history or found during clinical examination:

- exercise intolerance
- general weakness during morning periods
- the heart rate is irregular or slow
- the heart murmur is heard
- heart sounds are muffled
- dyspnea in the absence of primary respiratory disease
- wet respiratory sounds are identified (lung edema associated with CHF)
- cyanosis

THORACIC RADIOGRAPHY

Thoracic radiography is one of the most commonly used and useful tools in the diagnostic workup of rabbits and rodents with cardiac disease (**Figs. 2–6**). It is used for differentiating animals with respiratory disorders of cardiogenic etiology from those with respiratory disorders associated with primary respiratory disease. The standard view for radiographic evaluation of the thorax is right lateral and left-lateral view and dorsoventral (DV) and ventrodorsal (VD) view.

Some animals permit a complete radiographic study with minimal restraint, but others will require sedation or anesthesia. Sedation with benzodiazepines is mostly recommended to alleviate anxiety and fear. Heavy sedation or general anesthesia might affect the radiographic interpretation because of possible artifacts of pulmonary or cardiac imaging, particularly the congestion of pulmonary parenchyma and partial atelectasis of the lung close to the cassette. Contrary, asymmetric positioning can make interpretation of the thoracic radiograph very challenging to almost impossible.

Thoracic radiographs should be made using a high kVp (above 40–16 kV) and low mAs techniques, which maximizes the latitude of contrast and allow the imager to separate vascular, interstitial, and bronchial structures. The highest mA and the fastest time should be used to minimize respiratory motion artifact and to avoid radiographic

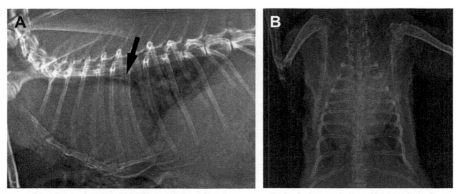

Fig. 2. Dorsoventral (*A*) and lateral (*B*) views of a rabbit with burn-out cardiomyopathy. Note the tracheal elevation due to cardiomegaly (*arrow*). (*Courtesy of* Jekl & Hauptman.)

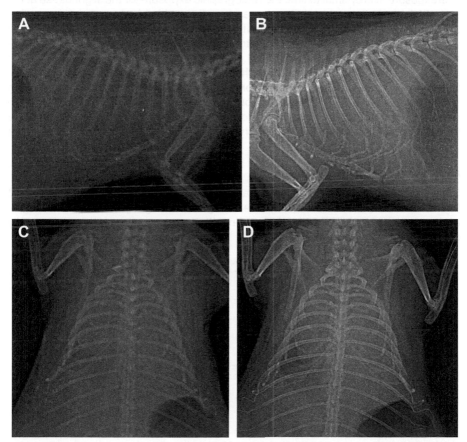

Fig. 3. Thoracic radiography of a guinea pig—right-left lateral view (*A*), left-right lateral view (*B*), dorsoventral (*C*), and ventrodorsal view (*D*). Cardiac borders are indistinct. A marked bronchointerstitial pattern is present in almost all the lung tissue, which is compatible with lung edema associated with congestive heart failure. (*Courtesy of* Jekl & Hauptman.)

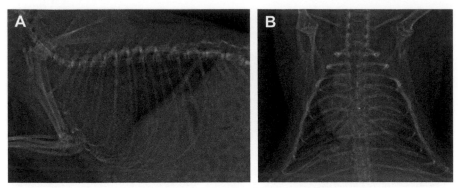

Fig. 4. Lateral (*A*) and dorsoventral (*B*) views of a chinchilla suffering from hypertrophic cardiomyopathy. Note enlarged heart silhouette and perihilar edema. (*Courtesy of* Jekl & Hauptman.)

overexposure. It is optimal to time the radiographic exposure for the slight pause at the end of full inspiration, which helps decrease radiographic blurring caused by motion and increases inherent thoracic contrast because of the increased volume of air. In rabbits and rodents with respiratory distress, timing the exposure relative to respiration is difficult. In the case of intubated animals, a radiograph taken in the assisted positive pressure inspiration could be helpful in differentiating subtle lung lesions. Overexposure gives the false impression of a pneumothorax or prevents recording subtle lung abnormalities. Rabbits and rodents (especially guinea pigs and chinchillas) with distended abdominal organs should be placed on x-ray cassette with elevated thoracic region; however, the thorax should be still in a parallel position with the cassette.

Positioning

Standard thoracic radiographic examinations include the right (left-right) lateral, left (right-left) lateral, DV, and VD views (see **Figs. 2–6**; **Fig. 7**).[22] The positioning is extremely important because any errors that occur cannot be subsequently compensated.

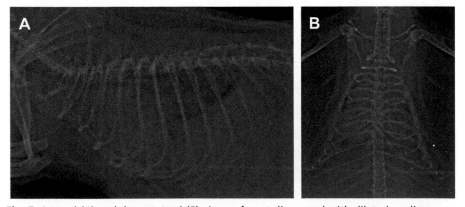

Fig. 5. Lateral (*A*) and dorsoventral (*B*) views of a rat diagnosed with dilated cardiomyopathy and congestive heart failure which resulted in lung edema and hydrothorax. Note severe generalized cardiomegaly, tracheal elevation, and increase in opacity of almost all the lung tissue. (*Courtesy of* Jekl & Hauptman.)

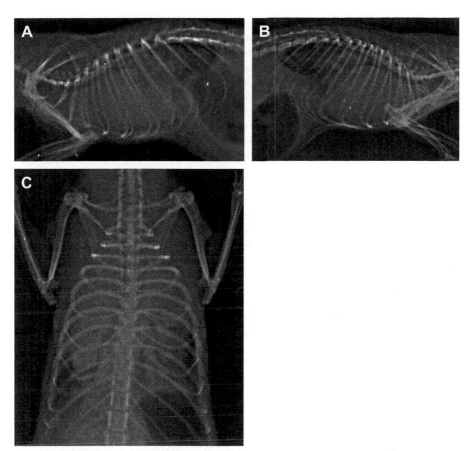

Fig. 6. Lef-right (*A*), right-left (*B*), and dorsoventral (*C*) views of a rat with intrathoracic soft tissue opacity mass. Trachea is elevated along the spine; only caudal parts of the lung lobes are aerated. (*Courtesy of* Jekl & Hauptman.)

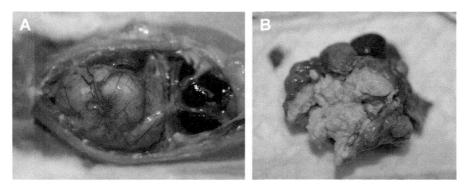

Fig. 7. Postmortal examination (*A*, *B*) of a rat (same as in **Fig. 6**) showed the presence of lung abscesses. Intrathoracic masses should be differentiated from cardiac disease using thoracic ultrasonography. (*Courtesy of* Jekl & Hauptman.)

The x-ray beam is centered in the mid-thorax. In technically adequate radiographs, coverage of the entire thorax, centered at the level of the cardiac silhouette, should be evident. The thoracic inlet to the caudal most extent of the caudodorsal lung field including the whole diaphragm should thereby be included in the field of view. The cervical portion of the trachea may be also included in the resulting image, or a separate radiograph of the cervical region is performed. In a radiograph made at peak inspiration, the caudodorsal aspect of the lung is caudal to the ninth thoracic vertebra; separation of the cardiac silhouette from the diaphragm is not commonly seen because of a fat localized in this region. x-Ray field should be enlarged to the second or third lumbar vertebra if all ribs should be evaluated.

DV and VD views

Significant respiratory compromise may occur if the animal is placed in dorsal recumbency when the stomach or caecum is greatly distended, so DV view is preferred. VD view is indicated for evaluation of the cranial mediastinum, the lungs, the caudal vena cava, and in case of pleural effusion. The standard view for the most accurate positioning[22] of the heart is the DV view, to ensure that the cardiac apex is in its normal position.

VD view is indicated for evaluation of the cranial and caudal mediastinum, the caudal vena cava, and the accessory lung lobe, and in cases of pleural effusion.

The front and hind limbs should be gently pulled forward and caudally, respectively, so that the soft tissues of the brachium and scapulas are not superimposed over the cranial thorax. Care should be taken to do not twist the legs to avoid scapulas superposition with the thorax. The spine must be superimposed with sternum throughout the entire length of the thorax. The spine should be in a straight line and ribs should be symmetrical in shape and location.

Lateral views

The front and hind limbs should be pulled slightly cranially and caudally, respectively. Care should be taken to maintain them parallel to avoid rotation of the thorax or spine. Conscious rabbits or rodents could respond to restraint with arching of the spine, which will result in thoracic misalignment. The spine and sternum must be parallel with the[22] cassette or table.

When a right versus left lateral radiograph is described, the terminology refers to the recumbent position of the patient during radiography. Selecting the appropriate patient position for the lateral radiographic view depends on the location of the expected pathology. If auscultation reveals abnormalities in particular thoracic quadrant, the patient should be positioned so that the more normal side is closed to the x-ray film. When the animal is in lateral recumbency, the lung parenchyma closer to the cassette cannot inflate completely due to the above structures compressing it. This results in suboptimal lung contrast due to the relative lung collapse and less parenchyma inflation. If no abnormalities are detected or a thorax is examined for suspected pulmonary parenchymal lesions, both left and right lateral views should be performed to avoid making a false-negative diagnosis and to assess even subtle pathologic changes.

In right lateral radiographs, the cardiac silhouette is typically more oval and relatively smaller than on left lateral radiographs.

In addition to changing the patient's position, the vertical x-ray beam can be oriented horizontally with the patient in a standing position in case of pleural effusion. Other radiographic views of the thorax that can be helpful include lateral oblique radiographs to evaluate ribs, mediastinal, or pleural abnormalities.

Radiograph interpretation

Rabbit or rodent thoracic radiographs can be challenging to evaluate and easy to over-interpret. The thoracic cavity is small in comparison with the large abdominal cavity. A good knowledge of normal thoracic anatomy is necessary to interpret rabbit and rodent thoracic radiographs.

On lateral radiographs, the retrosternal lucency, that is, the cranial lung lobes are very small, making evaluation of the pulmonary opacity in the cranial thorax difficult. The accessory lobe of the right lung is also very small. Large amounts of intrathoracic fat are often present, which increases thoracic opacity.

Rabbit, guinea pig, chinchilla, and rat lungs have no septa. The cranial lung lobes in rabbits, guinea pigs, and chinchillas are small and are commonly superimposed with mediastinal fat and the caudal lung lobes have a pronounced vasculature. The cranial border of the heart, which is localized between second(third) and fifth(sixth) intercostal spaces, is less distinct because of the presence of thymus, which persists in rabbits throughout the life.

Cardiac size can be evaluated based on vertebral heart score (for normal published values see **Table 1**). Vertebral heart size/scale (VHS) is measured on lateral thoracic radiographs. The long axis of the heart is measured from the carina to the heart apex; the short axis is perpendicular to the long axis and spans the width of the heart at its widest point. The sum of the long and short axes of the heart are expressed as VHS, when aligned to the vertebral column, with cranial portion starting at the cranial edge of the body of the fourth thoracic vertebra.[23] VHS is then measured in increments of one-fourth of vertebral body size.

COMPUTED TOMOGRAPHY

The most important advantage of computed tomography (CT) when compared with conventional radiography is the capability to provide images without the superimposition of adjacent anatomic structures. CT images of the thorax are evaluated as plain Ct or using contrast. CT is superior to traditional radiographs for the diagnosis of intrapulmonary diseases, such as abscesses in rabbits and rats, or lung metastases. They can be visualized in detail, providing a higher-quality diagnosis and prognosis.[24] Absolute and relative measurements of thoracic organs, heart, aorta, pulmonary arteries, and veins were also published.[25] Vertebral heart score can be also measured using CT and is more accurate when compared with radiography, where overinterpretation can be an issue.[26]

ELECTROCARDIOGRAPHY

ECG is a common, relatively simple, painless, and feasible procedure that records electrical impulses of the heart. The main use of ECG is to detect and identify

Table 1
Vertebral heart score of healthy rabbits, chinchillas, and rats

Species	Right Lateral View	Reference
Rabbit (<1.6 kg BW)	7.55 (6.9–8.1)	Onuma et al.[50] 2010
Rabbit (>1.6 kg BW)	7.99 (7.0–8.7)	Onuma et al.[50] 2010
Rabbit (New Zealand White)	7.6 (7.0–8.1)	Moarabi et al.[51] 2015
Chinchilla	8.9 (7.5–10.2)	Doss et al.[26] 2017
Rat	7.7 (7.0–8.5)	Dias et al.[52] 2021
Rat	7.4 (6.3–8.5)	Dorotea[53] 2016

arrhythmias. ECG may also give some information about chamber enlargement, pericardial effusion, and electrolyte abnormalities; however, this information should not be overinterpreted, and other diagnostic methods (echocardiography, blood analyses) must be used to confirm the diagnosis. Monitoring ECG during anesthesia is very valuable. When it is used simultaneously with other techniques like oximetry or capnography, it can record possible hypoxic episodes that may be shown as arrhythmia presence and/or ST or T wave changes during the anesthetic time.[27,28]

ECG Waves

ECG gives basic information as rate and rhythm of the heart, pacemaker origins, and impulse conduction. As in other species, small mammals ECG is sinus in origin. P wave represents atrial electrical activity. PQ (PR) interval assesses the conduction time between atria and ventricles. QRS complexes are associated with ventricular excitation (the Q wave is the first negative deflection being the septal depolarization, the R wave is the first positive deflection produced by ventricular depolarization. The S wave represents the depolarization of the posterior basal region of the left ventricle). T wave comes after describes heart repolarization. Owing to higher heart rates and small waves in small mammal ECG, interpretation is improved if recorded at a speed of 50 to 100 mm/s and an amplitude of 2 cm/mV (**Fig. 8**). Normal selected ECG parameters for rabbits, ferrets, and rats are summarized in **Table 2**.

The Lead System

The ECG lead system is composed of bipolar standard limb leads I, II, and III, augmented limb leads aVR, aVL, and aVF, and unipolar precordial (thoracic) leads; V1 to V15, but CV6LL (V2), CV6LU (V4), CV5RL (rV2) and V10 are traditionally used. The combination of limb leads and augmented unipolar leads produces the basic six-lead system called Bailey's hexaxial lead system. This also helps to build the mean electrical axis (MEA), which is the estimation of the average direction and

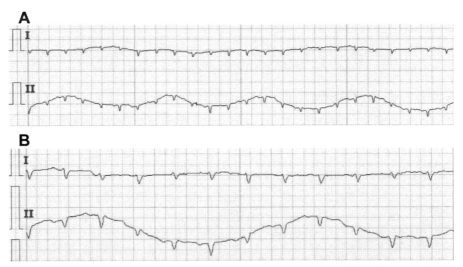

Fig. 8. ECG traces form a rabbit (lead I and II). (*A*) P waves are very difficult to see and QRS complexes are very small. Moreover, a breathing movement artifact is also present (base line is not straight). Paper speed 50 mm/s, 1 cm = 1 mV. (*B*) Same ECG at faster speed and higher amplitude to improve ECG analysis. Paper speed 100 mm/s, 2 cm = 1 mV.

Table 2
Normal ECG parameters in rabbits, guinea pigs, and rats[7]

Species	Heart Rate	Lead II Time Interval (S)				Lead II Amplitude (S)				
		P	PR	QRS	QT	P	Q	R	S	T
Rabbit	190–330	0.25–0.4	0.5–0.8	0.10–0.15		0.05–0.20	0.0	0.30–0.80	0.05–0.30	0.05–0.30
Guinea pig	200–300	0.022–0.048	0.046–0.077	0.020–0.030	0.110–0.185	0.10–0.22	0.0–0.11	0.82–2.63	0.0–0.58	0.08–0.38
Rat	228–600	0.010–0.016	0.033–0.050	0.012–0.026	0.038–0.080	0.02–.020	0.0	0.22–1.50	0.0–0.05	0.05–0.30

magnitude of the ventricular depolarization. Electrodes should be placed just below the olecranon and above the patella. In practice, at least a single lead placed anywhere is enough for arrhythmia detection. Right lateral recumbency is the standard position for ECG recording but as in other species, standing, sternal, or other positioning does not affect arrhythmia detection nor interval time but largely axis direction and waves amplitude.[4]

In general, ECG interpretation consists of 5 steps: to (1) determine heart rate; (2) determine heart rhythm; (3) calculate MEA; (4) estimate duration and amplitude of waves and intervals; and (5) determine right ventricular involvement. For further details, readers are encouraged to consult any of the excellent veterinary ECG literature elsewhere.[7–9,27,28]

Rabbit ECG

Rabbits can be positioned in sternal recumbency without sedation or anesthesia (after a brief period of acclimatization).[4,29,30] Heart rate in rabbits varies from 150 to 250 bpm,[31] but in general, it is very fast even in sedated animals. Polarity of waves is similar to those recorded in dogs, cats, and ferrets. The T wave is usually positive[29,32] (**Fig. 9**). However, one author claims that rabbits' high potassium and low-sodium diet may cause peaked T waves and a longer S–T segment relative to carnivores.[33] In contrast to ferrets, sinus arrhythmia is not a common feature because of a lack of influence of breathing on the autonomous innervation. Although relatively rare, arrhythmias such as AF and VPCs have been identified in pet rabbits with underlying cardiomyopathies and CHF (**Fig. 10**).[4]

As a prevention of anesthesia-induced bradycardia, glycopyrrolate may be more effective than atropine in increasing heart rate, in large part because some rabbits produce atropinesterases.[29]

Guinea Pig ECG

Several ECG values in guinea pigs are derived from cardiac electrophysiological safety assessment studies in humans because both species share similar cardiac physiology. P waves are positive and very small as well QRS complexes (small q, large R and small S waves, and T waves)[7] (see **Fig. 5**). The ST segment is present and usually isoelectric in limb leads. T waves are positive and concordant in the standard limb

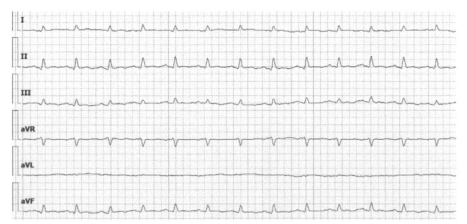

Fig. 9. Rabbit ECG. Six-lead trace ECG with prolonged P waves and QRS complexes (approximately 0.04 s each) in a patient with cardiomyopathy. Paper speed 100 mm/s, 2 cm = 1 mV.

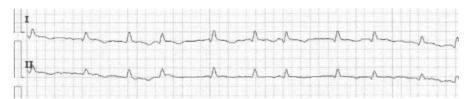

Fig. 10. Rabbit ECG with diagnosed hypertrophic cardiomyopathy and atrial fibrillation. Lead I and II showing irregular heart rhythm, lack of P waves (instead of f waves), and prolonged QRS complexes (0.05 s each). Paper speed 100 mm/s, 2 cm = 1 mV.

leads.[34] ECG patterns can be different according to the body weight and fat deposit, causing cardiac changes that can be seen in the ECG,[34] for instance, lower waves amplitude. Spontaneous acquired arrhythmias were still to now unreported in the literature, despite the presence of echocardiographic evidence of heart disease.

Rat ECG

In rats, the most prominent feature is a very fast heart rate (228–600 bpm).[35] In general, the P wave is normally positive in leads I, II, III, and aVF, negative in aVR, and flat or negative in aVL (Detweiler 2010). There is a lack of Q wave in most leads[35] while R is prominent, and S may be either prominent or absent.[7] All features may differ among studies because of different experimental settings, such as the age and strain of animals and the type of anesthesia used. The ST segment is absent and the S-wave termination in bipolar leads is often difficult to separate from the onset of T. The T wave is usually positive and concordant with QRS in leads II and III, but may be negative and discordant in lead I (Detweiler 2010). Prolongation of the P wave may be associated with increased susceptibility to supraventricular arrhythmias in Wistar rats after myocardial infarction.[35]

In general, ECG wave changes in rats can be seen as in other mammal species (**Fig. 11**). Sinus arrhythmia (50%), second atrioventricular block (about 7%), and ventricular premature complexes (about 8%) (**Fig. 12**) can be normal variations.[7]

ECHOCARDIOGRAPHY

Echocardiography offers a noninvasive view of the heart in many animals and is the method of choice for diagnosing structural and functional cardiac abnormalities. Echocardiography is more effective than radiography in the identification of heart chambers or great vessels enlargement. In general, the degree of chamber enlargement or secondary cardiac remodeling parallels disease severity.[36]

Echocardiography requires little preparation. The rapid heartbeat and the small size of some mammals nevertheless require equipment with transducers with small footprint and higher frequencies (7 MHz and more) and a high frame rate ultrasound machine. In some very small-sized patients, a linear transducer can be of help (Reese 2011). Authors (CA, VJ, and KH) recommend to clip hair in all cases, but it is a preference of the examiner. A padded or "echo" table is useful but not necessary. Sedation may be useful to obtain a quality examination, but initial stabilization with cage rest, oxygen, diuretics, and other supportive care is indicated if the patient is unstable. If anesthesia is advocated, effects on cardiac function should be considered. For example, myocardial contractility in rabbits is described to be higher under isoflurane anesthesia.[37] Based on the experience of the authors of the presented article, only little influence of isoflurane anesthesia in combination with midazolam premedication is

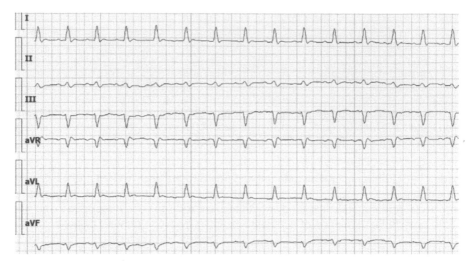

Fig. 11. Rat ECG. A. Six-lead trace ECG with normal P waves QRS complexes (according to reference 22). Paper speed 100 mm/s, 2 cm = 1 mV.

seen and echocardiography interpretation is based on repeated measurements on same individuals with different pathologies. The preferred method of examination is with patient in lateral recumbency from a dorsal approach as the heart is then very close to the thoracic wall and there is no substantial alteration of examination technique as was also described in ferrets.[38] The echocardiographic anatomy is similar as in other animals and windows and views are in general adopted from the reported from dogs and cats.[39] The technique should contemplate M-mode that provides information of chamber dimensions, wall thickness, wall and valve motion, and indices of systolic function (**Fig. 13**); also, the B-mode technique is used for examination of the anatomic details of the heart and adjacent structures. Doppler echocardiography permits to study direction, velocity, and time of blood flow. In very small patients, Doppler assessment of blood flow has to be performed in views from the right because the left apical view can result very difficult; however, the operator should respect ultrasound physics when obtaining images.

In small mammal species reported here, the left atrial diameter to aortic root is 1 to 1.6 cm, both aorta and pulmonary artery have similar size, and the left ventricular posterior wall thickness is alike to the interventricular septum thickness. The thickness of the right ventricular wall and its diameter are one-third to one-half of the left ventricle. An important feature when performing B mode in the short-axis view at the level of papillary muscles is the fact that presumably small mammals may have more cardiac

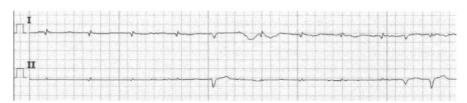

Fig. 12. Rat ECG with diagnosed hypertrophic cardiomyopathy. Lead I and II showing VPCs at 5th, 10th, and 11th complexes from left to right. Paper speed 50 mm/s, 0.5 cm = 1 mV.

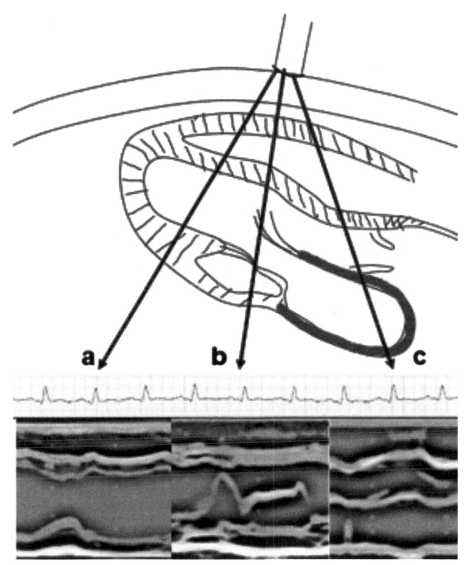

Fig. 13. Echocardiographic schema of the main right parasternal long-axis views from a dorsal approach related with ECG. (A) At the level of papillary muscles; (B) at the level of the mitral valve; and (C) at the level of aorta and left atrium.

twisting than other species, and for that reason rotation of the image is shifted more to left. Echocardiography can also help in diagnosis and therapy of intrathoracic masses, effusion, and lung ultrasound that can give additional information in a dyspneic patient in relation or not with heart disease.

Rabbit

One important indication for echocardiography in rabbits is that anterior mediastinal masses or increased mediastinal fat can have a similar appearance to cardiomegaly in radiographs. Rabbits have a large mediastinum, which can make the cranial cardiac border difficult to distinguish.[37] For that reason, echocardiographic windows are located cranially on both sides. Myocardial disease has been diagnosed very often and in lesser proportion valvular disease (same description as in other species). The most common disease seems to be dilated cardiomyopathy (DCM), but hypertrophic cardiomyopathy (HCM) and restrictive cardiomyopathy have been also reported but in lesser proportion[4] (**Figs. 14** and **15**). Detomidine and ketamine/xylazine administration has been associated with myocardial necrosis and fibrosis in New Zealand White rabbits leading to cardiomyopathy.[37] Rabbits subjected to intermittent crowding developed apparent stress-induced cardiomyopathy, which was fatal in 34 of 44 experimental animals.[4,29] This may be related to the Takotsubo cardiomyopathy, also reported in human and cats. Congenital heart disease is rarely reported in rabbits.[4]

The coronary sinus, which receives blood from the coronary veins and the left cranial vena cava, is very large and easily identified on the echocardiogram. This apparently dilated coronary sinus, circling around the AV junction, should not be interpreted as a congenital defect or as a sign of right-sided heart failure associated with elevated right atrial pressures.[29] Valvular insufficiencies were associated with primary valve degeneration, cardiomyopathy, or infection.[4] The mitral valve is affected more than the tricuspid valve; however, the tricuspid valve affection can be insufficient also under normal conditions.[30] Progression of the condition leads to volume overload and potential CHF.

Chinchilla

Reports on cardiology methods or cases in chinchillas are very scarce. Tricuspid valve regurgitation and HCM have been diagnosed on echocardiography (**Fig. 16**). Cardiomyopathy and valvular disease have been seen on postmortem examination of chinchillas presenting with heart failure and acute dyspnea.[40] Most of the observed pathologies at the authors' clinic were diagnosed as possible HCM.

Guinea Pigs

Echocardiography has been used for several years in this species because it has been frequently used as an experimental model in cardiovascular research. However, a recent study studied pet guinea pigs and established reference values.[41] The technique and procedure are performed alike other species (**Fig. 17**). Particularly, RV examination is difficult as others also found.[42] Also, the spectral Doppler of mitral and tricuspid valves may be challenging in demonstrating distinct E and A waves despite sometimes anesthesia reduces heart rate.[41] (see **Fig. 15**). We have observed cases of

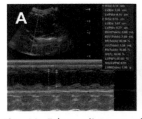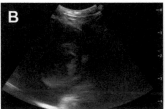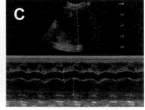

Fig. 14. Echocardiogram of a rabbit with dilated cardiomyopathy. (*A*) Right parasternal short axis view in B and M-mode tracing of the left ventricle demonstrating left ventricular enlargement, decreased contractility, and possibly volume overload. (*B*) One of the features of congestive heart failure is pericardial effusion. (*C*) Same view as A. Left atrial enlargement.

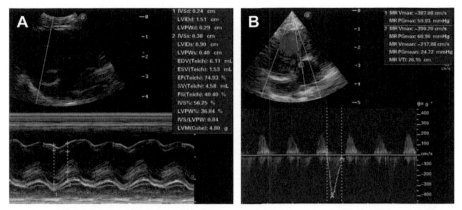

Fig. 15. Rabbit patient with hypertrophic cardiomyopathy. (*A*) Right parasternal short axis view in B and M-mode displaying measurements of interventricular septum (IVS) and left ventricular posterior wall (LVPW) with hypertrophy. (*B*) Modified left apical view recording mitral regurgitation. Also, note LA enlargement.

DCM and HCM frequently in CHF that can be seen as venous congestion, lung lobe atelectasis, and/or pericardial effusion (**Fig. 18**).

Rat

The same windows and techniques for echocardiography can be used as in other species. The ratio data such as fractional shortening and ejection fraction are similar in rats and humans except for mitral valve E peak, tissue E′, and pulmonary vein diastolic velocities which are 20% to 50% lower.[43] Reference ranges are derived from young laboratory individuals.[43] Rats can also suffer from cardiomyopathies that may lead to CHF (**Fig. 19**).

OXYGEN SATURATION MEASUREMENTS

Oxygen saturation can also be measured, mostly using the pulse oximetry. The sensor can be placed on ear, scrotal skin, toes, tail (where present), or shaved skin on flanks. An SpO_2 measurement of less than 94% is compatible with a hypoxemic state and requires oxygen supplementation.[17] SpO_2 may be underestimated when sensor is

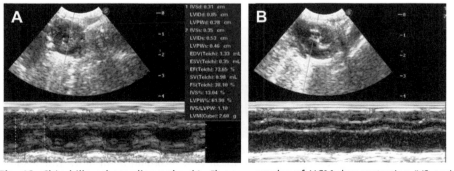

Fig. 16. Chinchilla echocardiography. (*A, B*) are examples of HCM demonstrating IVS and LVPW hypertrophy and left atrial enlargement.

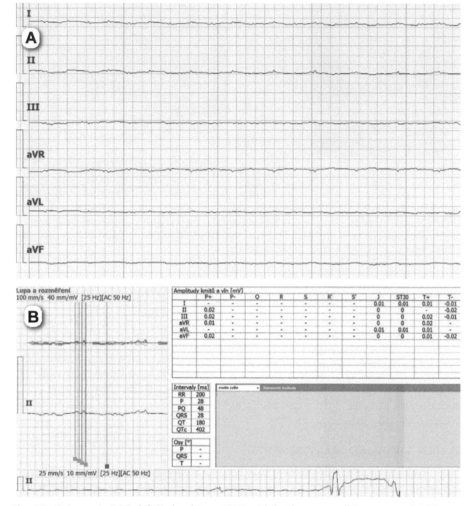

Fig. 17. Guinea pig ECG. (*A*) Six-lead trace ECG with both very small P waves and QRS complexes. (*B*) Simultaneous digital superimposition of all leads with automatic calculations on the right that makes easier interpretation. Paper speed 50 mm/s, 2 cm = 1 mV.

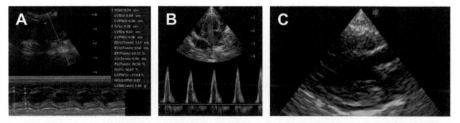

Fig. 18. Guinea pig with HCM. (*A*) Right parasternal short axis view in B and M-mode exhibiting IVS and LVPW hypertrophy. (*B*) Left apical view recording mitral flow, where still is possible discern between E and A waves. Also, note LA enlargement. (*C*) Pericardial effusion after CHF in the same patient.

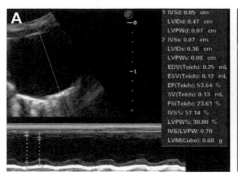
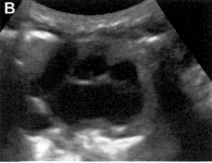

Fig. 19. Pet rat with echocardiographic findings of DCM. (*A*) Right parasternal short axis view in (*B*) and M-mode exhibiting left ventricular enlargement, decreased contractility, and possibly volume overload and B. Left atrial enlargement with surrounding lung lobes with atelectasis.

placed on pigmented skin or in cases of vasoconstriction, hypothermia, hypoperfusion, severe anemia, and other conditions caused by poor perfusion.[17]

BLOOD PRESSURE MEASUREMENTS

Blood pressure measurements can be performed in pet rabbits as well in small rodents; however, the accuracy of the measurement is not always achieved. Indirect blood pressure measurement can be performed using Doppler ultrasound and oscillometer devices.[44–46] However, most of the devices are used to monitor blood pressure during anesthesia. Sites for indirect blood pressure measurement include femoral artery, medial saphenous artery, dorsal pedal artery, radial artery, ventral coccygeal artery, and the auricular artery.[45–47]

Normal ranges of blood pressures in rabbits consist of systolic arterial pressures between 90 and 130 mm Hg and diastolic arterial pressures between 80 and 90 mm Hg.[48] Normal systolic blood pressure in guinea pigs is 91.8 to 96.2 mm Hg and a diastolic blood pressure of 46.8 to 50 mm Hg.[47] Normal cardiovascular parameters of the rat include a mean systolic blood pressure of 116 mm Hg and a diastolic blood pressure of 90 mm Hg.[12]

CARDIOVASCULAR MONITORING DURING ANESTHESIA

Cardiovascular function evaluation during anesthesia is one of the most important parts of patient monitoring.[49] As the prevalence of cardiac disease is increasing, importance is given to recognition of the heart disease before the surgery.

DISCLOSURE

The authors have nothing to disclose.

REFERENCES

1. Pignon C, Sanchez-Migallon Guzman D, Sinclair K, et al. Evaluation of heart murmurs in chinchillas (Chinchilla lanigera): 59 cases (1996-2009). J Am Vet Med Assoc 2012;241(10):1344–7.
2. Minarikova A, Hauptman K, Jeklova E, et al. Diseases in pet guinea pigs: a retrospective study in 1000 animals. Vet Rec 2015;177(8):200.

3. Herman E, Eldridge S. Spontaneously occurring cardiovascular lesions in commonly used laboratory animals. Cardio-Oncology 2019;5:6.
4. Orcutt C, Malakoff R L. Cardiovascular disease. In: Quesenberry KE, Orcutt C, Mans Ch, et al, editors. Ferrets, rabbits, and rodents. Clinical medicine and surgery. 4th edition. Elsevier; 2021. p. 250–7.
5. Rey F, Bulliot C, Bertin N, et al, REMORA Team. Morbidity and disease management in pet rats: a study of 375 cases. Vet Rec 2015;176(15):385.
6. Mäkitaipale J, Harcourt-Brown FM, Laitinen-Vapaavuori O. Health survey of 167 pet rabbits (Oryctolagus cuniculus) in Finland. Vet Rec 2015;177(16):418.
7. Detweiler DK. The mammalian electrocardiogram: comparative features. In: Macfarlane PW, van Oosterom A, Pahlm O, et al, editors. Comprehensive electrocardiology. London: Springer; 2010. p. 1909–47. https://doi.org/10.1007/978-1-84882-046-3_42.
8. Jekl V, Hauptman K, Jeklová E, et al. Blood sampling from the cranial vena cava in the Norway rat (Rattus norvegicus). Lab Anim 2005;39(2):236–9.
9. Williams WR, Kendall LV. Blood collection in the guinea pig (Cavia porcellus). Lab Anim (Ny) 2015;44(6):207–8.
10. Cruise LJ, Brewer NR. Anatomy. In: The biology of the laboratory rabbit. 2nd edition; 1994. p. 47–61. https://doi.org/10.1016/b978-0-12-469235-0.50009-9.
11. Maxwell MP, Hearse DJ, Yellon DM. Species variation in the coronary collateral circulation during regional myocardial ischaemia: a critical determinant of the rate of evolution and extent of myocardial infarction. Cardiovasc Res 1987;21(10):737–46.
12. Heatley JJ. Cardiovascular anatomy, physiology, and disease of rodents and small exotic mammals. Vet Clin North Am Exot Anim Pract 2009;12(1):99–113.
13. Sisk DB. Physiology. In: Wagner JE, Manning PJ, editors. The biology of the Guinea pig. San Diego: Academic Press; 1976. p. 63–92.
14. Pignon C, Mayer J. Guinea pigs. In: Quesenberry KE, Orcutt C, Mans Ch, et al, editors. Ferrets, rabbits, and rodents. Clinical medicine and surgery. 4th edition. Elsevier; 2021. p. 270–97.
15. Mans C, Donnelly T. Chinchillas. In: Quesenberry KE, Orcutt C, Mans Ch, et al, editors. Ferrets, rabbits, and rodents. Clinical medicine and surgery. 4th edition. Elsevier; 2021. p. 298–322.
16. Frohlich J. Rats and Mice. In: Quesenberry KE, Orcutt C, Mans Ch, et al, editors. Ferrets, rabbits, and rodents. Clinical medicine and surgery. 4th edition. Elsevier; 2021. p. 345–67.
17. Huynh M, Boyeaux A, Pignon C. Assessment and care of the critically Ill rabbit. Vet Clin North Am Exot Anim Pract 2016;19(2):379–409.
18. Ardiaca MG, Barceló AM, Bonvehí Nadeu C, et al. Respiratory diseases in guinea pigs, chinchillas and degus. Vet Clin North Am Exot Anim Pract 2021;24(2):419–57.
19. Potter G, Jones WMDC, Hermann CL. The circulatory system of the guinea pig. Bios 1958;29(1):3–13.
20. Javorka K, Calkovská A, Petrásková M, et al. Cardiorespiratory parameters and respiratory reflexes in rabbits during hyperthermia. Physiol Res 1996;45(6):439–47.
21. Di Girolamo N, Toth G, Selleri P. Prognostic value of rectal temperature at hospital admission in client-owned rabbits. J Am Vet Med Assoc 2016;248(3):288–97. PMID: 26799108.

22. Jekl V. Principles of radiography. In: Harcourt-Brown FM, Chitty J, editors. BSAVA manual of rabbit imaging, surgery and dentistry. Gloucester: BSAVA; 2013. p. 39–58.
23. Buchanan JW, Bücheler J. Vertebral scale system to measure canine heart size in radiographs. J Am Vet Med Assoc 1995;206(2):194–9.
24. Capello V, Lennox AM. Diagnostic imaging of the respiratory system in exotic companion mammals. Vet Clin North Am Exot Anim Pract 2011;14(2):369–89.
25. Müllhaupt D, Wenger S, Kircher P, et al. Computed tomography of the thorax in rabbits: a prospective study in ten clinically healthy New Zealand White rabbits. Acta Vet Scand 2017;59:72.
26. Doss GA, Mans C, Hoey S, et al. Vertebral heart size in chinchillas (Chinchilla lanigera) using radiography and CT. J Small Anim Pract 2017;58(12):714–9.
27. Smith F, Tilley L, Oyama M, et al. Manual of canine and feline cardiology. 5th edition. Saunders; 2015. p. 472.
28. Ware W, Bonagure J. Cardiovascular disease in companion animals. do, cat and horse. CRC Press; 2021. p. 966.
29. Pariaut R. Cardiovascular physiology and diseases of the rabbit. Vet Clin North Am Exot Anim Pract 2009;12(1):135–44, vii.
30. Giannico AT, Garcia DAA, Lima L, et al. Determination of normal echocardiographic, electrocardiographic, and radiographic cardiac parameters in the conscious New Zealand white rabbit. J Exot Pet Med 2015;24:223–34.
31. Varshney JP. Electrocardiography in other species. In: Varshney JP, editor. Electrocardiography in veterinary medicine. 1st edition. Springer; 2020. p. 263–91.
32. Lord B, Boswood A, Petrie A. Electrocardiography of the normal domestic pet rabbit. Vet Rec 2010;167(25):961–5.
33. Orcutt CJ. Cardiovascular disease. In: Meredith A, Lord B, editors. BSAVA manual of rabbit medicine. BSAVA; 2014. p. 205–13.
34. Botelho AFM, Oliveira MS, Soto-Blanco B. Computerized electrocardiography in healthy conscious guinea pigs (Cavia porcellus). Pesquisa Veterinária Brasileira 2016;36.1203–8
35. Konopelski P, Ufnal M. Electrocardiography in rats: a comparison to human. Physiol Res 2016,65(5):717–25.
36. DeFrancesco TC. Management of cardiac emergencies in small animals. Vet Clin North Am Small Anim Pract 2013;43(4):817–42.
37. Redrobe S. Ultrasonography. In: Harcourt-Brown F, Chitty J, editors. BSAVA manual of rabbit surgery, dentistry and imaging. BSAVA; 2013. p. 94–106.
38. Wagner RA. Ferret cardiology. Vet Clin North Am Exot Anim Pract 2009;12(1): 115–34, vii.
39. Reese S. Small mammals. Sonoanatomy. In: Krautwald-Junghanns ME, Pees M, Reese S, et al, editors. Ultrasonography diagnostic imaging of exotic pets: birds, small mammals, reptiles. 1st edition. Schlütersche; 2011.
40. Goodman G. Rodents: respiratory and cardiovascular system disorders. In: Keeble E, Meredith A, editors. BSAVA manual of rodents and ferrets. BSAVA; 2011. p. 142–9.
41. De Silva M, Mihailovic A, Baron Toaldo M. Two-dimensional, M-mode, and Doppler echocardiography in 22 conscious and apparently healthy pet guinea pigs. J Vet Cardiol 2020;27:54–61.
42. Cetin N, Cetin E, Toker M. Echocardiographic variables in healthy guineapigs anaesthetized with ketamine-xylazine. Lab Anim 2005;39(1):100–6.
43. Watson LE, Sheth M, Denyer RF, et al. Baseline echocardiographic values for adult male rats. J Am Soc Echocardiogr 2004;17(2):161–7.

44. Ypsilantis P, Didilis VN, Politou M, et al. A comparative study of invasive and os-cillometric methods of arterial blood pressure measurement in the anesthetized rabbit. Res Vet Sci 2005;78(3):269–75.
45. Harvey L, Knowles T, Murison PJ. Comparison of direct and Doppler arterial blood pressure measurements in rabbits during isoflurane anaesthesia. Vet Anaesth Analg 2012;39(2):174–84.
46. Calero Rodriguez A, van Zeeland YR, Schoemaker NJ, et al. Agreement between invasive and oscillometric arterial blood pressure measurement using a high-definition oscillometric device in normotensive New Zealand White rabbits using two different anaesthetic protocols. Vet Anaesth Analg 2021;48(5):679–87.
47. Kuwahara M, Yagi Y, Birumachi J, et al. Non-invasive measurement of systemic arterial pressure in guinea pigs by an automatic oscillometric device. Blood Press Monit 1996;1(5):433–7.
48. Comolli J, d'Ovidio D, Adami C, et al. Technological advances in exotic pet anes-thesia and analgesia. Vet Clin North Am Exot Anim Pract 2019;22(3):419–39.
49. Lichtenberger M, Ko J. Critical care monitoring. Vet Clin North Am Exot Anim Pract 2007;10(2):317–44.
50. Onuma M, Ono S, Ishida T, et al. Radiographic measurement of cardiac size in 27 rabbits. J Vet Med Sci 2010;72(4):529–31.
51. Moarabi A, Mosallanejad B, Ghadiri A, et al. Radiographic Measurement of verte-bral heart scale (VHS) in New Zealand white rabbits. Iran J Vet Surg 2015;10(1):37–42.
52. Dias S, Anselmi C, Espada Y, et al. Vertebral heart score to evaluate cardiac size in thoracic radiographs of 124 healthy rats (Rattus norvegicus). Vet Radiol Ultra-sound 2021;62(4):394–401.
53. Dorotea SB. Standardization of radiographic and ultrasonographic features and measurements in two small mammal pet-species: domestic rat (Rattus norvegi-cus) and mixed breed dwarf rabbit (Oryctolagus cuniculus). Doctoral thesis. Uni-versity of Padova; 2016.

Cardiology in Rabbits and Rodents–Common Cardiac Diseases, Therapeutic Options, and Limitations

Kerstin Müller, PD Dr, Dipl ECZM[a],*,
Elisabetta Mancinelli, DVM, CertZooMed, Dipl ECZM (Small Mammal)[b]

KEYWORDS

• Cardiology • Rabbits • Guinea pig • Rodents • Heart disease • Therapeutics

KEY POINTS

- Cardiac disease has been increasingly diagnosed in rabbits and rodents, although reports of spontaneous disease are still sporadic.
- A thorough history, including details of husbandry and diet, past, and present medical history, should be collected in all cases of suspected cardiac disease.
- Clinical signs in rabbits and guinea pigs may include tachypnea or dyspnea, lethargy, weight loss, reduced appetite, and anorexia.
- Little is known about effective treatment of naturally occurring disease in these species, and often protocols are extrapolated from other more common companion species.

CARDIAC DISEASE IN RABBITS

In contrast to dogs and cats, cardiac disease occurs less frequently in pet rabbits. Only a few case reports and case series are published, and no larger scientific studies are available. The median age of rabbits with cardiac diseases reported in the literature was 4.4 years (range: 0.17–9.7 years).[1–15] Despite the suspicion that large breeds might be overrepresented,[6,16] reports are mainly about smaller rabbit breeds with a median weight of 1.7 kg (range: 0.4–4 kg).[1,3–5,7–9,11,13,14] No sex disposition is obvious in the reported cases (15 intact females, 6 castrated females; 10 intact males, 10 castrated males).[1–4,7–15]

HEART FAILURE

Systolic (myocardial performance) and diastolic (abnormal filling during diastole) dysfunction or both can lead to heart failure. Congestion/edema are caused by

[a] Small Animal Clinic, Freie Universität Berlin, Oertzenweg 19b, Berlin 14163, Germany;
[b] Valley Exotics, Valley Veterinary Hospital, Gwaelod y Garth Ind Est., Cardiff CF15 9AA, UK
* Corresponding author.
E-mail address: Kerstin.Mueller@fu-berlin.de

Vet Clin Exot Anim 25 (2022) 525–540
https://doi.org/10.1016/j.cvex.2022.01.006
vetexotic.theclinics.com

backward failure of the right and/or the left heart side; while circulatory failure is caused by forward heart failure (low output).[17] In rabbits mainly congestive heart failure (CHF) has been described.

Congestive Heart Failure

Congestive heart failure (CHF) is a clinical syndrome caused by decompensation of many, but not all, heart diseases.[18] In this condition, decompensated cardiac dysfunction of the left and/or right side leads to accumulation and retention of sodium and water, causing pulmonary edema (left-sided failure), peritoneal effusion, hepatomegaly, thoracic effusion, subcutaneous edema (right-sided failure), or all of these conditions.[17–19]

CHF was described in rabbits with various cardiac diseases.[3,4,12,13] Clinical signs of CHF can be unspecific and may include lethargy, weight loss,[4] inappetence,[3] dyspnea, and hind limb weakness.[4] Cyanosis is often seen in animals with congenital heart defects, where oxygen-poor blood from the right side of the heart shunts to the left side.[10,12] Heart murmur[13] and irregular heart rhythm[4,13] might be obvious during clinical examination.

Diagnosis of CHF is made by clinical examination, radiography, and echocardiography. Sonography of the abdomen may rule out hepatomegaly and peritoneal effusion.

Treatment of CHF is always symptomatic and aims to improve quality of life of the patients. The goal is to improve cardiac output, reduce and prevent edema or effusions, reduce the cardiac workload, and control arrhythmias. In addition, negative effects on other organs such as kidneys should be reduced. No controlled studies are available for rabbits; therefore drugs, dosages, and dosage intervals are extrapolated from small animal medicine (**Table 1**). Further to this, most drugs are not licensed to use in this species and are used "off label."

In acute stages of CHF, oxygen supply and application of parenteral diuretics (furosemide) are the first steps. Diuretics are the key point of CHF and are used to reduce hypervolemia in decompensated patients. Indications for the use of diuretics in cardiac diseases are CHF, lung edema, and thoracic effusion caused by cardiac insufficiency.[25] Furosemide is the first-choice diuretic for patients suffering CHF. High dosages and intervals (see **Table 1**) are used in animals with cardiac failure, and lower dosages (but at least 1 mg/kg) are used to reduce volume overload. For a fast effect in emergency, furosemide should be given intravenously, as it acts within 5 minutes with a peak at 30 minutes.[25] A better diuresis can be achieved with constant rate infusion (0.6–1 mg/kg). Because loop diuretics have a sigmoidal dose-responsive effect, dosages smaller than the threshold have no or little diuretic effect.[26] The threshold depends also on the clinical condition of the patient, as patients with renal impairment may need higher dosages. Threshold dosages for small mammals are unknown. Loop diuretics also have a ceiling effect at which the highest effect is reached.[26] Similar to the threshold effect, the ceiling dose can vary with clinical situations, and renal, liver, and cardiac disease can lead to shift of the ceiling dose.

If a patient in CHF can be stabilized, furosemide dosage may be reduced to 1 to 2 mg/kg once daily (SID) or 3 times daily (TID) orally (PO), depending on the clinical signs.

The diuretic effect of torsemide, another loop diuretic, was proved in rabbits in experimental studies but no studies for the use of torsemide in cardiac diseases of small mammals or exotic pets were found.[27,28]

Thiazides, such as hydrochlorothiazide or benzothiadiazine, do not have such a distinct effect as loop diuretics and are often used only in combination with furosemide.[25]

Table 1
Selected drugs and dosages mentioned in the literature for the use in therapy for cardiac diseases in rabbits and rodents

Drug	Rabbits	Rodents	Indication	Remarks
Diuretics				
Furosemide	1–4 mg/kg IV, SC, PO BID–QID[22]	1–5 mg/kg SC, IM, PO SID–BID[20]	Edema[21]	Some references recommend 2–10 mg/kg PO, SC, IM BID in hamsters, mice, rats[22]
Vasodilator				
Nitroglycerin 2% ointment	1/8 inch transdermal BID–QID[16]	Not mentioned	Reduction of preload in heart failure[21]	
Inodilator				
Pimobendan	0.1–0.3 mg/kg PO SID–BID[22,23]	0.2–0.4 mg/kg PO BID[20,22]	CHF, DCM[21]	Dosages/intervals for rabbits and rodents differ from dogs of unknown reasons; no studies available
ACEI				
Enalapril	0.25–0.5 mg/kg PO SID or every 2nd day[22]	0.5–1.0 mg/kg PO q24h[22]	CHF, hypertension[21]	Dosages/intervals for rabbits and rodents differ from dogs of unknown reasons, no studies available
Ramipril	0.125 mg/kg PO SID[3]	Not mentioned	CHF, hypertension[21]	
Imidapril	0.125 mg/kg PO SID[2]	0.125–0.25 mg/kg PO SID[20]	CHF, hypertension[21]	
Benazepril	0.25–0.5 mg/kg PO SID[22,23]	0.05–0.1 mg/kg PO SID[20]	CHF, hypertension[21]	Dosages/intervals for rabbits and rodents differ from dogs of unknown reasons; no studies available
Calcium channel blockers				
Diltiazem	0.5–1.0 mg/kg PO SID–TID[22]	0.5–1.0 mg/kg PO BID–SID[20,22]	Supraventricular arrhythmias, atrial fibrillation, atrial flatter, hypertrophic cardiomyopathy, other forms of tachycardia[21]	

(continued on next page)

Table 1
(continued)

Drug	Rabbits	Rodents	Indication	Remarks
Other cardiotherapeutics				
Digoxin	0.005–0.01 mg/kg PO SID–BID[22]	0.005–0.01 mg/kg PO SID–BID[20]	Supraventricular arrhythmias[21]	In hamsters dosages recommended as high as 0.05–0.1 mg/kg PO SID–BID for use in DCM,[20,22] but this indication is probably obsolete as pimobendan may be safer.
Taurine	100 mg/kg PO SID[24]	100 mg/kg PO BID 8 wk[20]	Positive effect on CHF in rabbits[24]	
Atenolol	Not mentioned	0.2–2 mg/kg PO SID[20]	Antiarrhythmic, decrease of sinus rate[21]	

Most drugs, dosages, and intervals are extrapolated from small animals or published without further explanation of their origin.
Abbreviations: ACEI, angiotensin-converting enzyme inhibitors; CHF, congestive heart failure; DCM, dilated cardiomyopathy; IM, intramuscular; IV, intravenous; PO, orally; SC, subcutaneous; SID, once daily; BID, 2 times daily; TID, 3 times daily; QID, 4 times daily.

In CHF, the inodilator pimobendan reduces the preload and afterload of the heart and increases the contractility of the heart muscles fibers.[29] It is used in small animals to treat CHF due to dilated cardiomyopathy (DCM) and myxomatous mitral valve disease.[17] Its compatibility was proved in ferrets,[30] but no studies are published for other small mammal species. Its use was mentioned in combination with diuretics and angiotensin-converting enzyme inhibitors (ACEI) in 2 rabbits with CHF.[29]

Transdermally applied nitroglycerin 2% ointment is sometimes used in emergency cases of CHF to reduce congestion[17] in rabbits (see **Table 1**).[16]

In rabbits, severe thoracic effusion can be seen in CHF,[4,13] and thoracocentesis might help to stabilize dyspneic patients. It is controversial if sedation may be helpful in dyspneic rabbits. The authors' experience is inconsistent. One of the authors (KM) found that in some patients, sedation with midazolam (0.2–0.5 mg/kg intramuscularly [IM]) combined with butorphanol (0.1–0.3 mg/kg IM) had an obvious calming and anxiety-reducing effect, but few animals collapsed and died. It remained unclear if sedation played a role in the death of the animals.

The use of some ACEI, such as enalapril,[7,29] ramipril,[3] or imidapril,[2] has been reported in rabbits with CHF.[21] ACEI cause relaxation of blood vessels and decrease blood volume, leading to lower blood pressure and lower oxygen demand of the heart. ACEI are often used in combination with furosemide and pimobendan. No scientific studies are available for the use of ACEI in small mammals.

In experimental studies, taurine (100 mg/kg SID orally) had a positive effect on rabbits with chronic CHF.[24]

In rabbits with CHF assisted feeding is often needed, because inappetence is a common clinical sign.

Clinical reevaluation (especially breathing type and rate, hydration status), radiographs, and laboratory analysis (eg, hematocrit, total protein, creatinine, sodium, potassium) will help to monitor patients' clinical condition and to adapt therapy.

The outcome of rabbits with CHF is guarded. Often patients are presented in end-stage disease, and survival might be only few hours or days.[4] Some treated patients are reported to live for some months.[29]

MYOCARDIAL DISEASES

Deeb and DiGiacomo[31] mentioned that cardiomyopathy is found regularly during postmortem examination of older rabbits. The median age of rabbits with cardiomyopathy reported in the literature is 7 years (range: 0.5–8.5 years).[1–5] In most published cases, affected animals are of smaller breeds, with a median body weight of 1.7 kg (range: 0.9–3.3 kg),[1–5] with no obvious sex disposition (6 intact females, 4 castrated females; 2 intact males, 5 castrated males).[1–5]

The cause of cardiomyopathies in pet rabbits remains often unknown.[2,3,5] Experimental studies showed that some infectious agents, such as *Pasteurella multocida*, *Salmonella*, *Clostridium piliforme*,[32] coronavirus,[33] and *Encephalitozoon cuniculi*,[34,35] can cause pathologic alterations of the myocardium, but these chances might not have influence on the cardiac function. Clinical reports of infectious agents causing heart failure in pet rabbits are lacking. Weber and Van der Walt[36] described stress caused by overcrowding leading to DCM and sudden death in rabbits. A case of congenital DCM was described by Romanucci and colleagues[1] in a 6-month-old female rabbit that died during anesthesia for ovariectomy.

DCM seems to occur more often[1,3,5] than hypertrophic cardiomyopathy (HCM).[4] No clinical case of restrictive cardiomyopathy in rabbits has been published so far.

Myocardial fibrosis was found in rabbits that underwent multiple anesthesias with high doses of ketamine/xylazine (8–10 times over a period of 1 year).[37] Myocardial fibrosis occurred also in rabbits that received detomidine alone and in combination with ketamine or diazepam.[38] Myocardial ischemia caused by reduced coronary blood flow was thought to cause this alteration.

Taurine deficiency is known to cause cardiomyopathy in cats and dogs[39,40] and is not reported for pet rabbits.

Interestingly, laboratory rabbits with low vitamin E serum concentrations were sensitive to develop cardiomyopathy after several anesthetic procedures with ketamine.[37] There is some evidence that hypovitaminosis E may cause myocardial disease in rabbits,[41] but other studies did not see any effect on the heart.[42] Nevertheless, before cardiac pathologies appear, severe alterations of the skeletal muscles with severe clinical symptoms will become obvious.[41] It is unlikely that hypovitaminosis E plays a role in normally kept and fed pet rabbits.

No special treatment and no consensus of treatment of occult DCM is available even for dogs.[43] If DCM is leading to CHF in rabbits, the aforementioned therapy steps can be undertaken. In dogs, pimobendan and ACEI are often used alone or in combination. ß-blockers are sometimes added.[43] Digitalis was used in older publications to increase the cardiac output in rabbits with DCM,[3] due to its positive inotropic action.

Carnitine was found to improve the clinical condition in some dog breeds with DCM.[40] Its use in rabbits is not reported.

Treatment of HCM is not described in rabbits and is complex in cats, as therapy depends on disease stage.[44] Appropriate literature should be consulted for more detailed information in specific cases. Off-label use of drugs should be considered.

VALVULAR DISEASES

Insufficiencies of the cardiac valves, especially the atrioventricular (AV) valves, can regularly be seen in rabbits.[16] Often the cause remains unknown. In dogs and cats, insufficiencies of cardiac valves can be caused by primary valvular disease, such as degenerative valve disease (valvular endocardiosis) or valvular malformation, endocarditis, ruptured mitral chordae tendineae, or myocardial disease, such as DCM, HCM, or other causes of dilation of the left ventricle.[45,46]

Fibrosis of the atrioventricular valves (endocardiosis) was mentioned in 7 rabbits examined echocardiographically by Kattinger and colleagues.[3] The definitive diagnosis of this condition can only be made by histopathology, which was not performed in that study. The thickening of the valves was mostly accompanied by AV insufficiency leading in some cases to ventricular dilation. Kattinger and colleagues[3] concluded that due to the broad variation of age in the rabbits with thickened valves, endocarditis may have been the cause of the thickening. Further studies are needed to confirm this hypothesis. Interestingly, fibrosis of the atrioventricular valves was not mentioned in pathologic reports. Endocarditis seems to be rare in rabbits, despite rabbits being used as model for bacterial endocarditis.[47] Only one case of atrioventricular endocarditis was published.[13] In that case, *Haemophilus parainfluenzae* caused endocarditis and aorto-cavitary fistula. The rabbit also suffered periodontal disease. If cardiac and dental condition were associated remained unclear.

Insufficiency of AV valves can also occur during other cardiac diseases, such as DCM and HCM, and was mentioned in several reports.[3,4,11]

There is no etiologic treatment of valve diseases.[46] Depending on the disease stage, diuresis (furosemide), and supporting of contractibility and vasodilation (pimobendan) will improve live quality. In cases of (suspected) endocarditis, intravenous antibiotics might be indicated, and the possible source of infection should be removed, if possible.[48]

Congenital Heart Diseases

Several congenital heart defects were reported in pet and laboratory rabbits, including chordae anomalia, aortic stenosis,[3] pulmonary valve stenosis,[49] cor triatriatum,[6] ventricular septal defect (VSD),[9–11,14,49,50] atrial septal defect (ASD),[7,8] right atrioventricular valvular dysplasia,[12] and DCM.[1] In one case, the VSD was leading to an Eisenmenger syndrome.[10] Only few of these cases were described more in detail,[7–10,12] so no further conclusions can be made. Rabbits with heart malformations are young (median age: 0.7 years; range: 0.17–1.5 years)[3,6–12,14] and of smaller breeds (median body weight: 1.2 kg; range: 0.38–3.8).[3,7–9,11,14] Four intact females and 4 intact males were reported.[3,7–12,14]

In rabbits, no specific therapeutic options are mentioned for these diseases. Mostly, therapy with furosemide was initiated to treat CHF.[4,7,8] In some cases, ACEI and some other drugs were added.[7] Surgical intervention was not described.

There is only one report of a rabbit with a VSD that survived for a longer period (6 years after diagnosis).[9] The small size of the defect (0.8 mm) caused a small shunt volume and no further effects. The animal received no therapy and died 6 years after diagnosis of an unrelated cause. If the VSD did possibly close during the rabbit's life, as described in humans,[51] it was not reevaluated.

Pericardial Effusion

In dogs and cats, many conditions can cause pericardial effusion, such as cardiovascular disease, neoplasm, infection, trauma, metabolic disease, intoxication, and coagulopathy. Idiopathic pericardial effusion is common in dogs.[52] In clinical reports of rabbits with cardiac disease, pericardial effusion was observed but did not lead to cardiac tamponade.[3,4,8] Pericardial effusions were observed in postmortems of rabbits with RHDV2-infection[53] and intoxication with avocado leaves (Persea americana).[54] No treatment was described.

If pericardial effusion is leading to cardiac tamponade with severe hemodynamic compromise, pericardiocentesis should be performed.[52] The patients should receive intravenous infusions. Because of the small size of rabbits, pericardiocentesis can be challenging. If the punctured fluid has a hemorrhagic appearance, aspiration should be stopped and the fluid should be watched several seconds for clotting. If no coagulation occurs, it is very likely that the pericardial effusion was punctured, if the fluid clots puncture of the heart or large vessels is very likely. Pericardiocentesis would be contraindicated in patients with coagulopathies or atrial tear,[55] which is not described in rabbits.

OTHER CARDIAC DISEASES

Pericarditis secondary to Pasteurella multocida infection has been mentioned in rabbits as well as abscesses in the heart caused by P multocida and Staphylococcus aureus.[32] Usually these diagnoses are made at necropsy, and no specific clinical signs or treatment options are reported. In dogs and cats with pericarditis, pericardectomy and systemic antibiotics might be indicated.[52]

In 4 rabbits, cor pulmonale was suspected based on echocardiographic findings.[2] The described parameters that were leading to this diagnosis (right ventricular enlargement, in parts thickening of the myocardium and septal flattening) seem not be sufficient to diagnose this condition.

Myocardial infarction, described as hypomotility of a myocardial area and increased creatinkinase activitiy (CK), was mentioned in a 2-year-old inappetent and lethargic rabbit.[2] Without further diagnostics, such as electrocardiogram, angiography, or pathology, it remains questionable if this diagnosis was appropriate. Increase of total CK activity is not a specific and sensitive parameter for diagnosis of myocardial disease.[56]

VASCULAR DISEASES
Arteriosclerosis

Spontaneously occurring arteriosclerosis has been described in rabbits of all breeds and purpose of use, such as pet,[15,57] laboratory, meat, and wild rabbits.[58] In pet rabbits, Deeb and DiGiacomo[31] mentioned that arteriosclerosis seem to occur mainly in older animals, but this condition was also found by other investigators in rabbits as young as 6 weeks.[59] Interestingly, Gaman and colleagues[58] did not observe age differences and no increase of severity with age in meat rabbits. Arteriosclerotic lesions can be found at the main arteries, such as the thoracic and abdominal aorta,[60] but were also found in the brachiocephalic trunk, subclavian, iliac, common carotid, and renal arteries.[57]

The cause of spontaneous arteriosclerosis is unknown. Genetic factors may play an important role.[59] In some cases arteriosclerosis was associated with hypercalcemia in rabbits with renal insufficiency.[61] Hypercalcemia induced by vitamin D oversupplementation was also leading to calcification of the aortic wall.[62,63] Spontaneous arteriosclerosis in rabbits has to be differentiated from experimental induced causes of arteriosclerosis, as it occurs for instance in heritable hyperlipidemic rabbits as described by Kondo and Watanabe.[64] Other factors may induce arteriosclerosis in rabbits under experimental settings; therefore, rabbits are used as model for that condition.[65,66]

In many cases of spontaneous occurring arteriosclerosis, no symptoms are obvious.[58] Some animals were presented with seizures.[57] No causative treatment is known. Fitzgerald and colleagues[29] provide a comprehensive overview of drugs that might have some benefit in animals with arteriosclerosis, such as ACEI, isoxsuprine, and pentoxifylline. Off-license use of drugs should be taken into consideration.

Cardiogenic Arterial Thromboembolism

Cardiogenic arterial thromboembolism is caused by several factors and is described especially in cats with HCM or other heart diseases.[67] Left atrial enlargement is one of the main factors leading to this complication. Thrombus formation seems to be rare in rabbits with cardiac disease. In one rabbit with cardiomyopathy a thrombus was found in the left atrium.[4] A mural thrombus on the endocardial surface of the left ventricular free wall was diagnosed in a rabbit with multifocal myocardial necrosis after anesthesia with ketamine and high-dose detomidine.[68] One thrombus was mentioned in a rabbit with DCM with no further description.[2]

Echocardiography could help diagnosing this condition in living patients. Enlarged left atrium, thrombus formation in the left atrium or left ventricle as well as echogenic "smoke" appearance of the blood (slower velocity of the blood in the left atrium) are signs of atrial disease and thromboembolism or the risk for it.[46] The use of heparin, clopridogrel, and aspirin may be indicated if these signs are present. Agents and dosages have to be extrapolated from other species, such as cats. Drugs's use is mostly off-license. Thrombolytics are not recommend in cats and should also not be used in small mammals.

ARRHYTHMIAS

Arrhythmias were reported in detail in 6 rabbits with cardiac disease, including three with myocardial disease (HCM,[4] unspecified cardiomyopathy)[4,5] and three with valvular disease.[3,13] Arrhythmias described were atrial fibrillation,[4,5,13] left bundle branch block,[13] right bundle branch block,[3] AV block,[3,15] and gallop rhythm.[4]

Only few information about the treatment and outcome of rabbits with arrhythmias have been published. In some cases, no treatment was initiated because the animals were in end-stage conditions.[4,5,13] Pacemaker implantation was described in a rabbit with AV block grade II and III.[15] Antiarrhythmic drugs mentioned in case reports included digitalis and diltiazem.[2] Treatment with lidocaine or Mexitil was not described. Rarely ß-blockers were used.[2] Treatment of arrhythmias should only be initiated if clinical signs are obvious.[69] Drugs and dosages have to be extrapolated from small animal medicine. Digoxin can be used for treatment of supraventricular tachycardias such as atrial fibrillation.[69] Digoxin can cause inappetence and ileus and should be carefully titrated. If the patient becomes inappetent, the dose should be reduced or treatment interrupted. It is recommended that digoxin serum levels are checked 6 to 8 hours after the last dose.[69] Diltiazem, a calcium channel blocker, can also be used to treat supraventricular tachycardia, but reduction of contractility followed by hypotension might be an unintended side effect.[69]

Ventricular tachyarrhythmias can be treated with intravenous lidocaine[69] as well as sotalol and mexiletine.[6]

SYSTEMIC HYPERTENSION

Rabbits are used as model for experimentally induced systemic hypertension,[70] but spontaneously occurring systemic hypertension seems to be very rare in this species. No reports about this condition in pet rabbits could be found. Blood pressure and other factors, different drugs, and management systems are used to treat canine and feline hypertension.[71] Mainly ACEI, angiotensin receptor blocker, calcium channel blocker, and cardio-selective beta-1 adrenergic blockers are used.[71] These drugs might also work for rabbits.

CARDIAC DISEASE IN GUINEA PIGS

Only sparse information is available about cardiac diseases in guinea pigs. An investigation of 1000 guinea pigs presented to a clinic reported cardiac disease in 12 animals (7 females, 5 males) of different age groups (5 up to 2 years, 4 between 2 and 5 years, 3 up to 5 years).[72] Another larger study found a prevalence of 4.24% of cardiac diseases and/or CHF in pet guinea pigs with an average age of 4.04 years.[73] No sex differences were observed. Some case reports are published about heart diseases in this species. The median age of these guinea pigs was 3.0 (range: 0.13–5 years),[74–82] and no sex differences were obvious (9 females, 6 males).[74–82]

Clinical symptoms in guinea pigs with heart disease, mainly dyspnea, lethargy[76,78–80] as well as weight loss,[74,76,77,81,83] are comparable to rabbits

The cardiac diseases more frequently described in guinea pigs include valvular heart diseases such as mitral or tricuspid valve dysplasia,[69] mitral or tricuspid valve insufficiencies,[73] DCM,[69,70,73] HCM,[73] pericardial effusion,[73,78–81,84] neoplasms,[75,77,81,83] and CHF.[73,79]

Pericardial effusion seems to be the main finding in guinea pigs with cardiac disease, regularly associated with cardiac tamponade.[73,78,80,82,85] The cause of cardiac effusion remains often unknown.[78,79,85] Infectious pericardial effusion was diagnosed in 2 guinea pigs.[80,82] DCM[76,78,85] or HCM was additionally found in guinea pigs with pericardial effusion.[77] Pericardiocentesis is the treatment of choice where tamponade is present; this was reported in 3 animals that underwent that procedure.[78,80,82] Two of the animals survived for more than 2 years postprocedure,[78,80] whereas one died 6 weeks later.[82] A case of infectious pericardial effusion associated with a multiresistant *Staphylococcus* was also treated with pericardiocentesis, antibiotics as well as ACEI and survived at least for 2 years.[80]

Intracardiac thrombus formation without further information was mentioned by Moreno and colleagues.[73]

Few reports describe spontaneously occurring tumors of the heart in guinea pigs, including a round cell sarcoma,[83] leiomyosarcoma,[77] and 4 mesenchymomas.[75] An ectopic thyroid carcinoma was found in another guinea pig at the base of the heart.[81] Guinea pigs with cardiac tumors have a median age of 1.75 years (range: 0.6–1.75)[75,77,83] and females seem predominantly affected (5 females, 1 male). A cause for this sex bias might be that all mesenchymomas were from females of one colony.[75] Lethargy, anorexia, dyspnoea,[77] and weight loss[77,83] were mentioned symptoms. Some animals were found dead without obvious symptoms.[75] In one animal the tumor was an incidental finding during postmortem.[75] Pericardial effusion, as described in dogs with heart tumors,[49] was not observed in affected animals. Survival times are either short or not reported.[77]

In addition, rhabdomyomatosis, a morphologic alteration of cardiac myocytes, was described in pathologic examinations but seems to have little or no clinical relevance.[86]

Hyperthyroidism is sometimes diagnosed in guinea pigs.[87] Guinea pigs with thyroid neoplasm (and unknown T4 concentration) were found to have, besides other organ alterations, also myocardial disease.[88] To date, it is not clear if hyperthyroidism in guinea pigs may cause cardiac effects as described in cats.[89]

Intoxication with *Nerium oleander* leaves caused arrhythmia with atrial premature complexes, ventricular premature complexes, and atrial fibrillation.[90]

Beside pericardiocentesis, therapy for cardiac diseases in guinea pigs, is not well described. Drugs and dosages published in the literature are usually extrapolated from small animals.[20,23,29] Depending on the diagnostic findings, furosemide, pimobendan, ACEI, as well as antibiotics (in cases of pericarditis) have been used, mostly off-license.[74,76–82] Arrhythmia (atrial premature complexes, ventricular premature complexes, atrial fibrillation) caused by intoxication with *N oleander* leaves was successfully treated with infusions, furosemide, and a ß-blocker (propranolol).[90] Within 35 minutes, a normal sinus rhythm was achieved. Four hours later atrial fibrillation reoccurred, but the condition of the animal stabilized without further intervention. The following 5 days propranolol was given PO TID, and the animal was discharged 10 days after admission.

Survival time of guinea pigs with cardiac diseases seems to be often very short,[74,81,85] and only few animals are reported to live for more than 2 years after admission.[78,80]

CARDIAC DISEASES IN OTHER RODENTS
Chinchilla

Heart murmurs are a regular clinical finding in chinchillas but not always a sign of cardiac disease.[91] Of 15 chinchillas with heart murmurs that were echocardiographically investigated, 8 chinchillas had cardiac alterations, such as mitral valve and tricuspid valve regurgitation, dynamic right ventricular outflow tract obstruction, hypertrophy of the left ventricle, and hypovolemia. Chinchillas with heart murmurs of grade 3 and higher were 29 times more likely to have echocardiographic abnormalities than chinchillas without a heart murmur.

To the authors' knowledge, no further publications regarding chinchillas' heart disease are available in the scientific literature. The occurrence of cardiomyopathy and valvular disease in chinchillas was mentioned in different text books.[92] Patients were presented with radiological signs of CHF, such as pleural effusion, pulmonary edema, and cardiomegaly.[92] Prognosis is generally poor. Echocardiographically diagnosed TV valve insufficiency and HCM were mentioned.[93] Papillary muscle dysplasia, mitral valve malformation, and ventricular septal defect were reported in a 3-year-old chinchilla that died suddenly 16 months after the heart murmur was detected.[94]

Degu

Cardiac disease seems to occur rarely in degus, as no animal with cardiac disease was reported in a large clinical study.[95] Sanchez and colleagues[96] describe a clinical case of a 2-year-old male degu with ventricular septal defect causing CHF. A cardiac murmur was audible during auscultation. On radiographs, severe cardiomegaly and an interstitial pulmonary pattern were seen. A VSD was diagnosed by echocardiography and confirmed by pathology. No other publications could be found on cardiac diseases in degus.

Hamster

Several cardiac diseases were described in laboratory hamster, including atrial thrombosis, valvular malformations, DCM, and myocardial mineralization.[97] Only a few cases of cardiac disease in pet hamsters are present in the literature[98] but no scientific report about symptoms, diagnosis, and treatment was found.

Rat

Laboratory rats are model for various cardiac and vascular diseases and develop some diseases with increasing age including myocardial degeneration. For pet rats, information available is very sparce. Besides the fact that cardiac diseases are mentioned in several textbooks and reviews about pet rats,[99] no scientific report about cardiac diseases in pet rats was found.

Gerbil

No reports about cardiac diseases in pet gerbils were found. Gerbils kept as laboratory animals suffer from arteriosclerosis and focal myocardial degeneration.[93]

SUMMARY

The domestic rabbit and many rodent species are often used as animal models for cardiovascular research. However, information derived from experimental settings is often not applicable to the management of a pet rabbit or rodent with cardiac disease. Therefore, despite advances in rabbit and rodent medicine, very little is known about incidence and treatment of cardiac disease in pets. This article reviews the major cardiovascular disease of pet rabbits and common rodent species with an emphasis on treatment options. Treatment of cardiovascular disease in these species is severely impaired by the lack of clinical data, and drug dosages and frequency of administration are often extrapolated from more common companion species.

CLINICS CARE POINTS

- Congestive heart failure (CHF) is a clinical syndrome caused by decompensation of many heart diseases, often leading to accumulation and retention of sodium and water, causing pulmonary edema (left-sided failure), peritoneal effusion, hepatomegaly, thoracic effusion, subcutaneous edema (right-sided failure), or all of these conditions.

- Diuretics, and furosemide in particular, are the first choice in CHF treatment and are used to reduce hypervolemia in decompensated patients.

- It is unclear whether sedation may help reducing anxiety and calming patient presented as an emergency with CHF.

DISCLOSURE

The authors have nothing to disclose.

REFERENCES

1. Romanucci M, Defourny SV, Massimini M, et al. Unexpected cardiac death during anaesthesia of a young rabbit associated with fibro-fatty replacement of the right ventricular myocardium. J Comp Pathol 2017;156(1):33–6.
2. Schuhmann B, Helmich K. Herzerkrankungen bei Kaninchen. Wien Tierärztl Monatsschr 2014;101:197–205.
3. Kattinger P, Ewringmann A, Weyland J, et al. Kardiologische untersuchungen beim kaninchen. Kleintierpraxis 1999;44:761–72.
4. Lord B, Devine C, Smith S. Congestive heart failure in two pet rabbits. J Small Anim Pract 2011;52(1):46–50.
5. Martin MW, Darke PG, Else RW. Congestive heart failure with atrial fibrillation in a rabbit. Vet Rec 1987;121(24):570–1.
6. Varga M. Textbook of rabbit medicine. Edinburgh: Butterworth-Heinemann; 2014.
7. Nakata M, Miwa Y, Chambers JK, et al. Ostium secundum type of atrial septal defect in a rabbit. J Vet Med Sci 2018;80(8):1325–8.
8. Di Girolamo N, Palmieri C, Baron Toaldo M, et al. First description of partial atrioventricular septal defect in a rabbit. J Exot Pet Med 2018;27(4):5–9.
9. Hildebrandt N, Leuser C, Miltz D, et al. [Restrictive ventricular septal defect in a dwarf rabbit]. Tierärztl Prax Ausg K Kleintiere Heimtiere 2016;44(1):59–64.
10. Li X, Murphy JC, Lipman NS. Eisenmenger's syndrome in a New Zealand white rabbit. Lab Anim Sci 1995;45(5):618–20.
11. Vörös K, Seehusen F, Hungerbühler S, et al. Ventricular septal defect with aortic valve insufficiency in a New Zealand white rabbit. J Am Anim Hosp Assoc 2011; 47:e42–9.
12. Reed SD, Blaisdell ME. Right atrioventricular valvular dysplasia in a New Zealand white rabbit. Case Rep Vet Med 2021;2021:6674024.
13. Martel-Arquette A, Tjostheim SS, Miller J, et al. Aortocavitary fistula secondary to vegetative endocarditis in a rabbit. J Vet Cardiol 2019;21:49–56.
14. Kanemoto I, Chimura S. Congenital heart disease of th rabbit. A case of ventricular septal defect. Adv Anim Electrocard 1983;16:52–6.
15. Kanfer S. Transvenous pacemaker implantation for complete heart block in a rabbit (Oryctolagus cuniculi). Annu Conf Assoc Exotic Mammal Vet.; 2013.
16. Orcutt CJ, Malakoff RL. Rabbits: cardiovascular disease. In: Quesenberry K, Orcutt CJ, Mans C, et al, editors. Ferrets, rabbits and rodents - clinical medicine and surgery. 4th edition. St. Louis: Elsevier; 2021. p. 250–7.

17. Barrett KA. Cardiac emergencies. In: Ettinger SJ, Feldman EC, editors. Textbook of veterinary internal medicine. 7th edition. Philadelphia: Saunders; 2010. p. 476–8.
18. Scolan KF, Sisson DD. Cardiovascular disease. Pathopysiology of the heart failure. In: Ettinger SJ, Feldman EC, Coté E, editors. Textbook of veterinary internal medicine. 8th edition. St. Louis: Elsevier; 2017. p. 1153–63.
19. Rozanski E. Diseases of the pleural space. In: Ettinger SJ, Feldman EC, Coté E, editors. Textbook of veterinary internal medicine. 8th edition. St. Louis: Elsevier; 2017. p. 1136–43.
20. Mayer J, Mans C. Rodents. In: Carpenter JW, editor. Exotic animal formulary. 5th edition. St. Louis: Elsevier; 2018. p. 459–93.
21. Papich MG. Papich handbook of veterinary drugs. 5th edition. St. Louis: Saunders; 2021.
22. Morrisey JK, Carpenter JW. Formulary. In: Quesenberry KE, Orcutt CJ, Mans C, et al, editors. Ferrets, rabbits, and rodents: clinical medicine and surgery. 4th edition. St. Louis: Elsevier; 2021. p. 620–30.
23. Fisher P, Graham J. Rabbits. In: Carpenter JW, editor. Exotic animal formulary. 5th edition. St. Louis: Elsevier; 2018. p. 494–531.
24. Takihara K, Azuma J, Awata N, et al. Beneficial effect of taurine in rabbits with chronic congestive heart failure. Am Heart J 1986;112(6):1278–84.
25. Schroeder NA. Diuretics. In: Ettinger SJ, Feldman EC, editors. Textbook of veterinary internal medicine. 7th edition. Philadelphia: Saunders; 2010. p. 1212–4.
26. Oh SW, Han SY. Loop diuretics in clinical practice. Electrolyte Blood Press 2015; 13(1):17–21.
27. Kim YC, Lee MG, Ko SH, et al. Effect of intravenous infusion time on the pharmacokinetics and pharmacodynamics of the same total dose of torasemide in rabbits. Biopharm Drug Dispos 2004;25(5):211–8.
28. Dubourg L, Mosig D, Drukker A, et al. Torasemide is an effective diuretic in the newborn rabbit. Pediatr Nephrol 2000;14(6):476–9.
29. Fitzgerald BC, Dias S, Martorell J. Cardiovascular drugs in avian, small mammal, and reptile medicine. Vet Clin North Am Exot Anim Pract 2018;21(2):399–412.
30. Hermans K, Geerts T, Cauwerts K, et al. Tolerability of pimobendan in the ferret (Mustela putorius furo). Vlaams diergeneeskd tijdschr 2008;78(1):53–5.
31. Deeb BJ, DiGiacomo RE. Respiratory diseases of rabbits. Vet Clin North Am Exot Anim Pract 2000;3(3):465–80.
32. Delong D. Rabbits. Bacterial diseases. In: Suckow MA, Stevens KA, Wilson RP, editors. The laboratory rabbit, guinea pig, hamster, and other rodents. London: Academic Press; 2012. p. 301–63.
33. Digiacomo RF, Maré CJ. Viral diseases. In: Manning PJ, Ringler DH, Newcomer CE, editors. The biology of the laboratory rabbit. San Diego: Academic Press; 1994. p. 171–204.
34. Koller LD. Spontaneous Nosema cuniculi infection in laboratory rabbits. J Am Vet Med Assoc 1969;155(7):1108–14.
35. Csokai J, Gruber A, Künzel F, et al. Encephalitozoonosis in pet rabbits (Oryctolagus cuniculus): pathohistological findings in animals with latent infection versus clinical manifestation. Parasitol Res 2009;104(3):629–35.
36. Weber HW, Van Der Walt JJ. Cardiomyopathy in crowded rabbits. Recent Adv Stud Cardiac Struct Metab 1975;6:471–7.
37. Marini R, Li X, Harpster N, et al. Cardiovascular pathology possibly associated with ketamine/xylazine anesthesia in Dutch belted rabbits. Lab Anim Sci 1999; 49 2:153–60.

38. Lipman NS, Zhao ZB, Andrutis KA, et al. Prolactin-secreting pituitary adenomas with mammary dysplasia in New Zealand white rabbits. Lab Anim Sci 1994;44(2):114–20.
39. Pion PD, Kittleson MD, Thomas WP, et al. Clinical findings in cats with dilated cardiomyopathy and relationship of findings to taurine deficiency. J Am Vet Med Assoc 1992;201(2):267–74.
40. Kittleson MD, Keene B, Pion PD, et al. Results of the multicenter spaniel trial (MUST): taurine- and carnitine-responsive dilated cardiomyopathy in American cocker spaniels with decreased plasma taurine concentration. J Vet Intern Med 1997;11(4):204–11.
41. Bragdon JH, Levine HD. Myocarditis in vitamin E-deficient rabbits. Am J Pathol 1949;25(2):265–71.
42. Goettsch M, Pappenheimer AM. Nutritional muscular dystrophy in the guinea pig and rabbit. J Exp Med 1931;54(2):145–65.
43. Stern JA, Meurs KM. Myocardial disease: canine. In: Ettinger SJ, Feldman EC, Coté E, editors. Textbook of veterinary internal medicine. 8th edition. St. Louis: Elsevier; 2017. p. 1269–77.
44. Chetboul V. Myocardial disease: Feline. In: Ettinger SJ, Feldman EC, Coté E, editors. Textbook of veterinary internal medicine. 8th edition. St. Louis: Elsevier; 2017. p. 1278–305.
45. Ljungvall I, Häggström J. Adult-onset valvular heart disease. In: Ettinger SJ, Feldman EC, Coté E, editors. Textbook of veterinary internal medicine. 8th edition. St. Louis: Elsevier; 2017. p. 1249–69.
46. Bonagura JD, Fuentes VL. Echocardiography. In: Mattoon JS, Sellon RK, Berry CR, editors. Small animal diagnostic ultrasound. 4 edition. St. Louis: Saunders; 2021. p. 230–354.
47. Fox JG, Lipman NS, Newcomer CE. Models in infectious disease research. In: Manning PJ, Ringler DH, Newcomer CE, editors. The biology of the laboratory rabbit. San Diego: Academic Press; 1994. p. 381–408.
48. Olsen LH, Häggström J, Petersen HD. Acquired valvular heart disease. In: Ettinger SJ, Feldman EC, Coté E, editors. Textbook of veterinary internal medicine. 8th edition. St. Louis: Elsevier; 2017. p. 1299–319.
49. Crary DD, Fox RR. Hereditary vestigial pulmonary arterial trunk and related defects in rabbits. J Hered 1975;66(2):50–5.
50. Redrobe S. Imaging techniques in small mammals. Sem Avian Exot Pet Med 2001;10(4):187–97.
51. Zhao QM, Huang GY. Spontaneous closure rates of ventricular septal defects (6,750 consecutive neonates). Am J Cardiol 2019;124(4):613–7.
52. MacDonald K. Pericardial diseases. In: Ettinger SJ, Feldman EC, Coté E, editors. Textbook of veterinary internal medicine. 8th edition. St. Louis: Elsevier; 2017. p. 1305–16.
53. Bonvehi C, Ardiaca M, Montesinos A, et al. Clinicopathologic findings of naturally occurring rabbit hemorrhagic disease virus 2 infection in pet rabbits. Vet Clin Pathol 2019;48(1):89–95.
54. Aguirre LS, Sandoval GV, Medina DM, et al. Acute heart failure in rabbits by avocado leaf poisoning. Toxicon 2019;164:16–9.
55. Schnellbacher R, Olson EE, Mayer J. Emergency presentations associated with cardiovascular disease in exotic herbivores. J Exot Pet Med 2012;21(4):316–27.
56. Taylor SM. Creatine kinase. In: Ettinger SJ, Feldman EC, Coté E, editors. Textbook of veterinary internal medicine. 8th edition. St. Louis: Elsevier; 2017. p. 263–5.
57. Shell LG, Saunders G. Arteriosclerosis in a rabbit. J Am Vet Med Assoc 1989; 194(5):679–80.

58. Gaman EM, Feigenbaum AS, Schenk EA. Spontaneous aortic lesions in rabbits. 3. Incidence and genetic factors. J Atheroscler Res 1967;7(2):131–41.
59. Brock K, Gallaugher L, Bergdall VK, et al. Mycoses and non-infectious diseases. In: Suckow MA, Stevens KA, Wilson RP, editors. The laboratory rabbit, guinea pig, hamster, and other rodents. London: Academic Press; 2012. p. 503–28.
60. Garbarsch C, Matthiessen ME, Helin P, et al. Spontaneous aortic arteriosclerosis in rabbits of the Danish Country strain. Atherosclerosis 1970;12(2):291–300.
61. Harcourt-Brown FM. Diagnosis of renal disease in rabbits. Vet Clin North Am Exot Anim Pract 2013;16(1):145–74.
62. Kamphues J, Carstensen P, Schroeder D, et al. Effekte einer steigenden Calcium- und Vitamin D-Zufuhr auf den Calciumstoffwechsel von Kaninchen. J Anim Physiol Anim Nutr (Berl) 1986;56(1–5):191–208.
63. Zimmerman TE, Giddens WE Jr, DiGiacomo RF, et al. Soft tissue mineralization in rabbits fed a diet containing excess vitamin D. Lab Anim Sci 1990;40(2):212–5.
64. Kondo T, Watanabe Y. A heritable hyperlipemic rabbit. Jikken Dobutsu 1975;24(3):89–94.
65. Jayo JM, Schwenke DC, Clarkson TB. Atherosclerosis research. In: Manning PJ, Ringler DH, Newcomer CE, editors. The Biology of the Laboratory Rabbit. San Diego: Academic Press; 1994. p. 367–80.
66. Getz GS, Reardon CA. Animal models of atherosclerosis. Arterioscler Thromb Vasc Biol 2012;32(5):1104–15.
67. MacDonald K. Myocardial disease: Feline. In: Ettinger SJ, Feldman EC, editors. Textbook of veterinary internal medicine. 7th edition. Philadelphia: Saunders; 2010. p. 1328–61.
68. Hurley RJ, Marini RP, Avison DL, et al. Evaluation of detomidine anesthetic combinations in the rabbit. Lab Anim Sci 1994;44(5):472–8.
69. Pariaut R. Cardiovascular physiology and diseases of the rabbit. Vet Clin North Am Exot Anim Pract 2009;12(1):135–44, vii.
70. Lerman LO, Kurtz TW, Touyz RM, et al. Animal models of hypertension: a scientific statement from the American Heart Association. Hypertension 2019;73(6):c87–120.
71. Ohad DG. Treatment of systemic hypertension. In: Ettinger SJ, Feldman EC, Coté E, editors. Textbook of Veterinary Internal Medicine. 8th edition. St. Louis: Elsevier; 2017. p. 666–71.
72. Minarikova A, Hauptman K, Jeklova E, et al. Diseases in pet guinea pigs: a retrospective study in 1000 animals. Vet Rec 2015;177(8):200.
73. Moreno AC, Guillon L, Ruel Y, et al. Cardiac disease in pet guinea pigs (Cavia porcellus): a retrospective study of 62 cases (2011-2016). Paper presented at: 3rd International Conference on Avia, Herpetological and Exotic Mammal Medicine; 25.-29.03.2017, 2017; Venice, Italy.
74. Dias S, Todo M, Planellas M, et al. Unusual presentation of cardiac disease in two Guinea pigs (*Cavia porcellus*). X Southern Europ Vet Conf; 2016.
75. McConnell RF, Ediger RD. Benign mesenchymoma of the heart in the guinea pig. A report of four cases. Pathol Vet 1968;5(2):97–101.
76. Franklin JM, Guzman DS-M. Dilated cardiomyopathy and congestive heart failure in a guinea pig. Exot DVM 2006;7(6):9–12.
77. Vogler BR, Vetsch E, Wernick MB, et al. Primary leiomyosarcoma in the heart of a guinea pig. J Comp Pathol 2012;147(4):452–4.
78. Dzyban LA, Garrod LA, Besso JG. Pericardial effusion and pericardiocentesis in a guinea pig (*Cavia porcellus*). J Am Anim Hosp Assoc 2001;37(1):21–6.
79. Cox I, Haworth P. Cardiac disease in guinea pigs. Vet Rec 2000;146(21):620.

80. Quinton J, Valentin S, Ruel Y. A case of infectious pericardial effusion and tampo-nade in a guinea pig (*Cavia porcellus*) associated with a multiresistant staphylo-coccus. Vet Rec Case Rep 2014;2:e000075.
81. Kondo H, Koizumi I, Yamamoto N, et al. Thyroid adenoma and ectopic thyroid carcinoma in a guinea pig (*Cavia porcellus*). Comp Med 2018;68(3):212–4.
82. Pouyol O, Vlaemynck F. Bacterial pericarditis in a guinea pig (Cavia porcellus). Paper presented at: 2nd International Conference on Avian, Herpetological and Exotic Mammal Medicine; 18.-23.04.2015, 2015; Paris, France.
83. Bender L. Sarcoma of the heart in a guinea pig. J Cancer Res 1925;9:384–7.
84. Heggem-Perry BH, Ramer C, Pariaut R, et al. Pericardial effusion, pericardocent-esis, and thoracocentesis in a Guinea pig (*Cavia porcellus*). San Francisco: As-sociation of Exotic Mammals Veterinarians; 2012. p. 48–9.
85. Quinton JF, Ruel Y, Guillon L. Three cases of pericardial effusion in guinea pigs. Paper presented at: 2nd International Conference on Avian, Herpetological and Exotic Mammal Medicine; 18.-23.04.2015, 2015; Paris, France.
86. Williams BH. Guinea pig. Non-infectious diseases. In: Suckow MA, Stevens KA, Wilson RP, editors. The laboratory rabbit, guinea pig, hamster, and other rodents. London: Academic Press; 2012. p. 685–704.
87. Künzel F, Hierlmeier B, Christian M, et al. Hyperthyroidism in four guinea pigs: clinical manifestations, diagnosis, and treatment. J Small Anim Pract 2013; 54(12):667–71.
88. Gibbons PM, Garner MM. Pathological aspects of thyroid tumors in Guinea pigs (*Cavia porcellus*). USA: Milwaukee; 2009.
89. Graves TK. Feline hyperthyreoidism. In: Ettinger SJ, Feldman EC, Coté E, editors. Textbook of veterinary internal medicine. 8th edition. St. Louis: Elsevier; 2017. p. 1747–57.
90. Ewringmann A, Weyland J, Skrodzki M, et al. Oleandervergiftung bei einem Meerschweinchen. Kleintierpraxis 1999;44:487–560.
91. Pignon C, Sanchez-Migallon Guzman D, Sinclair K, et al. Evaluation of heart mur-murs in chinchillas (*Chinchilla lanigera*): 59 cases (1996-2009). J Am Vet Med As-soc 2012;241(10):1344–7.
92. Hoefer HL, Crossley DA. Chinchillas. In: Meredith A, Redrobe SP, editors. BSAVA manual of exotic pets. 4th edition. Gloucester: BSAVA; 2002. p. 65–75.
93. Goodman G. Rodents: Respiratory and cardiovascular sxstem disorders. In: Keeble E, Meredith A, editors. BSAVA manual of rodents and ferrets. Glucester: BSAVA; 2009. p. 142–9.
94. Donnelly T. Disease problems of chinchillas. In: Quesenberry KE, Carpenter JW, editors. Ferrets, rabbits, and rodents: clinical medicine and surgery. 2th edition. St. Louis: Saunders; 2002. p. 255–65.
95. Jekl V, Hauptman K, Knotek Z. Diseases in pet degus: a retrospective study in 300 animals. J Small Anim Pract 2011;52(2):107–12.
96. Sanchez JN, Summa NME, Visser LC, et al. Ventricular septal defect and congestive heart failure in a common degu (*Octodon degus*). J Exot Pet Med 2019;31:32–5.
97. Schmidt RE, Reavill DR. Cardiovascular disease in hamsters: review and retro-spective study. J Exot Pet Med 2007;16(1):49–51.
98. Beaufrère H, Schilliger L, Pariaut R. Cardiovascular system: current therapy in exotic pet practice. In: Mitchell M, Tully T, editors. Current therapy in exotic pet practice. Saunders; 2016. p. 151–220.
99. Heatley JJ. Cardiovascular anatomy, physiology, and disease of rodents and small exotic mammals. Vet Clin North Am Exot Anim Pract 2009;12(1):99–113.

Ferret Cardiology

Yvonne R.A. van Zeeland, DVM, MVR, PhD, Dip ECZM (Avian, Small mammal), CPBC,
Nico J. Schoemaker, DVM, PhD, Dip ECZM (Small mammal, Avian)*

KEYWORDS

- Arrhythmia • Cardiomyopathy • Cardiac disease • Dirofilariasis • Echocardiography
- Electrocardiography • *Mustela putorius furo* • Valvular disease

KEY POINTS

- Cardiac disease is seen most often in middle-aged to older ferrets, with dilated cardiomyopathy and endocardiosis being the most common cardiac abnormalities to be diagnosed.
- Clinical signs are often recognized only in advanced stages of disease and may involve signs of congestion (eg, pleural effusion, respiratory distress, and/or ascites) or decreased cardiac output (eg, hind limb weakness, syncope, exercise intolerance).
- Diagnostic workup will usually involve (a combination of) echocardiography, electrocardiography, and/or radiographs, with the method of choice being dependent on the type of clinical signs presented by the ferret.
- Therapeutic options and dosing regimen largely follow guidelines such as those established in dogs and cats and are aimed at alleviating sign of congestion, improving cardiac output, and reducing preload and afterload.

INTRODUCTION

Cardiac disease is relatively common in pet ferrets, particularly in middle-aged to older ferrets, and may comprise either problems with conduction, contractility, or outflow.[1–4] These problems may arise from anatomic and/or physiologic disorders of varying causes.

In practice, ferrets are more commonly presented with heart failure, which is the end result of severe (systolic and/or diastolic) cardiac dysfunction and *only* occurs when severe cardiac disease is present. Resulting clinical signs arise either from increased venous pressure and congestion (ie, *backward failure*) or from low cardiac output and poor tissue perfusion (ie, *forward failure*). Less frequently, ferrets are diagnosed with cardiac disease in the absence of heart failure, which, dependent on the condition, may or may not require therapy, and may or may not ever progress to heart failure.[1,4]

To work up a cardiac ferret case in practice, knowledge of the diagnostic and therapeutic options as well as the cardiac diseases/conditions themselves is needed. This

Division of Zoological Medicine, Department of Clinical Sciences, Faculty of Veterinary Medicine, Utrecht University, Yalelaan 108, Utrecht 3584 CM, The Netherlands
* Corresponding author.
E-mail address: N.J.Schoemaker@uu.nl

Vet Clin Exot Anim 25 (2022) 541–562
https://doi.org/10.1016/j.cvex.2022.01.007   **vetexotic.theclinics.com**

article provides an overview of the diagnostic tools and treatment options, and different cardiac conditions reported in ferrets, including specifics regarding their diagnosis, treatment, and outcome.

DIAGNOSING CARDIAC DISEASE
Physical Examination

Clinical signs in ferrets with heart disease are often nonspecific and may include lethargy, exercise intolerance, weight loss, and anorexia. Other signs include tachypnea, cough (albeit rare), weakness in the hind limbs, and syncope (the latter specifically in bradyarrhythmic animals).[1,3,4]

During the physical examination, special attention should be paid to the heart, arterial, venous, and capillary systems. As a result of reduced output, mucous membranes can become pale or cyanotic, with a prolonged capillary refill time (CRT; **Fig. 1**).[3,4] In addition, a weak or irregular pulse may be palpated (**Fig. 2**). Auscultation of the heart is performed between the sixth and eighth intercostal space to evaluate whether heart murmurs, bradycardia, tachycardia, arrhythmias, or muffled heart sounds is present (**Fig. 3**).[5] Lungs should also be auscultated to evaluate the presence of moist rales or crackles, muffled lung sounds, or increased bronchovesicular sounds, indicative of pleural effusion or lung edema.[1,4] Venous tension cannot easily be determined in ferrets. The abdomen should be checked for the presence of ascites, though.

Diagnostic Workup

To diagnose cardiac disease, an echocardiogram, thoracic radiographs, electrocardiogram (ECG), blood pressure measurement, blood work (complete blood count + biochemical profile), and/or urinalysis may be required. In areas where heartworm (*Dirofilaria immitis*) is endemic, specific testing is indicated. Thoracocentesis or abdominocentesis can be performed when fluid is present. This will not only provide material for cytologic, biochemical, and/or bacteriologic examination but also alleviate the associated dyspnea and discomfort.[1,3,4]

Findings obtained during the physical examination will largely determine which diagnostic test to pursue. For example, when abnormal sounds are auscultated, an echocardiogram is the first-choice diagnostic technique, whereas ECG is most useful when an abnormal rhythm or pulse frequency is detected. In the case of coughing, tachypnea, and/or dyspnea, the radiograph will be the method of choice, followed by an echocardiogram in the case of pleural effusion or heart enlargement.[4]

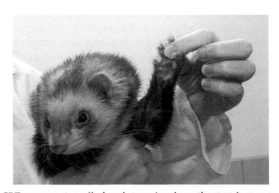

Fig. 1. In ferrets, CRT can most easily be determined on the unpigmented foot pads.

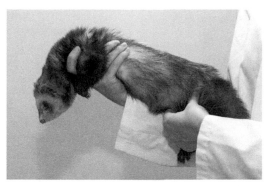

Fig. 2. In ferrets, the femoral pulse is easiest to palpate while the ferret's body rests on the forearm of the examiner.

Echocardiography

Echocardiography is ideal for identifying structural and/or functional abnormalities of the heart.[6,7] Sedation is often preferred to be able to perform accurate measurements and obtain accurate M-mode registrations and color-flow Doppler examinations (**Fig. 4**).

The routine echocardiogram (B-mode) is performed with the ferret in right and left lateral recumbency using imaging planes similar to those obtained in other species. Reference ranges for common cardiac measurements are summarized in **Table 1**. During the examination, the cardiac size is assessed, as well as contractility of the heart and leakage of the valves. M-mode measurements and Doppler echocardiography provide information on chamber dimensions, wall thickness, and systolic function, and blood flow velocity, and turbulence (indicative of, eg, valvular regurgitation), respectively (**Fig. 5**). Ultrasonography may also reveal the presence of effusion in the pericardium, thorax, or abdomen, as well as hepatomegaly or splenomegaly owing to congestion.[7]

Radiography

Thoracic radiographs are useful to detect lung edema or pleural effusion (signs of congestive heart failure; **Fig. 6**). The best-positioned, standard 2-view thoracic radiographs are often obtained in the sedated or anesthetized animal. However, sedation

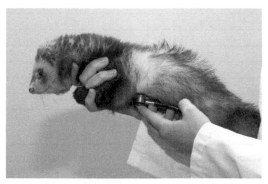

Fig. 3. In ferrets, because of the more caudal position of the heart, auscultation is performed at the level of the sixth to eighth intercostal space.

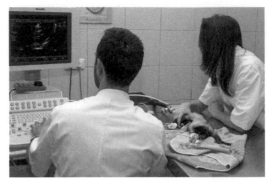

Fig. 4. Ferrets frequently are so mobile that performing a proper echocardiography is not possible without sedation. For this purpose, the use of short-acting injectables and/or inhalant anesthetics is recommended. Just as in the other companion animals, ultrasound should best be performed on both sides of the thorax. However, in the case of severe dyspnea, it may be best to place the ferret in sternal recumbency.

can decrease the inspiratory volume, thereby hindering accurate evaluation of the lungs.[4]

The heart size is evaluated using a modified vertebral heart score, for which different methods exist.[9] However, if the heart size is increased, these methods do not allow for distinction between pericardial effusion or cardiomegaly nor the type of cardiomegaly (dilated or hypertrophic cardiomyopathy) leading to the size increase. Echocardiography therefore remains the preferred diagnostic tool for evaluating cardiac disease.

Electrocardiography

ECGs are predominantly used in ferrets suspected of an abnormal heart rate or rhythm.[7,10–12] As electrical conduction is altered in the case of cardiac chamber

Table 1
Echocardiographic reference values obtained in 29 ferrets anesthetized with isoflurane

Parameter	Mean ± SD	Range	Median
IVSd (mm)	3.4 ± 0.4	2.5–4.4	3.4
IVSs (mm)	4.4 ± 0.6	3.3–5.4	4.4
LVIDd (mm)	9.8 ± 1.4	6.8–12.7	9.6
LVIDs (mm)	6.9 ± 1.3	4.5–9.7	6.9
LVWd (mm)	2.7 ± 0.5	1.8–3.7	2.7
LVWs (mm)	3.8 ± 0.8	2.4–5.9	3.8
FS (%)	29.5 ± 7.9	13.9–48.7	28.0
Ao (mm)	4.4 ± 0.6	3.3–6.0	4.2
LAAD (mm)	5.8 ± 0.9	3.2–7.3	5.7
LAAD/Ao	1.3 ± 0.2	1.0–1.8	1.3
EPSS (mm)	1.2 ± 0.6	0–2.2	1.2

Abbreviations: Ao, aorta diameter; EPSS, E-point to septal separation diameter; FS, fractional shortening; IVSd and IVSs, interventricular septum thickness in diastole and systole; LAAD, left atrium appendage diameter; LVIDd and LVIDs, left ventricular internal diameter in diastole and systole; LVWd and LVWs, left ventricular wall thickness in diastole and systole; SD, standard deviation.
(Derived from Vastenburg et al, 2004).[8]

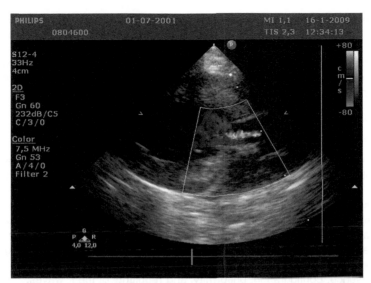

Fig. 5. Color-flow Doppler can be used to assess the velocity of the blood flow and potential presence of turbulence, indicative of, for example, valvular regurgitation. Flow toward the transducer is depicted in red, whereas flow away from the transducer is shown in blue. In the case of turbulent flow, both colors are mixed, as can be seen in this ferret with an aorta valve insufficiency.

enlargement, pericardial and/or pleural effusion, ECGs can be helpful for the diagnosis of these conditions. In addition, ECGs can be indicated for monitoring the progression of cardiac disease and effects of cardioactive drugs, or for monitoring cardiac function during anesthesia.[7]

Physiologic and pathologic arrhythmias that have been identified in ferrets include sinus bradycardia and tachycardia, atrial and ventricular premature contractions, atrial fibrillation, first-, second-, and third-degree atrioventricular (AV) blocks.

Bradycardia or bradyarrhythmia can be due to metabolic causes (eg, hypokalemia or hyperkalemia, hypoglycemia) and may be vagally mediated. A so-called atropine

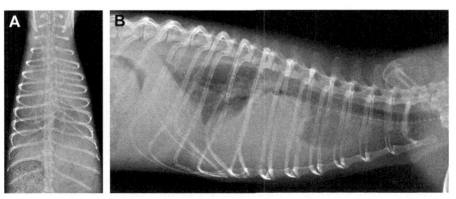

Fig. 6. Dorsoventral (*A*) and lateral (*B*) radiographs of a ferret with severe pleural effusion. Fluid accumulation obscures the heart shadow and compresses the lungs, which, similar to the trachea, show up as radiolucent structures dorsal in the thorax, owing to the presence of air.

response test, during which atropine is administered intravenously (IV), intramuscularly (IM), or subcutaneously (SC) at 0.02 to 0.05 mg/kg, can be performed to evaluate vagal involvement.[4] In vagally mediated bradycardia, increased heart rates or improved SA and AV node conduction can be within 15 to 30 minutes following atropine administration (**Fig. 7**). Incomplete responses may necessitate a repetition of the procedure.

Electrocardiogram Interpretation

ECG interpretation is done according to a standardized protocol:

1. Calculate the heart rate (in beats per minute, bpm) by counting the number of QRS complexes over a length of 7.5 cm (equaling 3 seconds) at a paper speed of 25 mm/s and multiply the number of complexes by 20.
2. Assess the heart rhythm through evaluation of the following parameters:
   a. Regularity of the rhythm, when marking 4 R waves on a piece of paper, the marks should continue to correspond to any and all R waves upon moving the paper with markings alongside the ECG (a variation of 10% in regularity is considered acceptable);
   b. Presence, configuration, uniformity, and regularity of the P waves;
   c. Presence, configuration, uniformity, and regularity of the QRS complexes;
   d. Presence of a relationship between P waves and following QRS complexes: evaluate (a) whether each P wave is followed by a QRS complex; and (b) whether each QRS complex is preceded by a P wave.

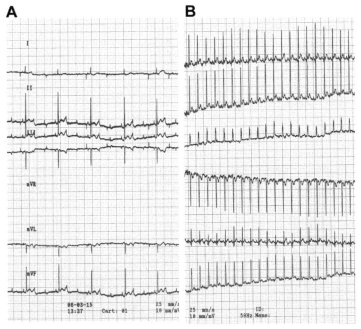

Fig. 7. An ECG of a ferret with a second-degree type II AV block (*A*). In type II blocks, the PR interval is constant, and there is a fixed relationship between the atrial and ventricular rate of, for example, 2:1, meaning 2 P waves to every QRS complex. Twenty minutes after administration of atropine (0.05 mg/kg IM), the block disappeared, and a fully normal ECG was seen (*B*).

3. Evaluate the duration and amplitude of each of the complexes and intervals in lead II. **Table 2** lists reference ranges for the different measurements.
4. Determine the mean electrical axis (MEA) through measuring net deflections in 2 leads (most often lead I and III; **Fig. 8**).

Blood Pressure Measurement

Because of the relative inaccessibility of peripheral arteries, direct arterial blood pressure measurement is not feasible in clinical practice for ferrets. Indirect systolic blood pressure measurements can be obtained using a Doppler and pressure cuff placed around the front limb, hind limb, or tail.[14] Proper cuff size, that is, approximately 40% of the circumference of the extremity, is important, as too large cuff sizes can result in underestimation of actual blood pressure. A study on the accuracy and precision of indirect arterial blood pressure measurement using high-definition oscillometry showed that the method can be used in ferrets. With adequate sedation (ie, butorphanol and midazolam, 0.2 mg/kg each), reference ranges were established at 95 to 155, 69 to 109, and 51 to 87 mm Hg for systolic, mean, and diastolic arterial pressure.[15]

GENERAL MANAGEMENT OF CARDIAC DISEASE IN FERRETS

Medical management of cardiac disease in ferrets is similar to that of dogs and cats.[1,3,4] In most instances, no specific pharmacokinetic or pharmacodynamic data are available for cardiac drugs in ferrets. Therefore, feline doses are often used as a starting point for therapy. **Table 3** provides an overview of drugs that can be indicated in ferrets with cardiovascular disease.[4]

Three mainstays in the treatment of acute congestive heart failure are as follows: (1) providing supplemental oxygen, for instance, in an incubator; (2) reducing the preload by giving diuretics (eg, furosemide, thiazide, spironolactone) or nitroglycerin (a venous dilator); and (3) reducing the afterload by giving angiotensin-converting enzyme (ACE) Inhibitors, which induce vasodilatation and decrease water and salt retention (thereby

Table 2
Electrocardiographic reference values obtained in 20 awake ferrets placed in dorsoventral position

Parameter	Mean ± SD	Range
Heart frequency (bpm)	220	175–265
Heart axis (°)	88.5 ± 5.5	85–102
Measurements in lead II		
P duration (s)	0.019 ± 0.003	0.01–0.02
P amplitude (mV)	0.11 ± 0.04	0.09–0.2
PR interval (s)	0.049 ± 0.009	0.04–0.07
QRS duration (s)	0.026 ± 0.006	0.02–0.04
QRS amplitude (mV)	2.9 ± 1.2	1.4–4.4
QT interval (s)	0.14 ± 0.02	0.11–0.16
ST segment (mV)	0.03 ± 0.01	0.02–0.05
T duration (s)	0.084 ± 0.018	0.06–0.11
T amplitude (mV)	0.26 ± 0.08	0.15–0.4

(derived from Zandvliet, 2004).[13]

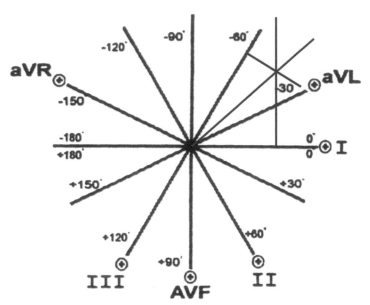

Fig. 8. To determine the mean electrical axis (MEA), the net deflections for the QRS complexes are measured in lead I and III and marked off from the zero point in the triaxial system. Next, perpendicular lines (blue) are drawn originating from the end points of the deflections until they intersect. A connecting arrow (red) is then drawn between the origin and the point of intersection, following which the MEA can be determined as the angle between the lead I axis (horizontal plane) and the connecting arrow. AVF, **augmented Vector Foot**; aVR, augmented Vector Right; aVL, augmented Vector Left.

also reducing the preload). In case of significant pleural effusion, thoracocentesis can be performed to alleviate dyspnea. In a stabilized animal with contractility dysfunction, pimobendan may be added to enhance inotropy.[4]

Beta-blockers (eg, atenolol) or calcium channel blockers (eg, diltiazem) can be used to reduce the heart rate and treat supraventricular and ventricular arrhythmias. In the case of ventricular tachycardias, IV lidocaine can be titrated to effect, whereas atropine may be indicated if bradycardia or bradyarrhythmia is present. However, as atropine only results in a short-term effect, long-acting parasympatholytic drugs (eg, propantheline) should be used for maintenance. Sympathomimetic drugs (metaproterenol, isoproterenol) have also been used in the medicinal therapy of third-degree heart block. However, if these are not effective, pacemaker implantation should be considered (**Fig. 9**).[16]

CARDIAC DISEASES
Congenital Heart Disease

In ferrets, the following congenital heart defects have been reported: (1) atrial and ventricular septal defects (n = 1 for both)[17,18]; (2) an AV canal defect (n = 1)[19]; (3) tetralogy of Fallot (n = 3)[20–22]; and (4) patent ductus arteriosus (PDA).[23]

Clinical signs
Congenital heart disease has been diagnosed in ferrets up to 6 years. Dependent on the size and type of defect, animals may be symptomless, or die before or shortly after birth. Growth retardation can be seen, and animals may develop pulmonary edema,

Table 3
Drugs to be used in the treatment of cardiovascular disease in ferrets[4]

Drug	Action	Dosage
Amlodipine	Calcium antagonist; afterload reduction	0.2–04 mg/kg po q12h
Atenolol	Beta-blocker for treatment of HCM	3.125–6.25 mg/kg po q24h
Atropine	Parasympatholytic drug for treatment of bradycardia	0.02–0.05 mg/kg SC/IM
Benazepril	ACE inhibitor; vasodilator	0.25–0.5 mg/kg po q24h
Captopril	ACE inhibitor; vasodilator	1/8 of 12.5 mg tablet/animal po q48h
Digoxin	Positive inotropic drug for treatment of DCM	0.005–0.01 mg/kg po q12–24h
Diltiazem	Calcium channel blocker for treatment of HCM, AF, or SVT	1.5–7.5 mg/kg po q12h
Dobutamine	Sympathomimetic drug used in treatment of heart failure and cardiogenic shock	5–10 µg/kg/min IV (canine dose)
Enalapril	ACE inhibitor; vasodilator	0.25–0.5 mg/kg po q24–48h
Furosemide	Loop diuretic for treatment of congestion	1–4 mg/kg po/SC/IM/IV q8–12h
Hydroclorothiazide	Diuretic for treatment of congestion; may be combined with spironolactone	1 mg/kg po q12–24h (cat dose)
Isoproterenol	Sympathomimetic drug for treatment of 3rd-degree AV block	40–50 µg/kg po/SC/IM q12h
Ivermectin	Broad-spectrum antiparasitic avermectin for treatment of heartworm	0.02 mg/kg po/SC (preventative) or 50 µg/kg SC q30d (treatment)
Melarsomine	Arsenical; adulticide used to treat heartworm disease	2.5 mg/kg IM at day 1, 30, 31
Metaproterenol	Sympathomimetic drug for treatment of 3rd-degree AV block	0.25–1 mg/kg po q12h
Milbemycin oxime	Broad-spectrum antiparasitic milbemycin; prevention of heartworm disease	1.15–2.33 mg/kg po q30d
Moxidectin	Broad-spectrum antiparasitic avermectin; used to treat heartworm (adulticide)	0.1 mL SC (single dose); use every 6 mo as preventative treatment
Nitroglycerin	Vasodilator	1/16–1/8 in per animal of a 2% ointment q12–24h, applied to shaved inner thigh or pinna
Pimobendan	Phosphodiesterase inhibitor; increase cardiac contractility in patients with DCM	0.5–1.25 mg/kg po q12h
Propanolol	Beta-blocker for treatment of HCM	0.2–1 mg/kg po/SC q8–12h

(continued on next page)

Table 3 *(continued)*		
Drug	**Action**	**Dosage**
Propantheline	Long-acting parasympatholytic for treatment of sinus bradyarrhythmia	0.25–0.5 mg/kg po 8–12 hours (canine dose)
Selamectin	Broad-spectrum antiparasitic avermectin; used as preventive treatment for heartworm	18 mg/kg topically
Spironolactone	Diuretic for treatment of congestion	1–2 mg/kg po q12h
Theophylline	Methylxanthine drug, which serves as a bronchodilator (relaxation of bronchial smooth muscles) and also has positive inotropic and chronotropic effects	4.25 mg/kg po q8–12h

pleural effusion, hepatomegaly, and/or ascites as a result of congestive heart failure, which may lead to dyspnea, tachypnea, cough, muscle wasting, and/or distended abdomen. On physical examination, a (holodiastolic, holosystolic, or continuous) cardiac murmur will often be audible. In addition, a tachycardia, faint pulse, cyanotic or pale mucous membranes, and/or prolonged CRT can be present.

Diagnosis
Echocardiography is the preferred technique to be used for diagnosing congenital heart abnormalities. Color Doppler ultrasonography may be useful to detect left-to-right or right-to-left shunting, or turbulent blood flow owing to stenosis or valvular insufficiencies (**Fig. 10**). Secondary cardiac changes (eg, atrial dilatation, concentric or eccentric ventricular hypertrophy) may also be noted.

Radiographs can reveal an enlarged cardiac silhouette and signs of congestive heart failure (eg, pulmonary edema, pleural effusion ascites).

Treatment
Mild congenital heart defects in asymptomatic ferrets may not require any treatment. However, regular monitoring is recommended so that developing congestive heart

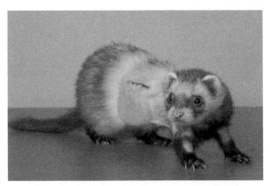

Fig. 9. A 6-year-old neutered female ferret with a recently placed transvenous pacemaker for management of a third-degree heart block.

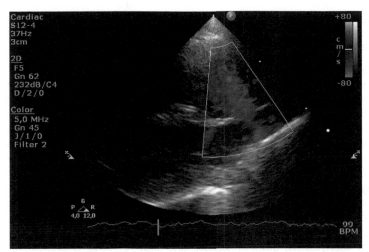

Fig. 10. Color-flow Doppler demonstrates a direct blood flow between both atria in a 2-year-old, male castrated ferret with an atrial septal defect. (Previously printed in Journal of Exotic Pet Medicine 2013 22 (1): 70 to 75.)

failure can be caught early and treated promptly. Treatment is indicated in animals with congestive heart failure (eg, furosemide, enalapril, pimobendan, digoxin, atenolol). Surgical intervention, which is performed in dogs with, for example, PDA, has not been described in ferrets.

Acquired Heart Disease

Dilated cardiomyopathy (DCM) and acquired valvular disease (AVD; endocardiosis or myxomatous valvular degeneration) are the most common acquired heart diseases to be encountered in ferrets.[3,4] Other, less frequently reported cardiac conditions include infectious diseases (such as fungal or bacterial myocarditis, endocarditis, or pericarditis, toxoplasmosis, heartworm disease or dirofilariasis, and Aleutian disease), neoplasia (eg, lymphoma, lymphosarcoma), hypertrophic cardiomyopathy (HCM), and pericardial effusion.[3,4,24]

Dilated Cardiomyopathy

(DCM is most common in middle-aged to older ferrets, with no sex predilection reported.[1-4] DCM is characterized by an increased diastolic dimension and systolic dysfunction of the left and/or right ventricles. Histologically, DCM is characterized by multifocal myocyte degeneration and necrosis, myofiber loss, and replacement fibrosis. Occasionally, inflammatory infiltrates may be present.[25] The exact cause is unknown, although nonconfirmed associations with taurine or carnitine deficiencies have been made. Preexisting endocrine disease, intoxications, or infectious disease (eg, viruses, cryptococcus),[26] as well as a genetic origin may also play a role in the development of the disease.[4]

Clinical signs
Clinical signs may develop from completely asymptomatic to lethargy, weakness, anorexia, weight loss, exercise intolerance, and respiratory distress (tachypnea, dyspnea, cough). Physical examination may reveal a weak pulse, pulse deficit, tachycardia (>250 bpm), (systolic) heart murmur, gallop rhythm/arrhythmia, hypothermia,

pallor, cyanosis, increased respiratory effort, muffled heart and lung sounds, moist rales or crackles, increased respiratory sounds, prolonged CRT, posterior paresis, hepato(spleno)megaly, or ascites.[1–4,27]

Diagnosis

Characteristic echocardiographic findings include thin ventricular walls, dilatation of the left ventricle with increase in end-systolic and end-diastolic dimensions, enlargement of the left atrium, and reduced fractional shortening (**Fig. 11**). Outflow tract velocities of the left ventricle can be normal or reduced. Dilatation of the right ventricle and atrium indicates involvement of the right side. In advanced stages, mitral valve and tricuspid insufficiency and regurgitation can be identified with Doppler ultrasound. Similarly, signs of pleural effusion, liver congestion, and/or ascites can be observed.[1,3,4]

Radiographs are useful to identify pleural effusion or pulmonary edema, or to rule out mediastinal lymphoma. If the abdomen is included in the radiograph, the presence of hepatomegaly or splenomegaly, or ascites can be evaluated.

ECG can be normal or reveal atrial and ventricular premature contractions, atrial or ventricular tachycardia, atrial fibrillation, and first- or second-degree heart block. Signs of left atrial or ventricular enlargement (eg, broadened P wave, reduced voltage, and/or widened QRS complexes) can also be present.[3,4]

Routine blood tests and urinalysis will generally not reveal abnormalities unless severe heart failure is present, resulting in prerenal azotemia, hyponatremia and increased ALT concentrations, or concurrent disease. B-type natriuretic peptide and N-terminal pro b-type natriuretic peptide levels are currently of limited clinical use.

Treatment/management

Initial treatment includes provision of oxygen, diuretics (eg, furosemide, thiazide, spironolactone), and thoracocentesis (if pleural effusion is present). Monitoring of the

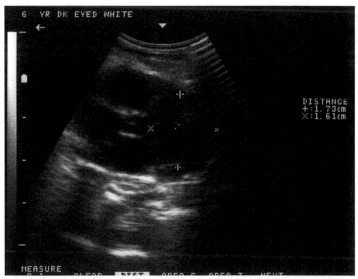

Fig. 11. Cardiac ultrasound of a 6-year-old ferret with DCM. The inner diameter of the left ventricle was 1.7 × 1.6 cm (reference <1.3 cm in ferrets). In addition to a dilated ventricle, a decreased wall thickness and decreased FS may also be observed. (Photo courtesy of Cathy Johnson-Delaney. Previously printed in Disorders of the cardiovascular system. Ferret Medicine and Surgery.)

respiratory rate and effort, and auscultating lung sounds are helpful to evaluate treatment response. Stress should be avoided at all costs, as this may lead to death.[3,4]

Following stabilization, the diuretic dose is adjusted, if needed, whereas ACE inhibitors, pimobendan and/or digoxin (in case of tachycardia), can be added to the treatment protocol. The dose of diuretics should be reduced to the lowest dose that prevents reaccumulation of pleural effusion and pulmonary edema, as overzealous administration of diuretics may result in dehydration and hypokalemia. ACE inhibitors (eg, enalapril) are recommended for long-term therapy to help reduce preload and afterload, improve cardiac output, and reduce congestion. Careful monitoring is recommended, as ferrets are suggested to be sensitive to the hypotensive effects of ACE inhibitors, thereby quickly becoming weak and lethargic. Pimobendan and digoxin are indicated to increase ventricular contractility. For severe systolic dysfunction, a combination of both drugs may be beneficial. Pimobendan acts as a positive inotrope and vasodilator, thereby helping to reduce preload and afterload. Digoxin is indicated (with or without propranolol) in ferrets with atrial fibrillation to slow down the heart rate to 180 to 250 bpm in resting state. The narrow therapeutic window warrants careful monitoring of serum concentrations (therapeutic range: 1–2 ng/mL 6–12 hours following oral administration) and clinical signs of toxicity (eg, anorexia, nausea, vomiting, and lethargy), especially in ferrets with renal insufficiency. Periodic monitoring is recommended, which should include a physical examination, echocardiography, electrocardiography, and measurement of urea or blood urea nitrogen, and electrolytes.[3,4]

Prognosis
If diagnosed in an early stage, prognosis appears fair, with ferrets often responding well to therapy and living a good quality of life for several months, up to 2 years. If disease is more advanced, prognosis is considered more guarded. Sudden death may occur because of life-threatening arrhythmias.

Heartworm Disease (Dirofilariasis)

Heartworm disease, caused by infection with *D immitis*, is an uncommon disease in ferrets.[28–30] Mosquitoes serve as a vector and intermediate host for the parasite. The susceptibility and life cycle of *D immitis* are similar to those in dogs.[31–34] Ferrets are considered aberrant hosts, with those that live (outdoors) in or originate from heartworm endemic areas (ie, along the Atlantic and Gulf coast, in tropical and semi-tropical areas) being most at risk to develop disease.

Worms can reside in the right ventricle, cranial vena cava, or main pulmonary artery and cause villous endarteritis. Even a single worm can lead to severe heart disease, and as few as 2 adult heartworms have resulted in fatal right-sided heart failure owing to mechanical obstruction of the blood flow.[3]

Clinical presentation
Clinical signs are similar to those observed in cats and may range from asymptomatic individuals to sudden death, resulting from pulmonary artery obstruction. Other clinical signs include anorexia, lethargy, weakness, depression, dyspnea, tachypnea, cyanosis, coughing, pale mucous membranes, abdominal distension, and rarely, melena.[3,28–31] Physical examination may reveal labored breathing, crackles, and moist rales in the case of pulmonary edema, or shallow breathing, decreased chest compliance, and muffled heart and lung sounds in the case of pleural effusion. Ascites, hepatomegaly, and splenomegaly may be present in the case of right-sided heart failure. Upon heart auscultation, a tachycardia and/or heart murmur can sometimes be heard. Occasionally, arrhythmias (most commonly atrial fibrillation) can be identified. Caval

syndrome, frequently leading to hemoglobinemia, hemoglobinuria, and hemolytic anemia, as well as renal and hepatic dysfunction, has been reported in ferrets and may be life threatening. Aberrant larval migration, with associated central nervous system signs, has also been documented in one ferret with a *D immitis* infection.[31]

Diagnosis
Because of the rapid progression of the disease, heartworm should be diagnosed as early as possible. Echocardiography is most useful in the diagnosis, as the adult worms may be visualized in the pulmonary artery, right ventricle, and/or right atrium as parallel, linear echodensities.[35] Right atrial and ventricular dilation can be noted. Doppler echocardiography may confirm the presence of pulmonary hypertension. Thoracic radiographs can reveal pleural effusion, ascites, and cardiomegaly.[34] Enlargement of the caudal vena cava, right atrium, and right ventricle are often seen, whereas peripheral pulmonary arterial changes are rare in ferrets.

Serologic tests that identify adult *D immitis* antigen are the first choice in diagnosing infection, although little is known regarding its sensitivity and specificity in ferrets. Because the test will only detect antigen that is shed by the adult female heartworms, and multiple worms are needed to produce enough antigen, false negative results may occur with low worm burdens (<5 worms). A modified Knott test can be performed to detect circulating microfilaria. However, peripheral microfilaremia only seems present in half of the affected animals, thereby limiting the usefulness of this test.[3,4]

Treatment
Ivermectin (0.05–0.1 mg/kg every 30 days SC) is the preferred drug of treatment and needs to be administered until resolution of the clinical signs and microfilaremia. Other protocols include the use of adulticides, such as melarsomine (Immiticide, Rhone Merieux; 2.5 mg/kg IM followed by 2 injections 24 hours apart 1 month later) and thiacetarsemide (0.22 mL/kg every 12 hours IV for 2 days). Moxidectin (0.1 mL SC) has anecdotally been suggested as an effective and safe adulticide.[36] If microfilaremia is present, a microfilaricide therapy should be initiated 4 to 6 weeks following adulticide therapy.[3,4] Microfilaricides that have been used include dithiazanine iodide (6–20 mg/kg by mouth) or milbemycin oxime (1.15–2.33 mg/kg by mouth every 30 days), although therapeutic efficacy of the latter has not been clearly documented. Transvenous heartworm extraction is nowadays also a viable option,[32] especially because adulticide therapy has fallen out of favor because of anecdotal adverse reactions, including sudden death and myositis at the injection site.

Complications may arise from worm emboli. As a result, prednisone (0.5–1 mg/kg every 12–24 hours by mouth) is often initiated concurrently with the adulticide treatment and continued for at least 4 months. Strict cage rest and restriction of exercise are advised for a minimum of 4 to 6 weeks following adulticide therapy.

Symptomatic ferrets may require stabilization and treatment for heart failure (including oxygen, furosemide, enalapril, and theophylline) before initiating adulticide treatment. Thoracocentesis is indicated in ferrets with pleural effusion.

A follow-up enzyme-linked immunosorbent assay for heartworm antigen can be performed approximately 3 months after initiating therapy. Testing is then repeated on a monthly basis until results are negative (usually 4 months following successful adulticide therapy). Further tests (eg, radiographs, echocardiography) may be warranted if test results remain positive.[3,4]

Prevention
Control is best achieved through monthly administration of a heartworm preventative. This includes the administration of ivermectin (0.05 mg/kg every 30 days by mouth or

SC), milbemycin oxime (1.15–2.33 mg/kg every 30 days by mouth), selamectin (18 mg/kg topically), or moxidectin (0.1 mL [single dose] SC, repeat every 6 months). Prevention should start 1 month before and continue until 1 month after the heartworm season. Housing ferrets indoors, particularly during the mosquito season, may also help to minimize exposure.[3,4]

Endocarditis

Endocarditis has rarely been documented in ferrets.[37,38] It is characterized by an inflammation of the endocardial tissues, that is, the valves (endocarditis valvularis), the wall (endocarditis parietalis), or chordae tendineae (endocarditis chordalis), and can be bacterial or nonbacterial origin.

Clinical presentation
Clinical signs may include lethargy, anorexia, weight loss, lameness, and pyrexia. Hemorrhage may occur if the animal develops diffuse intravascular coagulation. A cardiac murmur may be heard upon auscultation.

Diagnosis
A bacterial endocarditis is usually diagnosed based on 2 or more positive blood cultures in addition to echocardiographic evidence of vegetations or valve destruction, or the documented recent onset of a (regurgitant) cardiac murmur. However, negative cultures do not rule out the possibility of bacterial endocarditis, and structural abnormalities and vegetations visualized during echocardiography will be difficult to differentiate from endocardiosis.

Nonbacterial endocarditis may present on echocardiography as an irregular thickening of the valve leaflets, with normal chamber dimensions and normal systolic function.[37]

Treatment
Bacterial endocarditis requires prolonged antibiotic treatment (ie, over the course of at least 4 weeks), using either a broad-spectrum antibiotic or one that is appropriate based on culture and sensitivity results. In addition, symptomatic treatment, aimed at alleviating the clinical signs, is initiated. However, survival seems poor, with none of the reported ferrets surviving for more than 3 days.

Hypertrophic Cardiomyopathy

HCM is a rare condition in (younger) ferrets.[1,3,4] The cause is currently unknown. HCM is characterized by concentric hypertrophy (ie, increased wall thickness) of the left ventricular wall and interventricular septum. Histologically, HCM is characterized by hyperplasia of the individual myofibers, primarily of the left ventricle.

Clinical presentation
Clinical presentation may range from an asymptomatic ferret to sudden death (especially during anesthesia) without preemptive signs.[2] Clinical signs are linked either to the reduced cardiac output resulting from the impaired ventricular filling (eg, weakness manifesting by paresis posterior, ataxia) or to the increased filling pressure in the left ventricle, which results in pulmonary congestion (left-sided heart failure). A physical examination may reveal a weak or irregular pulse, tachycardia, (S3 or S4) gallop rhythm, arrhythmias, and/or systolic heart murmur. In the case of pulmonary congestion, increased respiratory sounds, moist rales, and/or crackles can be heard.[3,4]

Diagnosis
Ultrasound may reveal (generalized or local) gross thickening of the interventricular septum and/or left ventricular free wall and decreased left ventricular dimensions. Fractional shortening may be normal or increased. Left atrial enlargement or systolic anterior mitral valve motion (associated with interventricular septum hypertrophy) can also be seen. Doppler echocardiographic evaluation may reveal turbulence in the left ventricular outflow tract secondary to dynamic obstruction and mitral regurgitation.[3,4]

Radiographs may reveal a normal to increased cardiac silhouette or, in the case of (left-sided) heart failure, signs of pulmonary edema or pleural effusion. Electrocardiography may reveal sinus tachycardia (>280 bpm) and, occasionally, atrial or ventricular premature contractions. Widened QRS complexes of increased amplitude, and signs of atrial enlargement (ie, broadened P wave) may also be noted.

Treatment
Treatment is aimed at eliminating heart failure (if present) and, following stabilization, improving the diastolic filling of the ventricles. Beta-blockers, for example, propranolol (0.2–1.0 mg/kg every 8–12 hours by mouth) or atenolol (3.1–6.2 mg every 24 hours by mouth), are commonly recommended to reduce heart rate and correct atrial and ventricular arrhythmias. In addition, calcium channel blockers (eg, diltiazem, 3.7–7.5 mg every 12 hours by mouth) can be administered to reduce heart rate, improve diastolic relaxation and ventricular filling, and induce vasodilatation, which helps to reduce preload and afterload and increase myocardial perfusion (through vasodilatation of the coronary arteries). Combined, the drugs help to reduce myocardial oxygen consumption and increase cardiac output, but careful monitoring is warranted, as overdosing may lead to significant bradycardia, hypotension, lethargy, and/or inappetence.

Treatment with diuretics and ACE inhibitors may be considered if heart failure is present. Positive inotropic drugs should be avoided. Aspirin or heparin therapy is not considered necessary because of the rare incidence of arterial thromboembolism in ferrets.[3,4]

Myocarditis

Myocarditis is a focal or diffuse inflammation of the myocardium with myocyte degeneration and/or necrosis, which results in reduced myocardial function, arrhythmias, and, in the end stages, replacement fibrosis. Myocarditis can occur as part of a systemic vasculitis, autoimmune disease, intoxication (eg, doxorubicin cardiotoxicosis), traumatic injury (eg, cardiac puncture or ischemic events), or parasitic, bacterial, fungal, or viral infection. Myocarditis may also occur secondary to an endocarditis or inflammatory process elsewhere in the body.[3,4]

Myocarditis is rarely diagnosed in ferrets. In those cases that have been described, a toxoplasma-like organism, Aleutian disease (a parvoviral infection), bacterial and fungal infections in the myocardium, have played a role.[39,40]

Clinical presentation
The clinical signs generally result from systolic dysfunction or pathologic arrhythmias that can occur, leading to classic signs of congestive left or right heart failure (eg, dyspnea, tachypnea, ascites), or sudden death owing to onset of ventricular tachycardia or ventricular fibrillation. Other signs include lethargy, anorexia, and fever. A heart murmur, resulting from mitral or tricuspid valve regurgitation, may be audible on auscultation, as well as an irregular heart rhythm.[3,4]

Diagnosis

The gold standard is histologic evaluation of the myocardium. However, obtaining cardiac biopsies is difficult, thereby hindering antemortem diagnosis. Diagnosis therefore usually is presumptive and based on exclusion of other causes. ECG may reveal atrial fibrillation or ventricular and/or atrial premature complexes, whereas chamber dilation and poor ventricular contractility with essentially normal valves may be noted on echocardiography. Leukocytosis, neutrophilia, and hyperfibrinogenemia can be noted in the hematologic and biochemical profile. Cardiac isoenzymes (creatinine kinase, lactate dehydrogenase, and troponin) are often increased. Serum cardiac troponin T (cTnT) and I (cTnI) are considered sensitive and specific indicators of myocardial damage (eg, owing to ischemia or inflammation) in humans and other animals and may thus be of use in ferrets. However, reference ranges (ie, 0.05–0.10 ng/mL) are below the detection limit of commercially available assays.[3] Combined with a lack of clinical trials or controlled studies, this limits the current clinical use of cTnT and cTnI in ferrets.

Treatment

Treatment is aimed at eliminating the primary cause and alleviating symptoms related to congestive heart failure and arrhythmias. Pimobendan or digoxin can improve the cardiac contractility, whereas furosemide helps to control signs of pulmonary edema, pleural effusion, or ascites. Corticosteroids may be considered in the absence of an infectious cause.

Neoplasia

Neoplasia involving the myocardium or pericardium is rare in ferrets, with only one case of an atrial tumor being reported in the literature.[2] In addition, the authors have diagnosed a ventricular sarcoma in a 5-year-old male ferret. This ferret presented with dyspnea of sudden onset as a result of pleural effusion. Upon auscultation, a gallop rhythm could be heard. As the ferret died shortly after presentation in the clinic, the diagnosis was only made at postmortem examination.[1]

Restrictive Cardiomyopathy

Restrictive cardiomyopathy, which is defined as a clinically normal-appearing left ventricle combined with left atrial enlargement, is rare in ferrets.[7] As a result of scar formation following inflammation, the heart muscle is stiffened and can no longer expand, preventing normal filling of the ventricles (ie, diastolic dysfunction).

Diagnosis

Definite diagnosis requires documentation of diastolic dysfunction during ultrasound (eg, using tissue Doppler imaging) or histologic evaluation of cardiac tissue.

Treatment

Treatment follows similar guidelines as those described for HCM. In cats, prognosis of restrictive cardiomyopathy appears guarded to poor, with animals rarely surviving for longer periods of time and often responding poorly to therapy. Prognosis in ferrets is likely similar.

Valvular Disease (Acquired) or Endocardiosis

AVD or endocardiosis is recognized with increasing frequency in middle-aged to older ferrets. It is characterized by degenerative changes and depositions of proteoglycans and glycosaminoglycans in the subendocardial valve leaflets and chordae tendineae.[3,4,7] The aortic and mitral valves appear most commonly affected. Gross lesions include opaque nodular thickening and shortening at the free edge and base of the valve leaflets. Secondary dilatation of the left atrium and ventricle may occur.[3,4]

Clinical presentation
Mitral valve regurgitation often results in a systolic murmur, which is best heard over the left apical region, whereas tricuspid valve regurgitation is best auscultated in the right parasternal location.[2] Aortic insufficiency, presenting as a diastolic murmur, is rarely heard on auscultation. Additional signs can be observed if congestive heart failure and may include a weak pulse, abdominal distension resulting from hepatosplenomegaly and/or ascites, dyspnea, tachypnea, coughing, increased respiratory sounds, moist rales or crackles, or muffled heart and lung sounds.[3,4]

Diagnosis
Echocardiographic findings may include cardiomegaly, atrial and/or (mild) ventricular dilatation, thickening of the valves, and a normal to increased fractional shortening with normal ventricular contractility and wall thickness. Valvular regurgitation can be identified and quantified using color-flow and/or pulse-wave Doppler. Note that small regurgitant jets of blood can occur in clinically healthy ferrets, which should not be mistaken for cardiac pathologic condition.[3,4]

Thoracic radiographs can be useful to evaluate cardiac size and establish whether signs of congestive heart failure (pulmonary edema, pleural effusion, ascites) are present. Electrocardiography is often unremarkable but may include signs of atrial enlargement (ie, broadened P wave) or atrial arrhythmias.[3,4]

Treatment
Therapy is not recommended as long as ferrets are asymptomatic. If signs of congestive heart failure are present, treatment may be initiated with furosemide and ACE inhibitors (eg, enalapril) to alleviate the neurohormonal activation of the Renin-Angiotensin-Aldosteorne System (RAAS) that occurs with advanced cardiac disease and congestive heart failure. In the case of impaired systolic function and/or supraventricular arrhythmias, positive inotropic drugs, such as pimobendan and digoxin, may be given once the ferret has stabilized.[3,4]

Pericardial Effusion and Pericarditis

Pericardial effusion is characterized by the presence of an abnormal amount of fluid between the heart and the pericardium and may result from inflammation of the pericardium (ie, pericarditis). Pericardial effusion can occur as a primary condition or secondary to other medical conditions (eg, viral or bacterial infections, neoplasia, uremia, autoimmune disease, trauma, coagulopathies, hypoalbuminemia, cardiomyopathy, and right-sided heart failure). Primary pericardial effusion without concurrent disease has thus far not been reported in ferrets.[4]

Clinical signs
Dependent on the amount of fluid present in the pericardial sac, clinical signs may be totally absent or result in significant disease owing to impaired filling of the ventricles (ie, cardiac or pericardial tamponade). If the pericardial effusion builds up slowly, the left ventricular function often remains intact, and only signs associated with right-sided heart failure (ie, hepatomegaly, ascites, pleural effusion with concurrent dyspnea, tachypnea and cough, and exercise intolerance) will develop. However, a rapidly developing pericardial effusion may compromise both left and right ventricular outflow, thereby resulting in severe shock, syncope, and potentially death. Animals with minor to moderate pericardial effusion can remain asymptomatic, with pericardial

effusion noted as a coincidental finding during echocardiography. Physical examination will often reveal a weak pulse and so-called pulsus paradoxus (a drop in arterial blood pressure concurrent with inspiration), as well as muffled cardiac sounds and tachycardia.[4]

Diagnosis
Echocardiography is used to identify the presence of excess fluid surrounding the heart, whereas ECG can reveal low-voltage QRS complexes and pulsus alternans (ie, changing amplitude of the QRS complexes).

Pericardiocentesis can help to identify the cause of the pericardial effusion. The collected fluid may be submitted for cytologic analysis, biochemical analysis, and/or (bacterial) culture.[4]

Treatment
Small pericardial effusions in asymptomatic animals often require no special treatment. For pericardial effusion owing to pericarditis or secondary to other diseases, treatment should be aimed at the initiating cause. Severe pericardial effusions with cardiac impairment warrant drainage by pericardiocentesis. In the case of recurrence and/or idiopathic pericardial effusion, pericardiectomy may be considered (although this has not yet been described in ferrets).[4]

Cardiac Arrhythmias and Conduction Disturbances

Cardiac arrhythmias and conduction abnormalities may occur as a result of changes in the electrical conduction system of the heart and can be physiologic or pathologic in origin. Sinus arrhythmia is the most common physiologic arrhythmia noted and may be caused by respiration or an increased vagal tone. Sinus tachycardia and second-degree AV block have also been reported to occur physiologically in healthy ferrets.[4,7]

Pathologic arrhythmias can result following stress, pain, hyperthermia, hypoxia, shock, electrolyte or metabolic disturbances (eg, hypercalcemia, hypokalemia, or hyperkalemia), infections (eg, sepsis), intoxications (eg, digoxin), anesthesia, endocrine disease (eg, hyperthyroidism), anemia, and cardiac abnormalities (eg, DCM, myocarditis).[4]

Clinical presentation
Cardiac arrhythmias and conduction abnormalities can largely remain undetected until they are discovered as a coincidental finding during a routine auscultation or electrocardiography. Dependent on the type of arrhythmia or conduction disturbance that is present, irregular pulse waves or pulse deficits may be palpated. (Life-threatening) bradycardia (<120 bpm), with subsequent lethargy, weakness, exercise intolerance, and syncope, may result from second- and third-degree AV blocks.[16,41] Congestive heart failure and hypoperfusion may develop once the heart rate consistently drops to less than 80 bpm. In animals with severe tachycardia (>300 bpm), similar signs may be noted, with ventricular tachycardias quickly resulting in death if not promptly treated.[4] Because of impaired cardiac filling and output, the pulse in these animals will often be weak.

Diagnosis
Electrocardiography is required to identify the type of arrhythmia or conduction disturbance and establish a definite diagnosis. Bradycardia warrants the use of an atropine response test to determine vagal involvement.[4] Other diagnostic tests (eg, echocardiography, radiography, hematology, and biochemistry) may be useful to rule out underlying disease.

Treatment
In the case of tachycardia or tachyarrhythmia, antiarrhythmic drugs, such as lidocaine, digoxin, or beta-blockers (eg, propranolol, atenolol), are indicated to lower the heart rate. Ferrets with clinical signs resulting from high-grade second-degree and third-degree AV block may benefit from anticholinergics (eg, propantheline), beta-adrenergics (eg, terbutaline, isoproterenol), and phosphodiesterase inhibitors (eg, aminophylline, theophylline), particularly if heart rate increased following atropine administration.[4] In animals with little response to aforementioned medications, pacemakers may be implanted.[16] Treatment furthermore comprises alleviation of the clinical signs as well as eliminating the underlying cause.

Prognosis
Most electrocardiographic abnormalities that have been identified in ferrets are discovered by coincidence and will not affect the animal in any way. Profound bradycardia (<80 bpm), as can be seen with high-degree second- or third-degree AV block, carries a poor prognosis if not treated promptly.

SUMMARY

While most common in middle-aged to older ferrets, cardiac disease should be considered in the differential diagnosis of any ferret displaying signs of weakness, lethargy or dyspnea. Commonly, heart failure results from dilated cardiomyopathy, but hypertrophic cardiomyopathy, valvular disease and other cardiac conditions may certainly also occur. Hence, geriatric patients may benefit from routine check-ups which include cardiac monitoring. If suspecting cardiac disease, diagnostic modalities such as ultrasound, radiographs and ECG may help establish a definitve diagnosis, which can serve as an important starting point for therapeutic intervention.

DISCLOSURE

The authors have nothing to disclose.

REFERENCES

1. Hoefer HL. Heart disease in ferrets. In: Bonagura JD, editor. Kirk's current veterinary therapy XIII: small animal practice. Philadelphia: WB Saunders Co; 2000. p. 1144–8.
2. Lewington JH. Cardiovascular disease. In: Lewington JH, editor. Ferret husbandry, medicine, and surgery. 2nd edition. Oxford: Butterworth-Heinemann; 2007. p. 275–84.
3. Morrisey JK, Malakoff RL. Ferrets: cardiovascular and other diseases. In: Quesenberry KE, Orcutt CJ, Mans C, et al, editors. Ferrets, rabbits, and rodents: clinical medicine and surgery. St. Louis: Elsevier; 2021. p. 55–70.
4. van Zeeland YRA, Schoemaker NJ. Disorders of the cardiovascular system. In: Johnson-Delaney CA, editor. Ferret medicine and surgery. Boca Raton: CRC Press; 2016. p. 127–57.
5. Powers LV, Perpinan D. Ferrets: basic anatomy, physiology, and husbandry of ferrets. In: Quesenberry KE, Orcutt CJ, Mans C, et al, editors. Ferrets, rabbits, and rodents: clinical medicine and surgery. St. Louis: Elsevier; 2021. p. 1–12.
6. Dudás-Györki Z, Szabó Z, Manczur F, et al. Echocardiographic and electrocardiographic examination of clinically healthy, conscious ferrets. J Small Anim Pract 2011;52:18–25.

7. Malakoff RL, Laste NJ, Orcutt CJ. Echocardiographic and electrocardiographic findings in client-owned ferrets: 95 cases (1994–2009). J Am Vet Med Assoc 2012;241:1484–9.

8. Vastenburg M, Boroffka S, Schoemaker NJ. Echocardiographic measurements in clinically healthy ferrets anesthetized with isoflurane. Vet Radiol Ultrasound 2004; 45:228–32.

9. Stepien RL, Benson KG, Forrest LJ. Radiographic measurement of cardiac size in normal ferrets. Vet Radiol Ultrasound 1999;40:606–10.

10. Bone L, Battles AH, Goldfarb RD, et al. Electrocardiographic values from clinically normal, anesthetized ferrets (Mustela putorius furo). Am J Vet Res 1988; 49:1884–7.

11. Bublot I, Randolph W, Chalvet-Monfray K, et al. The surface electrocardiogram in domestic ferrets. J Vet Cardiol 2006;8:87–93.

12. Smith SH, Bishop SP. The electrocardiogram of normal ferrets and ferrets with right ventricular hypertrophy. Lab Anim Sci 1985;35:268–71.

13. Zandvliet MMJM. Electrocardiography in psittacine birds and ferrets. Semin Avian Exot Pet Med 2005;14:34–51.

14. Lichtenberger M, Ko J. Anesthesia and analgesia for small mammals and birds. Vet Clin North Am Exot Anim Pract 2007;10:293–315.

15. van Zeeland YRA, Wilde A, Bosman IH, et al. Non-invasive blood pressure measurement in ferrets (Mustela putorius furo) using high definition oscillometry. Vet J 2017;228:53–62.

16. Sanchez-Migallon Guzman D, Mayer J, Melidone R, et al. Pacemaker implantation in a ferret (Mustela putorius furo) with third-degree atrioventricular block. Vet Clin North Am Exot Anim Pract 2006;9:677–87.

17. Di Girolamo N, Critelli M, Zeyen U, et al. Ventricular septal defect in a ferret (Mustela putorius furo). J Small Anim Pract 2012;53:549–53.

18. Van Schaik-Gerritsen KM, Schoemaker NJ, Kik MJL, et al. Atrial septal defect in a ferret (Mustela putorius furo). J Exot Pet Med 2013;22:70–5.

19. Agudelo CF, Jekl V, Hauptman K, et al. A case of a complete atrioventricular canal defect in a ferret. BMC Vet Res 2021;17:45.

20. Dias S, Planellas M, Canturri A, et al. Extreme tetralogy of Fallot with polycythemia in a ferret (Mustela putorius furo). Top Companion Anim Med 2017;32:80–5.

21. Laniesse D, Hébert J, Larrat S, et al. Tetralogy of Fallot in a 6-year-old albino ferret (Mustela putorius furo). Can Vet J 2014;55:456–61.

22. Williams JG, Graham JE, Laste NJ, et al. Tetralogy of Fallot in a young ferret (Mustela putorius furo). J Exot Pet Med 2011;20:232–6.

23. Wagner RA. Ferret cardiology. Vet Clin North Am Exot Anim Pract 2009;12: 115–34.

24. Burns R, Williams ES, O'Toole DO, et al. Toxoplasma gondii infections in captive black-footed ferrets (Mustela nigripes), 1992–1998: clinical signs, serology, pathology, and prevention. J Wildl Dis 2003;39:787–97.

25. Heatley JJ. Ferret cardiomyopathy. Compendium's Stand Care Emerg Crit Care Med 2007;8:7–11.

26. Greenlee PG, Stephens E. Meningeal cryptococcosis and congestive cardiomyopathy in a ferret. J Am Vet Med Assoc 1984;184:840–1.

27. Lipman NS, Murphy JC, Fox JG. Clinical, functional and pathologic changes associated with a case of dilatative cardiomyopathy in a ferret. Lab Anim Sci 1987;37:210–2.

28. Miller WR, Merton DA. Dirofilariasis in a ferret. J Am Vet Med Assoc 1982;180: 1103–4.

29. Moreland AF, Battles AH, Nease JH. Dirofilariasis in a ferret. J Am Vet Med Assoc 1986;188:864.
30. Parrott TY, Greiner EC, Parrottt JD. Dirofilaria immitis infection in three ferrets. J Am Vet Med Assoc 1984;184:582–3.
31. Antinoff N. Clinical observations in ferrets with naturally occurring heartworm disease and preliminary evaluation of treatment with ivermectin with and without melarsomine. Proc Symp Am Heartworm Soc Recent Adv Heartworm Dis 2002;45–7.
32. Bradbury C, Saunders AB, Heatley JJ, et al. Transvenous heartworm extraction in a ferret with caval syndrome. J Am Anim Hosp Assoc 2010;46:31–5.
33. McCall JW. Dirofilariasis in the domestic ferret. Clin Tech Small Anim Pract 1998; 13:109–12.
34. Supakorndej P, McCall JW, Jun JJ. Early migration and development of *Dirofilaria immitis* in the ferret, *Mustela putorius furo*. J Parasitol 1994;80:237–44.
35. Sasai H, Kato T, Sasaki T, et al. Echocardiographic diagnosis of dirofilariasis in a ferret. J Small Anim Pract 2000;41:172–4.
36. Cottrell DK. Use of moxidectin (ProHeart 6) as a heartworm adulticide in 4 ferrets. Exot DVM 2004;5:9–12.
37. Kottwitz JJ, Luis-Fuentes V, Micheal B. Nonbacterial thrombotic endocarditis in a ferret (*Mustela putorius furo*). J Zoo Wildl Med 2006;37:197–201.
38. Paiva RMP, Garcia-Guasch L, Gaztañaga R, et al. Aortic endocarditis in a ferret. ExoticDVM 2010;12:17–23.
39. Daoust PY, Hunter DB. Spontaneous Aleutian disease in ferrets. Can Vet J 1978; 19:133–5.
40. Thornton RN, Cook TG. A congenital toxoplasma-like disease in ferrets (*Mustela putorius furo*). N Z Vet J 1986;34:31–3.
41. Menicagli F, Lanza A, Sbrocca F, et al. A case of advanced second-degree atrioventricular block in a ferret secondary to lymphoma. Open Vet J 2016;6:68–70.

Moving?

Make sure your subscription moves with you!

To notify us of your new address, find your **Clinics Account Number** (located on your mailing label above your name), and contact customer service at:

Email: journalscustomerservice-usa@elsevier.com

800-654-2452 (subscribers in the U.S. & Canada)
314-447-8871 (subscribers outside of the U.S. & Canada)

Fax number: 314-447-8029

Elsevier Health Sciences Division
Subscription Customer Service
3251 Riverport Lane
Maryland Heights, MO 63043

*To ensure uninterrupted delivery of your subscription, please notify us at least 4 weeks in advance of move.

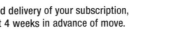